Emergency Medicine Simulation Workbook

Emergency Medicine Simulation Workbook

A Tool for Bringing the Curriculum to Life

SECOND EDITION

Edited by

Traci L. Thoureen

MD, MHS-CL, MMCi, FACEP
Associate Professor
Division of Emergency Medicine
Duke University Medical Center
Durham, NC

Sara B. Scott

MD, FACEP
Assistant Professor
Division of Emergency Medicine
Department of Surgery and Perioperative Care
University of Texas at Austin, Dell Medical School
Austin, TX

WILEY Blackwell

Registered Offices
John Wiley & Sons, Inc., 111 River Street, Hoboken, NJ 07030, USA
John Wiley & Sons Ltd, The Atrium, Southern Gate, Chichester, West Sussex, PO19 8SQ, UK

Editorial Office
9600 Garsington Road, Oxford, OX4 2DQ, UK

For details of our global editorial offices, customer services, and more information about Wiley products visit us at www.wiley.com.

Wiley also publishes its books in a variety of electronic formats and by print-on-demand. Some content that appears in standard print versions of this book may not be available in other formats.

Library of Congress Cataloging-in-Publication Data

Names: Thoureen, Traci L., editor. | Scott, Sara B., editor.
Title: Emergency medicine simulation workbook : a tool for bringing the
    curriculum to life / edited by Traci L. Thoureen, Sara B. Scott.
Description: Second edition. | Hoboken, NJ : Wiley-Blackwell, 2022. |
    Includes bibliographical references and index.
Identifiers: LCCN 2021058895 (print) | LCCN 2021058896 (ebook) | ISBN
    9781119633877 (paperback) | ISBN 9781119633914 (adobe pdf) | ISBN
    9781119633938 (epub)
Subjects: MESH: Emergency Medicine–education | Simulation Training |
    Emergencies | Teaching Materials | Case Reports | Outline
Classification: LCC RC86.7 (print) | LCC RC86.7 (ebook) | NLM WB 18.2 |
    DDC 616.02/5–dc23/eng/20220204
LC record available at https://lccn.loc.gov/2021058895
LC ebook record available at https://lccn.loc.gov/2021058896

Cover Design: Wiley
Cover Image: © Microgen/Shutterstock

Set in 10.5/13pt STIXTwoText by Straive, Pondicherry, India

SKYBFC164BE-CAA9-473A-9DC2-1E702DB82EB7_030422

Contents

Contributors

Afrah A. Ali, MBBS
Department of Emergency Medicine
University of Maryland School of Medicine
Baltimore, MD, USA

Michael Billet, MD
Department of Emergency Medicine
University of Maryland
Baltimore, MD, USA

Mark J. Bullard, MD, MS-HPEd
Department of Emergency Medicine, Carolinas Simulation Center
Carolinas Medical Center, Atrium Health
Charlotte, NC, USA

Michele Callahan, M.D
Department of Emergency Medicine
University of Maryland School of Medicine
Baltimore, MD, USA

Wan-Tsu W. Chang, MD
Department of Emergency Medicine
University of Maryland School of Medicine
Baltimore, MD, USA

Daa'iyah R. Cooper, MD
Department of Emergency Medicine
University of Maryland School of Medicine
Baltimore, MD, USA

Ashley C. Crimmins, MD
Department of Emergency Medicine
University of Maryland School of Medicine
Baltimore, MD, USA

Moira Davenport, MD, CAQSM
Temple University School of Medicine
Philadelphia, PA, USA

Sarah B. Dubbs, MD, FAAEM, FACEP
Department of Emergency Medicine
University of Maryland School of Medicine
Baltimore, MD, USA

Donald T. Ellis II, MD
Duke Children's Hospital and Health Center
Durham, NC, USA

Jeffrey N. Heimiller, MD
Department of Emergency Medicine
Vanderbilt University Medical Center
Nashville, TN, USA

Rupal Jain, MD
Department of Emergency Medicine
University of Maryland School of Medicine
Baltimore, MD, USA

Danya Khoujah, MBBS, MEHP
Emergency Medicine
MedStar Franklin Square Hospital
Baltimore, MD, USA

Diane Kuhn, MD, PhD
Department of Emergency Medicine
University of Maryland Medical Center
Baltimore, MD, USA

Charles Lei, MD
Department of Emergency Medicine
Vanderbilt University Medical Center
Nashville, TN, USA

Brittany N. Muller, MD
Temple University School of Medicine
Pittsburgh, PA, USA

Nur-Ain Nadir, MD, MEHP, FACEP
Department of Emergency Medicine
Kaiser Permanente Modesto Medical Center
Modesto, CA, USA

Andrew Ortega, MD
Department of Emergency Medicine
Kaiser Permanente Modesto Medical Center
Modesto, CA, USA

Ashley Pickering, MD, MPH
Department of Emergency Medicine
University of Maryland School of Medicine
Baltimore, MD, USA

Joseph R. Sikon, MD
Department of Emergency Medicine
Vanderbilt University Medical Center
Nashville, TN, USA

Catherine M. Wares, MD
Department of Emergency Medicine
Carolinas Medical Center, Atrium Health
Charlotte, NC, USA

Abbreviations

CLINICAL COMPETENCIES

ICS	interpersonal and communication skills
MK	medical knowledge
PBL	practice-based learning and improvement
PC	patient care
PC	professionalism
SBP	systems-based practice

ABC	airway, breathing, and circulation
ACE	angiotensin-converting enzyme
ACGME	Accreditation Council of Graduate Medical Education
ACLS	Advanced Cardiovascular Life Support
AF	atrial fibrillation
AHA	American Heart Association
AIS	acute ischemic stroke
AKI	acute kidney injury
ALT	alanine aminotransferase
ARDS	acute respiratory distress syndrome
AST	aspartate aminotransferase
BIPPV	non-invasive positive pressure ventilation
BVM	bag–valve mask
BVM	bag-valve-mask
CIWA	Clinical Institute Withdrawal Assessment
CNS	central nervous system
CPR	cardiopulmonary resuscitation
CRP	C-reactive protein
CSF	cerebrospinal fluid
CT	computed tomography
CTA	computed tomography angiography
D5W	5% dextrose in water
DC	direct current
DCV	direct current synchronized cardioversion
DIC	disseminated intravascular coagulation

DRC	Democratic Republic of the Congo
ECG	electrocardiogram
ED	emergency department
eFAST	extended Focused Assessment with Sonography in Trauma
EMS	emergency medical services
EVD	Ebola virus disease
FAST	Focused Assessment with Sonography in Trauma
FDA	Food and Drug Administration
FEU	fibrinogen-equivalent units
FFP	fresh frozen plasma
GABA	γ-aminobutyric acid
GCS	Glasgow Coma Scale
GI	gastrointestinal
HAPE	high-altitude pulmonary edema
hpf	high power factor
HPV	human papillomavirus
HSP	Henoch–Schönlein purpura
HUS	hemolytic uremic syndrome
ICH	intracerebral hemorrhage
ICU	intensive care unit
IM	intramuscular
INR	international normalized ratio
IO	intraosseous
IO	intraosseous
ITP	immune thrombocytopenic purpura
IV	intravenous
KCl	potassium chloride
LDH	lactate dehydrogenase
lpf	low power factor
LR	lactated Ringer's solution
LRINEC	laboratory risk indicator for necrotizing fasciitis
LVO	large vessel occlusion
MAC	multilumen access catheter
MAHA	microangiopathic hemolytic anemia
MCA	middle cerebral artery
MCV	mean corpuscular volume
MRI	magnetic resonance imaging
MRSA	methicillin-resistant Staphylococcus aureus
MTP	massive transfusion protocol
NAAT	nucleic acid amplification test
NEC	necrotizing enterocolitis
NICU	neonatal intensive care unit
NIHSS	National Institutes of Health Stroke Scale
NMDA	N-methyl-D-aspartate

NPO	nil per os (by mouth)
NSAID	nonsteroidal anti-inflammatory drug
PCC	prothrombin complex concentrate
PCR	olymerase chain reaction
PEA	pulseless electrical activity
PEEP	positive end-expiratory pressure
PICU	pediatric intensive care unit
PICU	pediatric intensive care unit
PPE	personal protective equipment
PPH	postpartum hemorrhage
PSI	percutaneous sheath introducer
PTT	partial prothromboplastin time
QRS	no expansion
qSOFA	Quick Sequential [Sepsis-related] Organ Failure Assessment
RA	right atrium
ROSC	return of spontaneous circulation
RSI	rapid sequence intubation
RVR	rapid ventricular rate
SAFE	sexual assault forensic examiner
SBP	systolic blood pressures
SCD	sickle cell disease
SCFE	slipped capital femoral epiphysis
SCORTEN	SCORe of toxic epidermal necrolysis
STI	sexually transmitted infections
SVT	supraventricular tachycardia
TEN	toxic epidermal necrolysis
TLS	tumor lysis syndrome
TTP	thrombotic thrombocytopenic purpura
TXA	tranexamic acid
VT	ventricular tachycardia
WPW	Wolff–Parkinson–White
μl	microliter (not mcl)

About the Companion Website

This book is accompanied by a companion website.

www.wiley.com/go/thoureen/simulation/workbook2e

This website includes:

- Video clips
- Imaging and laboratory results – presented in Powerpoint format for easy download

Introduction

Simulation has become increasingly prevalent in healthcare education, and particularly in emergency medicine education, over the past few decades [1]. It is a way to provide a safe environment for the application of knowledge and is therefore useful for undergraduate and graduate medical education, as well as for continuing professional development for physicians. Nurses and allied health professionals also use simulation-based learning as an educational tool [2].

Simulation-based learning has been shown to have positive effects on the growth of complex skills across many domains of higher education [3]. Competencies that are frequently taught with simulation include procedural skill acquisition, patient safety, communication, and interprofessional team training [2]. One meta-analysis found that simulations with high authenticity have greater effects than simulations with low authenticity [3]. It is therefore important to design realistic simulations with appropriate competency acquisition in mind.

The goal of this workbook is to help educators perform realistic simulation experiences with practical learning objectives for students, junior and postgraduate learners. The workbook was designed with the basic clinical competencies of emergency medicine physician trainees in mind, but the cases throughout may be incorporated into a curriculum for nurses, physician assistants, or paramedics. The chapters incorporate topics listed by the American Board of Emergency Medicine as included in the certification examination. Each chapter includes three individual simulation cases that highlight subject material pertinent to the chapter topic. Changes for the second edition of this book include almost entirely new case content, the addition of one pediatric case per chapter, and, when applicable, alternative options to make cases adaptable for prehospital provider education.

For ease of use, the presentation format for each individual simulation case is uniform. Each case starts with specific educational objectives and suggested critical actions. For those working within the United States postgraduate training system, the relevant Accreditation Council of Graduate Medical Education (ACGME) clinical competencies are included. These are (together with the abbreviations used in the chapters) medical

Emergency Medicine Simulation Workbook: A Tool for Bringing the Curriculum to Life,
Second Edition. Edited by Traci L. Thoureen and Sara B. Scott.
© 2022 John Wiley & Sons Ltd. Published 2022 by John Wiley & Sons Ltd.
Companion website: www.wiley.com/go/thoureen/simulation/workbook2e

knowledge (MK), patient care (PC), systems-based practice (SBP), professionalism (P), interpersonal and communication skills (ICS), practice-based learning and improvement (PBL).

Following the critical actions, you will find an outline for the case set-up. This includes a description of the physical environment, mannequin, props, distractors, and actors recommended for each simulation. An online resource is provided, which includes imaging and laboratory studies pertinent to each case. These multimedia images can be shown in real time on computer screens/monitors during the simulation session.

Next, you will find a brief narrative of the case. There is a description of the initial mannequin conditions and a case narrative, which details the changes in condition that occur after a specific time interval or in response to learner actions. Accompanying flow diagrams also outline the general sequence of actions for each case. In many of the cases, alternative options are described for use with varying levels of learners (e.g. a simple scenario for junior learners with a more difficult scenario for advanced learners).

At the end of each case you will find information to aid in debriefing. Instructor notes provide preceptors with basic background information about each specific case topic. There is also a list of potential questions for your learners to discuss during debriefing. Finally, you will also see a list of selected readings and/or references for each case. These can be distributed to learners either prior to or following the simulation.

We hope that you find this workbook useful for your emergency medicine simulation curriculum. Keep in mind that each simulation case is dynamic and can be modified in a variety of ways to best suit your learners and/or the fidelity of your mannequin.

REFERENCES

1 Okuda, Y., Bond, W., Bonfante, G. et al. (2008). National growth of simulation training within emergency medicine residency programs 2003-2008. *Acad. Emerg. Med.* 15 (11): 1113–1116.

2 Qayumi, K., Pachev, G., Zheng, B. et al. (2014). Status of simulation in health care education: an international survey. *Adv. Med. Educ. Pract.* 5: 457–467.

3 Chernikova, O., Heitzmann, N., Stadler, M. et al. (2020). Simulation-based learning in higher education: a meta-analysis. *Rev. Educ. Res.* 90 (4): 499–541.

CHAPTER 1

Abdominal/Gastroenterology Emergencies

Michele Callahan

Department of Emergency Medicine, University of Maryland School of Medicine, Baltimore, MD, USA

NECROTIZING ENTEROCOLITIS

Educational Goals

Learning Objectives

1. Demonstrate focused examination of a neonate (MK, PC).
2. Differentiate between normal neonatal behavior and pathological signs/symptoms that require further workup (MK, PC).
3. Recognize the need for imaging (MK, PC)
4. Demonstrate appropriate care for necrotizing enterocolitis (*NEC*) including nil per os (*NPO*) status and initiation of intravenous (IV) fluids and IV antibiotics (MK, PC).
5. Communicate effectively with team members to facilitate patient care (ICS, P).
6. Identify need for intensive care and pediatric surgery consultations (MK, P, SBP).
7. Demonstrate empathy and maintain family involvement when treating a pediatric patient (P, ICS).

Emergency Medicine Simulation Workbook: A Tool for Bringing the Curriculum to Life,
Second Edition. Edited by Traci L. Thoureen and Sara B. Scott.
© 2022 John Wiley & Sons Ltd. Published 2022 by John Wiley & Sons Ltd.
Companion website: www.wiley.com/go/thoureen/simulation/workbook2e

Critical Actions Checklist

- ☐ Obtain a full set of vital signs (PC)
- ☐ Obtain heelstick glucose (PC)
- ☐ Order appropriate blood tests and imaging studies to evaluate for obstruction, free air, and sepsis (MK).
- ☐ Early resuscitation with IV fluids and IV antibiotics (PC, MK).
- ☐ If no IV access, recognition that intraosseous (*IO*) is also an option (MK, PC).
- ☐ Appropriate consultation with pediatric surgery and critical care team (MK, SBP).

Simulation Set-Up

Environment: Emergency department

Mannequin: Newborn simulator mannequin, wearing a diaper with a onesie over top. Diaper is smeared with activated charcoal to simulate black stool. The simulator may have a weak cry, if this option is available.

Props: To be displayed on a computer/TV screen in the room, or printed out and handed to learners throughout the simulation. Should only be offered to learners if ordered/requested:

- Images (see online component for NEC, Scenario 1.1 at https://www.wiley.com/go/thoureen/simulation/workbook2e):
  - Abdominal x-ray showing distended bowel with early intraluminal gas (Figure 1.1).
  - Abdominal ultrasound showing pneumatosis (Figure 1.2).
  - Radiology interpretation of abdominal x-ray concerning for NEC (Figure 1.3).
  - Radiology interpretation of abdominal ultrasound showing pneumatosis (Figure 1.4).

> Imaging that is not provided but is requested by learners can be reported as normal.

- Laboratory tests (see online component as above):
  - Heelstick glucose (Table 1.1).
  - Complete blood count (Table 1.2).
  - Basic metabolic panel (Table 1.3).
  - Liver function panel (Table 1.4).
  - Lipase (Table 1.5).
  - Coagulation panel (Table 1.6).
  - Lactic acid (Table 1.7).

- C-reactive protein (Table 1.8).
- Troponin (Table 1.9).
- Urinalysis (Table 1.10).
- Urine microscopy (Table 1.11).

Available supplies:

- Pediatric code cart and basic airway supplies, including supplies for intubation.
- Pediatric length-based tape.
- Medications:
  - IV fluid bags: 0.9% saline, lactated Ringer's solution (*LR*), PlasmaLyte®.
- Pre-labeled bags:
  - Vasopressors (e.g. norepinephrine, dopamine, vasopressin).
- Pre-labeled syringes:
  - Dextrose (10 and 25%) in water.
  - Morphine.
  - Antiemetic.
  - Antibiotics (broad spectrum).
  - Intubation medications (sedatives and paralytics of choice at your facility).
- IO device (optional).

Distractor(s): None.

Actors

- Patient's parent provides history.
- Emergency department (ED) nurse: can help to place the patient on monitor, obtain IV access (IO should be done by learners, if needed), and administer medications/fluids. May cue learners if needed.
- Respiratory therapy (available when requested in ED).
- Pediatric/neonatal intensive care (PICU/NICU) team member via phone consultation.
- Pediatric surgery consultant via phone consultation.

Case Narrative

Scenario Background

A four-week-old preterm, female infant born by spontaneous vaginal delivery at 33 weeks of gestation, (birth weight 4 lbs (1.81 kg) presents to the ED for lethargy, decreased feeding, and vomiting with feeds. The patient was in NICU for four weeks but discharged to home three days ago. The patient's hospital stay was complicated by neonatal jaundice and temperature dysregulation, both of which were resolved prior to discharge. For the past two days, the patient's mother has noticed increased difficulty with feeding (formula fed), decreased PO intake, vomiting after feeds, and general sleepiness.

Chief complaint:	Lethargy, decreased feeding, vomiting.
Patient's medical history:	Ex-33 week, four-day preemie (current age 37 weeks of gestational age, actual age 4 weeks 3 days).
Surgical history:	None.
Allergies:	None.
Medictions:	Vitamin D supplementation.
Social history:	Not in daycare, lives at home with mom; no siblings.
Family history:	None.

Initial Scenario Conditions

Parent is holding the neonate. Patient has a weak cry.

Vital signs:	T 102.4°F (39.1°C) rectal, HR 215, RR 60, BP 70/35, SpO$_2$ 97% on room air.
Weight:	2.7 kg.
Head:	Atraumatic, normocephalic, fontanelle soft.
Eyes:	Pupils 4 mm bilaterally and reactive to light.
Neck:	Supple, full range of motion, no meningismus.
Heart:	Tachycardic, regular, no murmurs/rubs/gallops.
Lungs:	Tachypnea, clear to auscultation bilaterally.
Abdomen:	Moderately distended with high-pitched bowel sounds; patient screams when abdomen is palpated in all quadrants. No palpable masses. Dark black soft stool in diaper (hemoccult positive, if asked).
Extremities:	No gross deformities; warm extremities with capillary refill two to three seconds.
Skin:	Warm, no rashes, no mottling.
Neurologic:	Moves all extremities spontaneously; weak cry that increases with palpation of the abdomen.

> Physical exam findings that are not available on your mannequin may be offered verbally to learners if they ask (e.g., rectal exam and hemoccult testing can be reported if specifically requested by learners).

See flow diagram (Figure 1.5) for further scenario changes described.

Case Narrative, Continued

During the initial minutes of the scenario, learners of all levels should collect a thorough history from the patient's parent/s and perform a complete physical exam. Initial lab tests and imaging studies should be ordered after this assessment is complete. All learners should request a heelstick glucose (prompted by the nurse if the learner fails to request it).

Over the next five minutes, the patient will deteriorate regardless of interventions, becoming less responsive with hypotension, increased respiratory rate, and hypoxia. Eventually, there will be episodes of bradycardia with short apneic episodes.

For novice learners, not trained to perform intubation on infants, the use of bag–valve mask (*BVM*) ventilation for supplemental oxygen will stabilize the patient until the NICU team arrives. They may consult anesthesiology as well.

For more advanced learners, intubation will be required because of impending respiratory failure and worsening lethargy.

If there is a delay in providing advanced airway interventions (BVM and/or intubation), the patient will progress into a pulseless electrical activity (*PEA*) rhythm and require cardiopulmonary resuscitation (*CPR*). After two minutes of appropriate pediatric CPR, the patient will regain pulses.

Advanced learners will need to initiate vasopressors for persistent hypotension. If the learners do not order vasopressors, the nurse may prompt them by mentioning that the blood pressure remains abnormally low and the full IV fluid bolus has already been given.

Once the airway and hypotension are addressed (or upon finishing CPR), the learners will receive any remaining results not yet reported. They should then communicate their concern for NEC with pediatric surgery as well as the NICU/PICU team for admission and intervention. The case will end upon appropriate consultation with these teams.

Instructor Notes

Epidemiology

- NEC is more common in premature neonates:
  - Only around 10% occurs in full-term neonates.
  - Higher risk in lower birth weights.
  - Timing of onset is the inverse of gestational age (e.g. born close to term presents earlier postnatally than if born more prematurely).

Pathophysiology

- Etiology unclear:
  - Possibly related to intestinal ischemia with an immature gut barrier that predisposes to infectious agents.
  - Cytokines and growth factor implicated in pathogenesis.

- Bacteria in intestinal lumen ferment carbohydrates and produce hydrogen gas that leads to pneumatosis and portal venous gas.

Clinical Features

- Variable presentation.
- Historical features:
  - Increasing lethargy.
  - Forceful/projectile vomiting.
  - Presence of bloody or bilious vomit [1].
- May present similar to sepsis:
  - Hypo/hyperthermia, lethargy, apneic episodes, bradycardia, hypotension, poor glucose regulation.
- Gastrointestinal signs/symptoms:
  - Abdominal distension, bloody stools, vomiting, a palpable abdominal mass (intestinal loops) or abdominal wall redness or crepitus.
  - Scrotal discoloration (males).

Differential Diagnosis for Vomiting Neonate

- Gastrointestinal causes:
  - Overfeeding.
  - Gastroenteritis.
  - Malrotation with midgut volvulus.
  - NEC.
  - Intussusception.
  - Intestinal atresia.
  - Gastroesophageal reflux.
  - Pyloric stenosis.
  - Hirschsprung disease.
- Non-gastrointestinal causes:
  - Central nervous system diseases.
  - Metabolic/endocrine disorders.
  - Trauma.

Diagnosis

- Laboratory abnormalities may include:
  - Thrombocytopenia.
  - Hyponatremia.
  - Metabolic acidosis with elevated lactate.
  - Neutropenia or leukocytosis.

- Abdominal radiographs (anteroposterior and lateral) may show:
  - Pneumatosis intestinalis.
  - Portal venous gas.
  - Non-specific gas-filled loops of bowel.

Management [2–5]

- NPO.
- Gastric decompression with an orogastric tube
- Broad-spectrum intravenous antibiotics.
- Intravenous fluids.
- Surgical intervention, if pneumatosis is present.
- Survival rates depend on disease severity:
  - Those requiring surgical management have worse outcomes with mortality, around 35%.
  - If treated medically, mortality is around 20%.

Debriefing Plan

Allow approximately 20–30 minutes for debriefing after this scenario.

Potential Questions for Discussion

- What are pertinent history and physical exam findings in a vomiting neonate/infant?
- What is the differential diagnosis of bilious compared with nonbilious vomiting in neonates?
- If unable to obtain peripheral IV access in an infant, what alternatives are available for fluid resuscitation?
- What is the management for an infant with NEC?

REFERENCES FOR NECROTIZING ENTEROCOLITIS

1. Shields, T.M. and Lightdale, J.R. (2018). Vomiting in children. *Pediatr. Rev.* 39 (7): 342–358.
2. Rich, B. and Dolgin, S. (2017). Necrotizing enterocolitis. *Pediatr. Rev.* 38 (12): 552–559.
3. Burge, D. (2016). The management of bilious vomiting in the neonate. *Early Hum. Dev.* 102: 41–45.
4. Frost, B., Modi, B., Jaksic, T. et al. (2017). New medical and surgical insights into neonatal necrotizing enterocolitis. *JAMA Pediatr.* 171 (1): 83.
5. Ratnayake, K. and Kim, T.Y. (2014). Evidence-based management of neonatal vomiting in the emergency department. *Pediatr. Emerg. Med. Pract.* 11 (11): 1–20.

ACUTE ASCENDING CHOLANGITIS

Educational Goals

Learning Objectives

1. Demonstrate focused history and physical examination skills (PC, MK).
2. Identify the need for blood work and imaging studies (MK).
3. Recognize signs and symptoms of sepsis (MK).
4. Initiate appropriate management of sepsis (MK, PC).
5. Demonstrate appropriate consultation for acute cholangitis (MK, ICS, P, SBP)
6. Demonstrate ability to obtain collateral history from family members, emergency medical services (EMS), and/or nursing home staff, for a patient who is unable to provide a history (ICS, P, SBP).

Critical Actions Checklist

- ☐ Obtain IV access (PC).
- ☐ Administer IV fluids (30 cc/kg IV fluid bolus) (MK, PC).
- ☐ Administer broad-spectrum IV antibiotics (MK, PC).
- ☐ Obtain computed tomography (CT) to evaluate for causes of acute abdominal pain and to rule out life-threatening pathology (MK, PC).
- ☐ Consult general surgery and/or gastroenterology (ICS, P, SBP).

Simulation Set-Up

Environment: Emergency department resuscitation room.

This scenario may begin on scene at the patient's home with EMS gathering information from family, then transition to the ED.

Mannequin: Adult male simulator mannequin, with wig (gray hair if possible), fully dressed. Sclera should be icteric; this can be moulaged using a yellow erasable marker or removable yellow translucent film.

Props: To be displayed on screen or given as handouts when asked for/ returned from lab:

- Images (see online component for acute cholangitis, Scenario 1.2 at `https://www.wiley.com/go/thoureen/simulation/workbook2e`):
  - Chest x-ray showing no active pulmonary disease (Figure 1.6).

- Radiology reading of chest x-ray (normal) (Figure 1.7).
  - Head CT (static image 1-cut) showing no intracranial abnormality (Figure 1.8).
  - Radiology read CT head (normal) (Figure 1.9).
  - Ultrasound of right upper quadrant (static image) showing biliary dilation (Figure 1.10).
  - Radiology read showing biliary dilation concerning for choledocholithiasis (Figure 1.11).
  - CT abdomen/pelvis with IV contrast (static image, 1-cut) showing grossly dilated common bile duct (Figure 1.12).
  - CT read concerning for acute cholangitis (Figure 1.13).
  - Electrocardiogram (ECG) showing sinus tachycardia (Figure 1.14).
- Laboratory tests (see online component as above):
  - Complete blood count (Table 1.12).
  - Basic metabolic panel (Table 1.13).
  - Liver function panel (Table 1.14).
  - Lipase (Table 1.15).
  - Lactic acid (Table 1.16).
  - Coagulation panel (Table 1.17).
  - Troponin (Table 1.18).
  - Type and screen (Table 1.19).
  - Urinalysis (Table 1.20).
  - Urine microscopy (Table 1.21).

Available supplies:

- Adult code cart with basic airway supplies.
- Central line kit (triple lumen).
- Medications:
  - 0.9% saline, LR IV bags.
  - Pre-labeled IV bags.
    - IV vasopressor infusion (norepinephrine or similar).
    - Broad-spectrum antibiotics.
  - Pre-labeled syringes:
    - Antiemetics (ondansetron, metoclopramide).
    - Analgesic medications (morphine, fentanyl, hydromorphone).
    - Rapid sequence intubation medications (sedative/paralytics typical to your institution).

Distractor: none

Actors

- The patient is slightly confused as to the timeline of events/illness, but able to answer some questions. Occasionally moans due to abdominal pain. May have dry heaving if no antiemetics are ordered.
- EMS to share information gathered from family regarding how long he has been sick, what symptoms they have noticed (significantly less energetic and interactive, slow to respond to basic questions).
- ED nurse can cue the learners if needed to progress the case.
- Family member (patient's adult child) available by phone.
- General surgery and/or gastroenterology available for phone consultation.
- Admitting physician available for phone consultation.

Case Narrative

Scenario Background

A 60-year-old man presents for gradually worsening confusion over the course of two to three days. He reports having mild diffuse abdominal pain that is most severe in the upper abdomen. Over the course of the past one to two days, pain has become worse and he has begun to have vomiting and increased confusion.

Chief complaint:	Confusion.
Patient's medical history:	Hypertension, diabetes, stroke.
Surgical istory:	Appendectomy, hernia repair.
Allergies:	None.
Social history:	Previous cigarette smoker; no alcohol or drug use.
Family history:	Non-contributory.
Medications:	Lisinopril, metformin, aspirin, clopidogrel.

Initial Scenario Conditions

A 60-year-old man is brought in by EMS from home. Patient is moaning due to abdominal pain, complaining of feeling sick.

Vital signs:	Temp 102.5°F (39.2°C), HR 125, RR 22, BP 80/60, SpO2 99% on room air.
Head:	Atraumatic, normocephalic.
Eyes:	Icteric sclerae; pupils 4 mm bilaterally and reactive to light; extra-ocular movement intact without nystagmus.
Ears/nose/mouth:	Dry mucous membranes, with subungual icterus (if asked).
Neck:	Supple, full range of movement, no meningeal signs.
Heart:	Tachycardic, regular, no murmurs/rubs/gallops.

Lungs:	Clear to auscultation bilaterally (patient reports worsening belly pain when taking deep breaths).
Abdomen:	Distended, with hypoactive bowel sounds. Tender to palpation in the upper abdomen, most significant in the right upper quadrant and epigastric region. No rebound. Voluntary guarding in all quadrants.
Extremities:	No edema, cyanosis, or clubbing.
Skin:	Warm to the touch.
Neurologic:	Alert and oriented to person and place, but not to time. Answers most questions appropriately but seems confused and takes a while to respond to simple questions. No focal deficits. Cranial nerves intact. No asterixis.

Physical exam findings that are not available on your mannequin may be offered verbally to learners if they ask (e.g. if unable to simulate icteric sclera, can verbally report the scleral exam to the learners if they specifically ask for this information).

See flow diagram (Figure 1.15) for scenario changes based on learner actions.

Case Narrative, Continued

For all learners, the case should begin with obtaining a complete history as well as performing a thorough physical exam. The nurse can help the learners to set the patient up on the monitor to obtain vital signs. This should also include obtaining a fingerstick glucose, in light of the patient's slightly altered mental state.

Learners should order initial labs, imaging, IV fluids and medications.

If there is inadequate fluid resuscitation, the patient's hypotension will worsen. Continued failure to appropriately fluid resuscitate will lead to PEA, requiring CPR.

For novice learners, administration of an appropriate fluid bolus (30 cc/kg) will cause the patient's blood pressure to increase to a mean arterial pressure greater than 65 mmHg and his heart rate will slowly lower. With these improvements, the patient's mental status will also improve. Laboratory tests and imaging will then be available for review and appropriate consultation should be made with general surgery/GI, as well as an admitting physician. The case will end after appropriate disposition and consultation have occurred.

For advanced learners, despite initiation of IV fluids and broad-spectrum antibiotics, the patient will continue to be hypotensive and altered, requiring initiation of vasopressors and intubation. Failure to do so will result in PEA arrest. Once intubation is performed and vasopressors are initiated, the patient will stabilize. Consultation with general surgery/GI and the intensive care admitting physician should then occur. The case will end after appropriate disposition and consultation have occurred.

Instructor Notes

Pathophysiology

- Acute (or ascending) cholangitis results from inflammation and infection of the biliary system, often related to a blockage of the bile ducts or hepatic ducts:
  - Biliary obstruction leads to bacterial growth within the bile and subsequent infection.
  - Common causes of blockage include choledocholithiasis, malignancy, strictures, primary sclerosing cholangitis, and AIDS-related cholangiopathy.
- Most frequent pathogens found in acute cholangitis include *Escherichia coli*, *Klebsiella spp.*, *Enterococcus spp.*, and *Enterobacter spp.*
- Anaerobes such as *Bacteroides fragilis* and *Clostridium perfringens* have also been accountable, often in elderly patients or those with prior biliary surgery [1].

Clinical Features

- Charcot's triad:
  - Fever, right upper-quadrant abdominal pain, and jaundice.
  - "Classic" presentation, although it is only around 25% sensitive for acute cholangitis to have all three, 80–90% of patients with acute cholangitis will have fever and/or abdominal pain [2].
- Reynold's pentad:
  - Charcot's triad plus hypotension and altered mental state.
  - Severe presentation, but only seen in 5–7% of cases [2].

Diagnosis

- Laboratory tests that may support diagnosis:
  - Leukocytosis (with neutrophilic predominance).
  - Transaminitis.
  - Hyperbilirubinemia (conjugated).
  - Elevated alkaline phosphatase.
  - Elevated gamma-glutamyl transferase level.
- Imaging:
  - Ultrasound:
    - Best initial study. Can detect dilation of the common bile duct, gallstones, and other evidence of pathology.
  - CT with IV contrast:
    - Helpful for looking at other potential causes of biliary obstruction.
    - May show complications such as hepatic abscesses.
    - CT findings that may support the diagnosis of cholangitis include dilation of intra- or extra-hepatic biliary ducts, thickening of the ductal walls, presence of gallstones.

- Magnetic resonance cholangiopancreatography:
  - Sensitive imaging modality
  - May not be readily available at all institutions.

Management

- Resuscitation:
  - IV fluid administration.
  - Broad-spectrum IV antibiotics (with Gram-negative and anaerobic coverage).
  - Vasopressor administration (if needed).
- Analgesia.
- Specialist consultation (general surgery and/or gastroenterology) for intervention:
  - The type of intervention will depend on etiology:
    - Endoscopic retrograde cholangiopancreatography for biliary drainage, sphincterotomy, stone extraction, biliary stent placement.
    - Open surgical drainage.
  - If a patient is initially seen at a facility without these consult services, transfer to the nearest facility that has these resources should be undertaken [2, 3].

Debriefing Plan

Allow approximately 20–30 minutes for debriefing after this scenario.

Potential Questions for Discussion

- What are signs that a patient may have sepsis?
- What is the appropriate management of a patient with sepsis?
- How can you assess for end-organ dysfunction in a patient with sepsis?
- What are the indications for vasopressor initiation in sepsis?
- What is Charcot's triad?
- What is Reynold's pentad?

REFERENCES FOR SEPSIS

1. Ahmed, M. (2018). Acute cholangitis – an update. *World J. Gastrointest. Pathophysiol.* 9 (1): 1–7.
2. Ely, R., Long, B., and Koyfman, A. (2018). The emergency medicine–focused review of cholangitis. *J. Emerg. Med.* 54 (1): 64–72.
3. Mayumi, T., Okamoto, K., Takada, T. et al. (2018). Tokyo Guidelines 2018: management bundles for acute cholangitis and cholecystitis. *J. Hepatobiliary Pancreat. Sci.* 25 (1): 96–100.

SIGMOID VOLVULUS

Educational Goals

Learning Objectives

1. Assess a patient presenting with acute abdominal pain, utilizing a focused history and physical exam (MK, PC).
2. Formulate a differential diagnosis for acute abdominal pain (MK).
3. Recognize the signs and symptoms of a possible intestinal obstruction (MK).
4. Demonstrate appropriate utilization of lab tests and imaging studies to evaluate abdominal pain (MK, PC).
5. Recognize an agitated patient and use verbal de-escalation and negotiation skills (ICS, P).
6. Demonstrate professionalism while treating a patient with behavioral issues (P, ICS).
7. Demonstrate appropriate surgical consultation (P, ICS, SBP).

Critical Actions Checklist

☐ Recognize clinical signs of obstruction (MK).
☐ Obtain appropriate IV access (PC).
☐ Obtain imaging (MK).
☐ Administer analgesic medication and antiemetics for patient's symptoms (PC).
☐ Recognize an abnormal bowel gas pattern (concerning for obstruction) on x-ray and/or CT (MK).
☐ Maintain a calm and professional composure while communicating with a difficult, disruptive patient (PC, ICS, P).
☐ Consult general surgery for emergent management of volvulus (P, ICS, SBP).

Simulation Set-Up

Environment: ED treatment room.

Mannequin: Adult, male, simulator mannequin moulaged to appear disheveled (e.g. clothes may be slightly dirty and/or torn or used in appearance).

Props:
- Images (see online component for sigmoid volvulus, Scenario 1.3 at https://www.wiley.com/go/thoureen/simulation/workbook2e):
  - Abdominal x-ray showing evidence of distended sigmoid colon (Figure 1.16).
  - Radiology report of abdominal x-ray (Figure 1.17).
  - CT abdomen/pelvis with IV contrast (static image 1-cut) (Figure 1.18).

- Radiology report of sigmoid volvulus (Figure 1.19).
- ECG showing sinus tachycardia (Figure 1.20).
- Laboratory tests (see online component as above):
  - Complete blood count (Table 1.22).
  - Basic metabolic panel (Table 1.23).
  - Liver function panel (Table 1.24).
  - Lipase (Table 1.25).
  - Lactic acid (Table 1.26).
  - Troponin (Table 1.27).
  - Coagulation panel (Table 1.28).
  - Urinalysis (Table 1.29).
  - Urine microscopy (Table 1.30).

Available supplies:

- Adult code cart with basic airway supplies.
- Medications:
  - 0.9% saline/LR IV bags.
  - Pre-labeled IV bags:
    - Broad-spectrum antibiotics.
  - Pre-labeled syringes:
    - Analgesic medications (e.g. morphine, fentanyl, hydromorphone)
    - Antiemetics (e.g. metoclopramide, ondansetron)
    - Antipsychotics (typical of your institution examples include haloperidol, risperidone, etc.)
    - Benzodiazepines (lorazepam, diazepam, midazolam).
  - Optional: emesis basin.

Distractor: The patient's behavior is a distractor and the learner must demonstrate de-escalation and redirection techniques to obtain history and physical exam.

Actors

- Patient has chronic, poorly controlled schizophrenia. He is uncooperative and agitated with all the questioning and will require redirection and verbal de-escalation throughout the scenario. He is difficult to obtain history from, stating: "I am sick of answering all these questions." Eventually he will comply with the team's treatment plan (i.e., IV access, imaging, etc.).
- ED nurse is experienced and can cue the learners as needed.
- EMS may be an actor or may provide report via the phone (as a radio call from the field).
- General surgery consultant available via phone consultation.

Case Narrative

Scenario Background

A 50 year-old-man presents with worsening abdominal pain for the past two days. It is associated with intractable nausea and vomiting. He has not had a bowel movement for the past three days, which is unusual for him. His group home called because he has been vomiting and his pain is getting worse. He has no reported fever, chest discomfort, shortness of breath, or urinary difficulties.

Patient's medical history:	Paranoid schizophrenia, hypertension, anxiety.
Surgical history:	Hernia repair, tonsillectomy as a child.
Allergies:	haloperidol.
Medications:	Risperidone, trazodone, lorazepam.
Social history:	Previous cigarette smoker, no alcohol or drug use. Patient lives in a group living environment.
Family history:	Non-contributory.

Initial Scenario Conditions

A 50 year-old man lying on a hospital stretcher is moaning in pain. Patient is occasionally retching into a basin.

Vital signs:	T 98.7°F (37.1°C), P 115, RR 14, BP 110/60, SpO^2 99% on room air.
Head:	Atraumatic, normocephalic.
Eyes:	Pupils equal and reactive, extraocular muscles intact.
Ears/nose/mouth:	Dry mucous membranes.
Neck:	Supple, full range of motion, no meningismus.
Heart:	Tachycardic, regular, no murmurs/rubs/gallops.
Lungs:	Clear to auscultation bilaterally, no wheezes/rales/rhonchi.
Abdomen:	Distended, with hyperactive bowel sounds. Tender to palpation in all quadrants, no rebound/guarding/rigidity. Moans with deep palpation.
Extremities:	No edema, cyanosis, or clubbing.
Skin:	Warm and well-perfused, no rashes.
Neurologic:	Alert and oriented to self, place, and time. No focal deficits. Cranial nerves intact. No nystagmus.
Psychiatric:	Patient very rude and uncooperative, with agitated affect. Denies SI/HI/active hallucinations.

See flow diagram (Figure 1.21) for scenario changes based on learner actions.

Case Narrative, Continued

For all learners, the case should begin with obtaining a complete history, and performing a thorough physical exam. The nurse can help the learners to set the patient up on the monitor.

The learners should order laboratories, imaging studies, and appropriate medications (such as IV fluids, antiemetics, and pain control).

Throughout the scenario, the patient will be very disagreeable to the plan of care. He will be difficult to obtain history from and will be angry during the examination, "because that hurts me!" He will also initially refuse IV access and will require discussion about why this is necessary. He will then become hostile about the possibility of needing a CT scan because, "Aren't you a doctor? Can't you just figure it out based on what I've told you?" Ultimately he will require multiple efforts at verbal de-escalation before agreeing.

After the learner discusses the diagnosis of volvulus and the need for surgical evaluation with the patient, he will become upset and frustrated. He will calm down if the learner takes the time to listen to him and acknowledge his frustrations.

The trigger for the end of the case will be consultation with surgery for intervention and admission.

Instructor Notes

Epidemiology

- Third leading cause of large bowel obstruction worldwide, following cancer and complications of diverticulitis [1].
- Risk factors:
  - Elderly.
  - Individuals with chronic constipation and/or a high fiber diet.
  - Nursing home or long-term care facility patients [2], including patients with chronic psychiatric disorders and dementia.

Pathophysiology

- Sigmoid colon becomes stretched, attachments to the abdominal wall loosen, allowing colon to twist.
- Ischemia occurs, which can progress to gangrene and perforation.

Clinical Features

- Common symptoms:
  - Abdominal pain.
  - Bloating.
  - Constipation/obstipation.
  - Nausea/vomiting (may be feculent).
- Exam findings:
  - Pain on palpation.
  - Abdominal distension.
  - High-pitched bowel sounds.

Diagnosis

- Lab tests not diagnostic.
- Imaging:
  - Abdominal radiographs:
    - Distended loops of colon with or without air-fluid levels
    - "Bent inner tube sign" of distended colon in a U-shaped pattern and extending from the pelvis toward the right upper quadrant.
    - Paucity of gas in the rectum.
    - Free air under the diaphragm, if perforation has occurred.
  - Abdominal CT:
    - Dilated loops of bowel with evidence of obstruction.
    - "Whirl sign" or twisting of the mesentery.
    - "Bird's beak" sign if rectal contrast has been given.
    - Absence of gas in the rectum.
    - Transition point within the bowel.
    - Late findings that may indicate bowel necrosis or perforation: pneumatosis intestinalis, portal venous gas, loss of bowel wall enhancement.

Management

- Analgesia.
- Antiemetics.
- IV fluid resuscitation.
- IV antibiotics:
Recommended for signs of peritonitis, perforation or sepsis.
  - Emergent surgical consultation:
    - Flexible sigmoidoscopy.

- Recommended initial treatment strategy.
- Can be both diagnostic and therapeutic unless patients have perforation or significant ischemia.
  - Laparotomy:
    - If detorsion with endoscopy is not able to be performed, may be required.

Debriefing Plan

Provide approximately 20–30 minutes for debriefing after this scenario.

Potential Questions for Discussion

- What are some helpful strategies for dealing with difficult patients or patients with behavioral issues?
- What are risk factors for sigmoid volvulus?
- What abnormalities can be seen on abdominal x-ray in a patient with sigmoid volvulus?
- What is the management for a patient diagnosed with sigmoid volvulus? Is surgery always required?

REFERENCES FOR SIGMOID VOLVULUS

1. Bauman, Z.M. and Evans, C.H. (2018). Volvulus. *Surg. Clin. North Am.* 98 (5): 973–993.
2. Gingold, D. and Murrell, Z. (2012). Management of colonic volvulus. *Clin. Colon Rectal Surg.* 25 (4): 236–244.

SELECTED READING FOR SIGMOID VOLVULUS

Vestal, H.S., Sowden, G., Nejad, S. et al. (2017). Simulation-based training for residents in the management of acute agitation: a cluster randomized controlled trial. *Acad. Psychiatry* 41 (1): 62–67.

APPENDIX

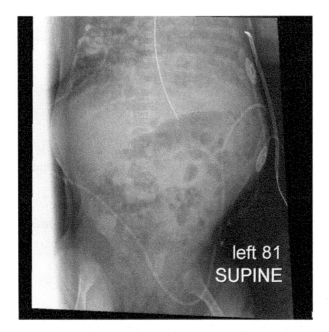

FIGURE 1.1   Abdominal x-ray showing distended bowel with early intraluminal gas.

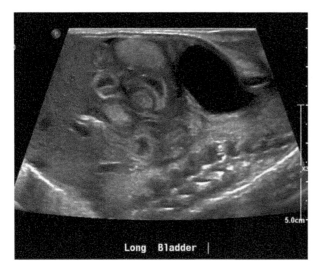

FIGURE 1.2   Abdominal ultrasound showing pneumatosis.

INDICATION: Nausea and vomiting, newborn

COMPARISON: None

TECHNIQUE: AP portable and lateral decubitus views of the chest and abdomen.

FINDINGS:

Lines and tubes: Nasogastric tube terminates in the stomach. ET tube is in the lower thoracic trachea. Left upper extremity PICC tip in the mid SVC.

Chest: Heart size is normal. Lungs are hypoinflated with diffuse coarse heterogeneous lung markings. Patchy airspace opacities in bilateral upper and left lower lobes with associated air bronchograms and left-sided volume loss (mediastinal shift and elevated left hemidiaphragm), compatible with atelectasis.

Abdomen: Abnormal bowel gas pattern demonstrating relative paucity of bowel gas with few distended bowel loops in the midabdomen and right lower quadrant. Bubbly lucencies in the right lower quadrant coalesce into intraluminal gas on the lateral decubitus view. Bubbly lucencies in the left mid abdomen on the supine view are not visible on the decubitus view. No portal venous gas or free air.

Osseous structures: Osteopenia without fracture.

IMPRESSION:

1. Abnormal bowel gas pattern with relative paucity of bowel gas. No free air, pneumatosis or portal venous gas.

FIGURE 1.3   Radiological interpretation of abdominal x-ray of concern for necrotizing enterocolitis.

INDICATION: Nausea/vomiting, prematurity

EXAMINATION: Abdominal sonogram with grayscale and color Doppler.

COMPARISON: None.

FINDINGS:

Liver: Normal contour and echotexure without cyst or mass. There is normal color-flow in the hepatic and portal veins. There is no biliary ductal dilation. No portal venous gas.
Gallbladder: Well distended without wall thickening. There are no gallstones. There is no pericholecystic fluid.

Spleen: Normal

Pancreas: Not well evaluated due to limited window.

Adrenals: Normal

Kidneys: Normal contour and echotexture without cyst or mass. There is no hydronephrosis or stone. Right kidney length 3.2 cm; left kidney length 2.9 cm

Diffusely hyperperistaltic bowel loops with echogenic content is noted. Complete evaluation of bowel peristals is limited in this study as a dedicated bowel ultrasound with focused cine images have not provided.

There are mild wall thickening at the of the bowel loops measuring up to 3 to 4 mm in thickness. Mild ascites. Although no significant convincing pneumatosis is appreciated in majority of bowel loops, I could see at least in one of the bowel loop nondependent foci along the wall (cine images performed at 10:26:33 AM) concerning for pneumatosis. Limited color Doppler images provided demonstrate some vascularity along the bowel wall at places.

Aorta/IVC: The aorta and inferior vena cava have normal caliber.

Bladder: The urinary bladder is appropriately distended without wall thickening.

IMPRESSION: Diffuse hypoperistalsic/aperistaltic bowel loops with mild wall thickening and possible pneumatosis at places. Mild ascites. Overall features are concerning for necrotizing enterocolitis. Recommend clinical correlation.

FIGURE 1.4   Radiological interpretation of abdominal ultrasound showing pneumatosis.

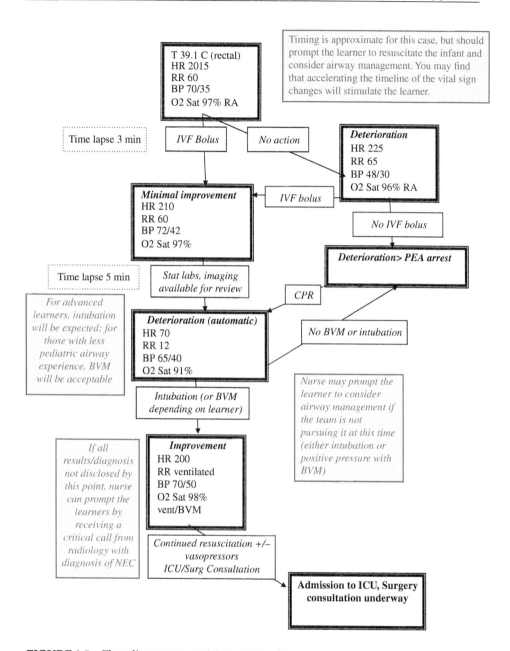

FIGURE 1.5 Flow diagram: necrotizing enterocolitis.

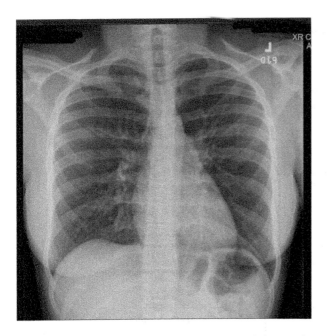

FIGURE 1.6 Chest x-ray showing no active pulmonary disease.

Clinical: Shortness of breath

TECHNIQUE: Single frontal view the chest

COMPARISON: None

FINDINGS:
No acute infiltrate, effusion, or pneumothorax. Cardiac mediastinal contours within normal limits. No evidence of acute osseous pathology. Visualized upper abdomen is unremarkable.

IMPRESSION:
As above

FIGURE 1.7 Radiological reading of chest x-ray (normal).

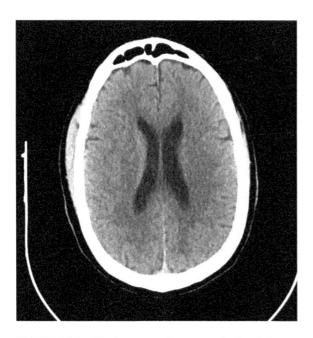

FIGURE 1.8   Head computed tomography (static image 1-cut) showing no intracranial abnormality.

CT HEAD WITHOUT CONTRAST.

INDICATION: Altered mental status

COMPARISON: CT, 04/07/2019

TECHNIQUE: Contiguous 3 mm axial noncontrast CT images of the brain were obtained along with 2-D multiplanar reformatted images in the coronal plane

This CT scan was performed with one or more of the following dose optimization techniques: iterative reconstruction, automatic exposure control, and/or manual adjustment of mAs and kVp according to the patients size.

FINDINGS:

The ventricles and cortical sulci are normal.

No evidence of hemorrhage, acute territorial infarction, mass effect, midline shift, hydrocephalus, or extra-axial collections.

No hyperdense arterial or venous sign.

Clear paranasal sinuses, mastoid air cells, and middle ear cavities.

The calvarium and overlying soft tissues are unremarkable.

IMPRESSION:

1. No acute intracranial process

FIGURE 1.9   Radiology read computed tomography of the head (normal).

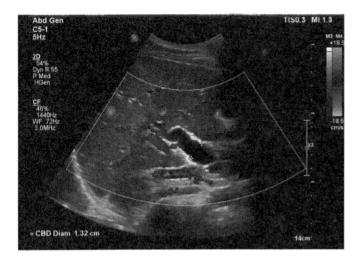

FIGURE 1.10   Ultrasound of right upper quadrant (static image) showing biliary dilation.

INDICATION: Abdominal Pain, confusion

TECHNIQUE: Grayscale and color Doppler ultrasound imaging of the right upper quadrant of the abdomen.

COMPARISON: None

FINDINGS:
Liver: Normal liver size and echogeniciy. it measures up to 14.9 cm in longest dimension. No fluid collections.
Main portal vein is patent.

Bile ducts: There is proximal dilatation of the common bile duct measuring 8 mm and continues to dilate distally
measuring up to 1.5 cm. There is also mild dilatation of central intrahepatic biliary radicals. No visualized stones
within the proximal duct. Distal most CBD is not well included in this provided image probably related to
technical limitaion.

Gallbladder: Multiple gallstones and gallbladder sludge with a positive Murphy sign. There is no pericholecystic fluid.
Suggestion of minimal gallbladder wall thickening.

Pancreas: The visualized pancreas is unremarkable.

Right kidney: There is a cystic lesion in the interpolar region of the right kidney with an internal echogenic focus.

IMPRESSION:

1. Gallbladder calculus and sludge with subtle wall thickening. The findings are somewhat equivocal for acute
cholecystitis. Recommend clinical correlation to rule out acute cholecystitis or cholangitis.

2. Dilated common bile duct concerning for a distal CBD calculus.

FIGURE 1.11   Radiology read showing biliary dilation concerning for choledocholithiasis.

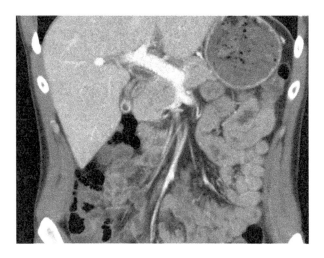

FIGURE 1.12 Computed tomography of the abdomen/pelvis with intravenous contrast (static image, 1-cut) showing grossly dilated common bile duct.

Indication: Abdominal pain, confusion

Exam Type: CT of the ABDOMEN and PELVIS

Technique: Multidetector CT axial images were obtained following the administration of nonionic intravenous contrast. Images were obtained in the portal venous phase. Sagittal and coronal reconstructions were subsequently obtained.

Findings:

Note that this was a single phase CT scan study. An arterial phase study was not performed, any vascular injury/active extravasation is not assessed in this study.

LOWER CHEST:
Normal.

ABDOMEN and PELVIS:
LIVER: No focal lesions. Normal size and density. Patent vasculature.
BILE DUCTS: The common bile duct measures up to 15 mm in diameter. The wall is thickened and enhancing.

GALLBLADDER: The gallbladder is contracted. There is wall enhancement, wall thickening and questionable mild pericholecystic fluid.

PANCREAS: Normal.

SPLEEN: Normal.

ADRENALS: Normal.

KIDNEYS/URETERS: Hypodense cyst in the midpole the right kidney measuring 10 mm without any septation and nodular component representing a simple cyst.

BLADDER: Normal.

BOWEL: The stomach is non distended. No evidence of bowel obstruction or wall thickening. The appendix is not visualized.

PERITONEUM/RETROPERITONEUM: Trace free fluid in the pelvis. No pneumoperitoneum.

LYMPH NODES: No adenopathy.

VESSELS: Normal.

ABDOMINAL WALL: Unremarkable.

IMPRESSION:

1. Contracted gallbladder with wall thickening and hyperenhancement, representing mild inflammation.
2. Minimal wall thickening and enhancement along the common bile duct concerning for acute cholangitis.
3. A simple cyst in the right kidney.

FIGURE 1.13 Computed tomography read concerning for acute cholangitis.

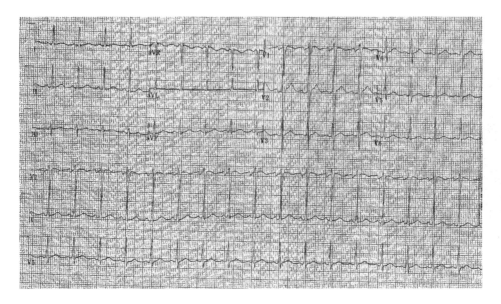

FIGURE 1.14 Electrocardiogram showing sinus tachycardia.

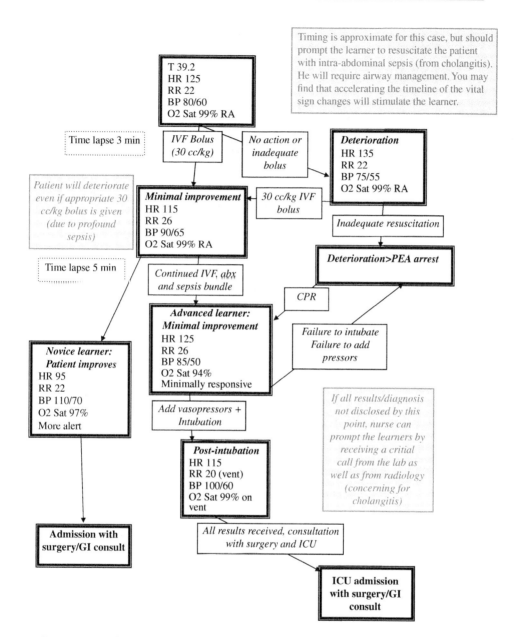

FIGURE 1.15 Flow diagram: ascending cholangitis.

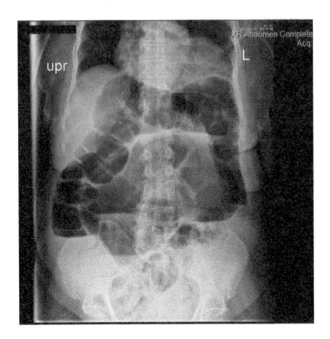

FIGURE 1.16   Abdominal x-ray showing evidence of distended sigmoid colon.

HISTORY: Bowel obstruction and volvulus.

EXAM: X-ray KUB.

COMPARISON: CT scan of the abdomen and pelvis from same day.

FINDINGS: An seen is marked distention of the sigmoid colon measuring approximately 7.7 cm. No definite transition zone is seen. There is no evidence of peritoneal free air or organomegaly or intra-abdominal calcifications. The visualized lung fields are clear. The cardiac silhouette is mildly enlarged.

IMPRESSION: Persistent marked distention of the colon. Recommend sigmoidoscopy and/or GI consultation.

FIGURE 1.17   Radiological report of abdominal x-ray.

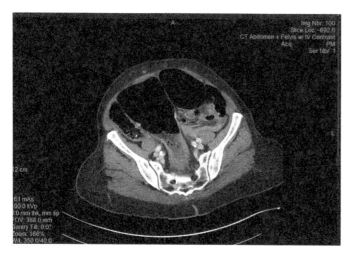

FIGURE 1.18 Computed tomography of the abdomen/pelvis with intravenous contrast (static image 1-cut).

CT ABDOMEN AND PELVIS WITH CONTRAST

CLINICAL HISTORY: Abdominal pain

COMPARISON: None.

TECHNIQUE: Multiple 3 mm axial images were obtained following the uneventful intravenous administration of 100 cc of Omnipaque 350. In addition, sagittal and coronal reformatted were also obtained.

This CT scan was performed with one or more of the following dose optimization techniques: iterative reconstruction, automatic exposure control, and/or manual adjustment of mAs and kVp according to the patient's size.

FINDINGS:

Mild bibasilar subsegmental atelectasis.
The heart is mildly enlarged.
Small hiatal hernia.

CT ABDOMEN:

The liver, spleen, pancreas, and adrenal glands are of normal size and attenuation. The gallbladder is normal in size without evidence of gallstones.
The kidneys are normal in size with a lobulated contour bilaterally.
Mild dilatation of the renal collecting systems bilaterally.
No evidence of nephrolithiasis or ureterolithiasis.
The aorta, IVC, and portal venous system are unremarkable.
No evidence of retroperitoneal hemorrhage or retroperitoneal lymphadenopathy.
There is twisting of the mesentery within the left lower quadrant with a large inverted distended U shaped segment of the sigmoid colon within the right upper quadrant that is consistent with a sigmoid volvulus.
Large amount of stool within the cecum and ascending colon.
No free air or free fluid within the peritoneal cavity.

CT PELVIS:

The bladder and rectum are unremarkable.
Mild degenerative changes of the spine.
The osseous structures demonstrate no acute abnormality.

IMPRESSION:

1. Sigmoid volvulus
2. No free air or free fluid

FIGURE 1.19 Radiological report of computed tomography showing sigmoid volvulus.

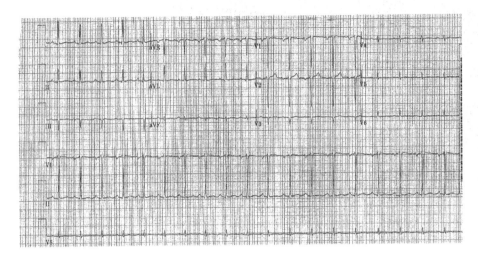

FIGURE 1.20   Electrocardiogram showing sinus tachycardia.

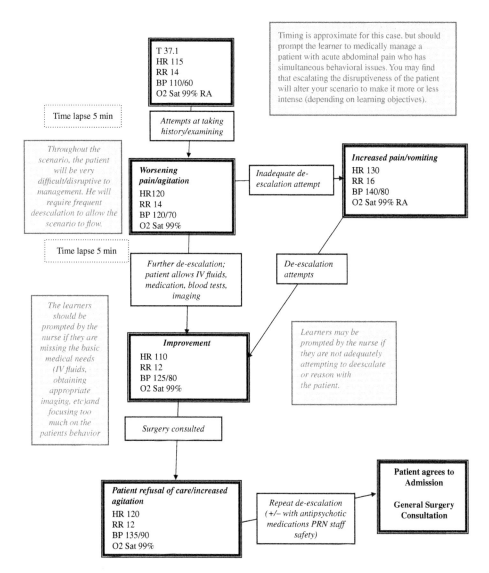

T 37.1
HR 115
RR 14
BP 110/60
O2 Sat 99% RA

Timing is approximate for this case, but should prompt the learner to medically manage a patient with acute abdominal pain who has simultaneous behavioral issues. You may find that escalating the disruptiveness of the patient will alter your scenario to make it more or less intense (depending on learning objectives).

Time lapse 5 min

Attempts at taking history/examining

Throughout the scenario, the patient will be very difficult/disruptive to management. He will require frequent deescalation to allow the scenario to flow.

Worsening pain/agitation
HR120
RR 14
BP 120/70
O2 Sat 99%

Inadequate de-escalation attempt

Increased pain/vomiting
HR 130
RR 16
BP 140/80
O2 Sat 99% RA

Time lapse 5 min

Further de-escalation; patient allows IV fluids, medication, blood tests, imaging

De-escalation attempts

The learners should be prompted by the nurse if they are missing the basic medical needs (IV fluids, obtaining appropriate imaging, etc)and focusing too much on the patients behavior

Improvement
HR 110
RR 12
BP 125/80
O2 Sat 99%

Learners may be prompted by the nurse if they are not adequately attempting to deescalate or reason with the patient.

Surgery consulted

Patient agrees to Admission

General Surgery Consultation

Patient refusal of care/increased agitation
HR 120
RR 12
BP 135/90
O2 Sat 99%

Repeat de-escalation (+/- with antipsychotic medications PRN staff safety)

FIGURE 1.21   Flow diagram: sigmoid volvulus.

TABLE 1.1   Heelstick glucose.

Test	Value	Reference range
Heelstick glucose (mg/dl)	80	70–100

TABLE 1.2   Complete blood count.

Test	Value	Reference range
White blood cells (× 10 000/μl)	26.8	4.5–10.6
Hemoglobin (g/dl)	11	13.7–15.6
Hematocrit (%)	39	41–47
Platelets (× 10^3/μl)	90	150–475

TABLE 1.3   Basic metabolic panel.

Test	Value	Reference range
Sodium (mmol/l)	132	136–145
Potassium (mmol/l)	3.1	3.5–5.1
Chloride (mmol/l)	95	98–107
CO_2 (mmol/l)	14	22–29
Blood urea nitrogen (mg/dl)	30	6–23
Creatinine (mg/dl)	1.2	0.7–1.2
Glucose (mg/dl)	78	70–100

TABLE 1.4   Liver function panel.

Test	Value	Reference range
Aspartate aminotransferase (iu/l)	35	5–40
Alanine aminotransferase (iu/l)	38	5–41
Alkaline phosphatase (iu/l)	100	40–129
Total bilirubin (mg/dl)	0.6	0.2–1
Albumin (g/dl)	3.2	3.5–4.2

TABLE 1.5   Lipase.

Test	Value	Reference range
Lipase (iu/l)	25	7–60

TABLE 1.6 Coagulation panel.

Test	Value	Reference range
Prothrombin time (seconds)	12	11.0–15.0
International normalized ratio	1	0–4
Partial thromboplastin time (seconds)	28	24.0–36.0

TABLE 1.7 Lactic acid.

Test	Value	Reference range
Lactic acid (mmol/l)	2.6	0–2

TABLE 1.8 C-reactive protein.

Test	Value	Reference range
C-reactive protein (mg/l)	12	0–3

TABLE 1.9 Troponin.

Test	Value	Reference range
Troponin (ng/ml)	< 0.01	0–0.4

TABLE 1.10 Urinalysis.

Test	Value	Reference range
Specific gravity	1.030	1.001–1.030
Ketones	3+	Negative
Bilirubin	Negative	Negative
Leukocyte esterase	Negative	Negative
Nitrite	Negative	Negative
Glucose	Negative	Negative
Urobilinogen (mg/dl)	1.0	0.2–1.0
Color	Dark	
Appearance	Yellow	
Protein	Negative	Negative
pH	7.0	5.0–8.0
Blood	Negative	Negative

TABLE 1.11   Urine microscopy.

Test	Value	Reference range
White blood cells (/hpf)	2	1–5
Red blood cells (/hpf)	Negative	1–5
squamous epithelial cells	Rare	None
Bacteria	Rare	Negative

TABLE 1.12   Complete blood count.

Test	Value	Reference range
White blood cells ($\times$ 10 000/μl)	22.5	4.5–10.6
Hemoglobin (g/dl)	12.8	13.7–15.6
Hematocrit (%)	41	41–47
Platelets ($\times$ 10^3/μl)	168	150 000–475

TABLE 1.13   Basic metabolic panel.

Test	Value	Reference range
Sodium (mmol/l)	142	136–145
Potassium (mmol/l)	3.1	3.5–5.1
Chloride (mmol/l)	97	98–107
CO_2 (mmol/l)	18	22–29
Blood urea nitrogen (mg/dl)	38	6–23
Creatinine (mg/dl)	1.9	0.7–1.2
Glucose (mg/dl)	80	70–100

TABLE 1.14   Liver function panel.

Test	Value	Reference range
Aspartate aminotransferase (iu/l)	65	5–40
Alanine aminotransferase (iu/l)	68	5–41
Alkaline phosphatase (iu/l)	165	40–129
Total bilirubin (mg/dl)	3.0	0.2–1
Albumin (g/dl)	4	3.5–4.2

TABLE 1.15 Lipase.

Test	Value	Reference range
Lipase (iu/l)	65	7–60

TABLE 1.16 Lactate.

Test	Value	Reference range
Lactic acid (mmol/l)	3.5	0–2

TABLE 1.17 Coagulation panel.

Test	Value	Reference range
Prothrombin time (seconds)	12	11.0–15.0
International normalized ratio	1	0–4
Partial thromboplastin time (seconds)	28	24.0–36.0

TABLE 1.18 Troponin.

Test	Value	Reference range
Troponin (ng/ml)	< 0.01	0–0.4

TABLE 1.19 Type and screen.

Test	Result
Blood type	AB+

TABLE 1.20   Urinalysis.

Test	Value	Reference range
Specific gravity	1.030	1.001–1.030
Ketones	1+	Negative
Bilirubin	Negative	Negative
Leukocyte esterase	Negative	Negative
Nitrite	Negative	Negative
Glucose	Negative	Negative
Urobilinogen	1.2	0.2–1.0
Color	Clear	
Appearance	Yellow	
Protein	Negative	Negative
pH	7.0	5.0–8.0
Blood	Negative	Negative

TABLE 1.21   Urine microscopy.

Test	Value	Reference range
White blood cells (/hpf)	Negative	1–5
Red blood cells (/hpf)	Negative	1–5
Squamous epithelial cells	Rare	
Bacteria	Rare	Negative

HPF, high power field.

TABLE 1.22   Complete blood count.

Test	Value	Reference range
White blood cells (× 10 000/µl)	11.2	4.5–10.6
Hemoglobin (g/dl)	14	13.7–15.6
Hematocrit (%)	41	41–47
Platelets (× 10³/µl)	450	150 000–475

TABLE 1.23 Basic metabolic panel.

Test	Value	Reference range
Sodium (mmol/l)	145	136–145
Potassium (mmol/l)	2.9	3.5–5.1
Chloride (mmol/l)	95	98–107
CO_2 (mmol/l)	20	22–29
Blood urea nitrogen (mg/dl)	38	6–23
Creatinine (mg/dl)	1.9	0.7–1.2
Glucose (mg/dl)	75	70–100

TABLE 1.24 Liver function panel.

Test	Value	Reference range
Aspartate aminotransferase (iu/l)	35	5–40
Alanine aminotransferase (iu/l)	38	5–41
Alkaline phosphatase (iu/l)	100	40–129
Total bilirubin (mg/dl)	0.6	0.2–1
Albumin (g/dl)	3	3.5–4.2

TABLE 1.25 Lipase.

Test	Value	Reference range
Lipase (iu/l)	25	7–60

TABLE 1.26 Troponin.

Test	Value	Reference range
Troponin (ng/ml)	< 0.01	0–0.4

TABLE 1.27   Lactic acid.

Test	Value	Reference range
Lactic acid (mmol/l)	2.1	0–2

TABLE 1.28   Coagulation panel.

Test	Value	Reference range
Prothombin time (seconds)	12	11.0–15.0
International normalized ratio	1	0–4
Partial thromboplastin time (seconds)	28	24.0–36.0

TABLE 1.29   Urinalysis.

Test	Value	Reference range
Specific gravity	1.030	1.001–1.030
Ketones	2+	Negative
Bilirubin	Negative	Negative
Leukocyte esterase	Negative	Negative
Nitrite	Negative	Negative
Glucose	Negative	Negative
Urobilinogen (mg/dl)	1.2	0.2–1.0
Color	Dark	
Appearance	Yellow	
Protein	1+	Negative
pH	7.0	5.0–8.0
Blood	Negative	Negative

TABLE 1.30   Urine microscopy.

Test	Value	Reference range
White blood cells (/hpf)	Negative	1–5
Red blood cells (/hpf)	Negative	1–5/
Squamous epithelial cells	Rare	
Bacteria	Rare	Negative

HPF, high power field

CHAPTER 2

Cardiovascular Emergencies

Mark J. Bullard and Catherine M. Wares

Department of Emergency Medicine, Carolinas Medical Center, Atrium Health, Charlotte, NC, USA

STABLE MONOMORPHIC VENTRICULAR TACHYCARDIA

Educational Goals

Learning Objectives

1. Recognize sustained, stable monomorphic ventricular tachycardia (*VT*) (MK, PC, PBL).
2. Formulate a differential diagnosis for sustained, stable monomorphic VT and initiate appropriate testing (MK, PBL, PC).
3. Appropriately cardiovert stable monomorphic VT (MK, PBL, PC).
4. Discuss care with patient and consultants (ICS, P, SBP).

Critical Actions Checklist

- ☐ Perform appropriate history and physical exam (PC)
- ☐ Order an ECG and identify abnormalities (MK, PC)
- ☐ Identify stable monomorphic VT (MK, PC)
- ☐ Order diagnostic testing for possible correctable causes (MK, PC)

Emergency Medicine Simulation Workbook: A Tool for Bringing the Curriculum to Life,
Second Edition. Edited by Traci L. Thoureen and Sara B. Scott.
© 2022 John Wiley & Sons Ltd. Published 2022 by John Wiley & Sons Ltd.
Companion website: www.wiley.com/go/thoureen/simulation/workbook2e

☐ Cardiovert VT prior to transfer:
   ☐ Pharmacologic compared with direct current (*DC*) (PC).
   ☐ Demonstrate appropriate use of the defibrillator (MK, PC).
☐ Discuss care with patient and family (ICS, P).
☐ Discuss care with consultant (ICS, P, SBP).

Critical actions can be changed to address the educational needs of learners (i.e.: emergency medical service (EMS) providers may have objectives related to therapies during transport; novice learners may DC cardiovert despite patient stability rather than attempting pharmacologic cardioversion).

Simulation Set-up

Environment: Emergency department (ED) resuscitation bay. This scenario may start "on scene" and transition to a hospital setting for EMS providers.

Mannequin: adult male simulator mannequin, sitting upright in ED stretcher.

Props: To be displayed on monitor or printed on handouts in scenario room when asked for:

- Images (see online component for stable monomorphic VT, Scenario 2.1 at https://www.wiley.com/go/thoureen/simulation/workbook2e):
  - Chest x-ray which is normal (Figure 2.1).
  - Electrocardiogram (ECG) showing wide complex tachycardia (Figure 2.2).
  - Previous ECG with normal sinus rhythm (Figure 2.3).
- Laboratory tests (see online component as above):
  - Complete blood count (Table 2.1).
  - Chemistry (Table 2.2).
  - Magnesium level (Table 2.3).
  - Troponin (Table 2.4).
  - Coagulation panel (Table 2.5).

Imaging or laboratory test values not provided can be verbally reported as "normal" if the learners order the study.

Available supplies:

- Airway and code cart.
- Defibrillator.

- Medications:
- Liter bags of 0.9% saline or lactated Ringers solution (*LR*).
- Pre-labeled in syringes:
  - Rapid sequence intubation medications (medications of choice for institution).
  - Sedative or procedural sedation medications.
  - Analgesic medication.
- Fiberoptic or video-assisted laryngoscope (optional).

Distractor: none

Actors

- EMS may be an actor.
- Patient voice is male.
- ED nurse can administer medications/fluids. The nurse may cue learners if needed.
- Cardiology consultant available by phone and may provide recommendations depending on the level of learner.

Case Narrative

Scenario Background

A 55-year-old man presents to the ED by EMS. The patient states that he has felt "funny" today and doesn't feel like himself. He has had one similar episode previously for which he was seen in the ED and discharged. He had a "normal" cardiac stress test, Holter monitor, and cardiac echo four years ago.

Patient's medical history:	Dyslipidemia, ventricular septal defect repair as a young child.
Medications:	Lipitor.
Allergies:	No known drug allergies.
Family history:	Mother living with hypertension. Father living with diabetes.
Social history:	No tobacco, drugs or alcohol use. Patient lives at home with his wife and two teenage children.

Initial scenario conditions

55-year old man brought in by EMS, no acute distress.

Case may start with EMS "on scene" evaluating stability, initiating treatment, and transporting according to local EMS protocols. EMS may then hand-off the patient to the ED care team. Alternatively, the case background may be presented by an EMS actor.

Vital signs: Temp 99.5°F (37.5°C), HR 180, RR 18, BP 98/60, SpO$_2$ 96% on room air.
Head: Normocephalic/atraumatic.
Eyes: Pupils 4 mm, reactive.
Neck: Supple, no lymphadenopathy, no thyromegaly.
Heart: Tachycardic, regular, distal pulses palpable.
Lungs: Clear breath sounds.
Abdomen: Soft, nontender, normal bowel sounds.
Extremities: No edema.
Skin: Normal.
Neurologic: Awake, oriented × 4.

> Physical exam findings not available on your mannequin can be reported verbally if asked for by learners. Visual findings can be presented via image.

See flow diagram (Figure 2.4) for scenario changes described.

Case Narrative, Continued

The patient is stable initially allowing for learners to develop a differential diagnosis and possible correctable causes for stable, sustained, monomorphic VT. The patient should be cardioverted prior to transfer.

Learners of all levels should initially perform a history and physical exam, obtain appropriate intravenous (IV) access and evaluate the ECG.

For novice learners, appropriate labs and imaging should be ordered and cardioversion should be initiated prior to transfer.

For advanced learners, pharmacologic cardioversion should be attempted given the patient's stability with the plan for synchronized DC cardioversion if pharmacologic cardioversion is unsuccessful.

If DC cardioversion is attempted, all learners should consider appropriate procedural sedation.

If pharmacologic or DC cardioversion does not occur, the patient will decompensate to ventricular fibrillation (*VF*) requiring defibrillation. Intubation can be done if that is an added learning objective.

The case ends when the patient is stabilized, care has been discussed with cardiology and the patient is admitted to a cardiac care center.

Instructor Notes

Pathophysiology

- Monomorphic VT:
  - Morphology does not change beat to beat.
  - Indicates a single focus.

- Stable substrate for reentrant circuit.
- Occurs in patients with and without structural heart disease.
- Polymorphic VT:
  - Continuously changing QRS morphology.
  - Patients with structural heart disease.
  - Ion channel disorders:
    - Brugada syndrome.
    - Long QT syndrome.
    - Catecholaminergic VT.
  - Myocardial ischemia is the most common etiology.

Diagnosis

- Regular, wide complex tachycardia QRS > 120 ms.
- Differential diagnosis for regular, wide complex tachycardia includes:
  - VT:
    - History of angina, myocardial infarction, congestive heart failure increase likelihood of VT.
    - Atrial–ventricular dissociation usually indicates VT.
    - QRS > 140 ms more indicative of VT.
    - Presence of fusion or capture beats is associated with VT:
      - Fusion: QRS arising from two different sources within the ventricle.
      - Capture: narrow complex sinus beat in the middle of tachycardia through normal conduction.
  - Supraventricular tachycardia (*SVT*) with aberrancy:
  - Patients younger than 35 years are more likely to have SVT with aberrancy.
  - Do not use hemodynamic status to differentiate between SVT and VT.
  - Irregularity usually indicates atrial fibrillation (*AF*) with antegrade preexcitation syndrome (Wolff–Parkinson–White, WPW).
  - Wide complex tachycardia with left or right bundle branch block morphology usually indicates SVT.
    - Pre-excitation syndrome: irregularity usually indicates AF with antegrade preexcitation syndrome (WPW).
    - Drug induced.
    - Electrolyte induced.

Management for Sustained Monomorphic Ventricular Tachycardia

- Treat reversible causes:
  - Electrolyte imbalances.

- Ischemia.
- Hypoxia.
- Drug toxicity.
- Stable VT:
  - Pharmacologic cardioversion.
    - Lidocaine:
      - Limited efficacy (approximately 30%) [1].
      - Less efficacious than procainamide [1, 2].
      - Works with ischemic myocardium.
    - Amiodarone:
      - Variable efficacy (approximately 25%) [2–4].
      - Onset of action slower than procainamide [5].
    - Procainamide:
      - More efficacious than amiodarone at VT cessation [2, 4].
      - Procainamide safer than amiodarone [4] – less hypotension, fewer major cardiac adverse events.
  - Synchronized cardioversion: energy per current Advanced Cardiovascular Life Support (ACLS) guidelines.
- Unstable VT:
  - Instability defined by: hypotension, pulmonary edema, ischemic chest pain, or altered mental status.
  - Manage with synchronized cardioversion, energy may vary depending on your defibrillator specifications and on current ACLS guidelines.

Debriefing Plan

Plan for approximately 30 minutes for discussion.

Potential Questions for Discussion

- What historical features help differentiate VT and SVT?
- What are contributory, reversible etiologies of sustained monomorphic VT?
- What are treatment options for stable, sustained monomorphic VT?
- What pharmacologic agents can be used for stable monomorphic VT and what is the efficacy of each therapy?
- How does one properly use the defibrillator?

REFERENCES FOR VENTRICULAR TACHYCARDIA

1. Komura, S., Chinushi, M., Furushima, H. et al. (2010). Efficacy of procainamide and lidocaine in terminating sustained monomorphic ventricular tachycardia. *Circ. J.* 74 (5): 864–869.

2. Long, B. and Koyfman, A. (2017). Best clinical practice: emergency medicine management of stable monomorphic ventricular tachycardia. *J. Emerg. Med.* 52 (4): 484–492.

3. Marill, K., deSouza, I., Nishijima, D. et al. (2010). Amiodarone or procainamide for the termination of sustained stable ventricular tachycardia: an historical multicenter comparison. *Acad. Emerg. Med.* 17 (3): 297–306.

4. Ortiz, M., Martín, A., Arribas, F. et al. (2016). Randomized comparison of intravenous procainamide vs. intravenous amiodarone for the acute treatment of tolerated wide QRS tachycardia: the PROCAMIO study. *Eur. Heart J.* 38: ehw230.

5. Roberts-Thomson, K., Lau, D., and Sanders, P. (2011). The diagnosis and management of ventricular arrhythmias. *Nat. Rev. Cardiol.* 8 (6): 311–321.

ATRIAL FIBRILLATION WITH RAPID VENTRICULAR RESPONSE

Educational Goals

Learning Objectives

1. Recognize AF on ECG and formulate a differential for recent-onset AF (MK, PBL, PC).
2. Demonstrate the appropriate management of AF with rapid ventricular rate (*RVR*) (MK, PBL, PC).
3. Demonstrate professionalism and good communication with the ED nurse, consultants, and patient (ICS, P).

Critical Actions Checklist

☐ Assess airway, breathing and circulation (PC).
☐ Place patient on cardiac monitoring (PC, MK).
☐ Perform focused history and exam (PC).
☐ Recognize AF on ECG (MK).
☐ Appropriately treat AF with RVR (MK, PC).
☐ Communicate effectively with patient and consultant (ICS, P).

> Critical actions can be changed to address the educational needs of the learner. For example, novice learners can address rate control, whereas more advanced learners may have an unstable patient requiring electrical cardioversion.

Simulation Set-up

Environment: ED treatment room.

Mannequin: Adult, male simulator mannequin in a hospital gown.

Props: To be displayed on monitor or printed out on handouts in scenario room when asked for:

- Images (see online component for AF Scenario 2.2 at https://www.wiley.com/go/thoureen/simulation/workbook2e):
  - ECG showing AF with RVR (Figure 2.5).
  - ECG showing AF normal rate (Figure 2.6).
  - ECG showing normal sinus rhythm (Figure 2.7).
  - Chest x-ray (normal) (Figure 2.1).
- Laboratory tests (see online component as above):
  - Basic metabolic panel (Table 2.6).
  - Complete blood count (Table 2.7).

- Troponin (Table 2.8).
- Cardiac brain natriuretic peptide (Table 2.9).
- Coagulation panel (Table 2.10).
- Lactate (Table 2.11).
- D-dimer (Table 2.12).
- Liver function tests (Table 2.13).
- Thyroid function tests (Table 2.14).
- Fingerstick glucose (Table 2.15).
- Urinalysis (Table 2.16).

Available supplies:

- Airway supplies, code cart, and defibrillator.
- Medications (labeled bags/syringes/IV bags):
  - Liter bags of 0.9% saline or LR.
  - Pre-labeled syringes:
    - Rate controlling medications (e.g., diltiazem, metoprolol, esmolol).
    - Sedation medications commonly used at your institution.
    - Anticoagulant (e.g., enoxaparin).
  - Pre-labeled IV bags:
    - Rate controlling medications (e.g., diltiazem, esmolol).
    - Anticoagulant medication (e.g., heparin).
    - Antiarrhythmics (e.g., procainamide, amiodarone).

Distractor: None.

Actors

- Patient voice is male, provides his own history and is interactive unless the facilitator makes the patient unstable and then is minimally conversant.
- Nurse can administer medications/fluids, assist with the defibrillator, and cue learners if needed.
- All consultants are available by telephone.

Case Narrative

Scenario Background

A 56-year-old man presents with palpitations, lightheadedness, and mild shortness of breath. Symptoms have been ongoing for a "few days" and were initially mild but have progressively worsened.

> Background can be presented by the nurse or provided by a triage sheet. For advanced learners, the patient states a clear onset of symptoms 18 hours ago while watching television.

Chief complaint: Palpitations
Patient's medical history: Hypertension, osteoarthritis of knees.
Medications: Hydrochlorothiazide, lisinopril, ibuprofen as needed.
Allergies: No known drug allergies.
Family history: Non-contributory
Social history: No tobacco, alcohol or drug use

Initial scenario conditions

The patient is alert and able to provide a full history.

> The case may start with EMS "on scene" as presented above while performing their objectives to identify and treat AF with RVR with stabilization, subsequent patient transport and communication with the accepting physician.

Vital signs: Temp 98.6°F (37°C), HR 142, RR 16, BP 142/68, SpO_2 99% on room air.
Head: Normocephalic and atraumatic.
Heart: Tachycardic, irregularly irregular with no murmurs, rubs, or gallops.
Lungs: Clear bilaterally.
Abdomen: Soft, nontender.
Extremities: Warm, well perfused.
Neurologic: Alert and oriented × 4, non-focal.

See flow diagram (Figure 2.8) for further scenario changes described.

Case Narrative, Continued

All learners should order an ECG and recognize AF with RVR. If AF is not recognized, the nurse can prompt the learner. Labs and imaging can be provided as requested.

Novice learners should initiate rate control.

For intermediate learners, the patient can present in unstable AF with RVR requiring synchronized cardioversion. If instability goes unrecognized, the patient will code.

For advanced learners, the patient can be stable and appropriate for ED cardioversion with subsequent discharge home.

The case ends when AF with RVR is rate controlled, and/or cardioverted, or the patient codes. The actual disposition is not critical and will depend on institutional culture and the facilitator's goals. Disposition should occur in consultation with another physician (for admission or discharge).

Instructor Notes

Pathophysiology

- AF is the most common sustained and clinically significant cardiac arrhythmia.
- Prevalence increases with advancing age.
- Symptoms result from:
  - Irregular or raised ventricular rate.
  - Loss of "atrial kick" to cardiac output.
- Common diagnoses associated with AF:
  - Acute myocardial infarction.
  - Pulmonary embolism.
  - Thyrotoxicosis.
  - Alcohol abuse.
  - Mitral valve disease.
  - Sympathomimetics.
  - WPW syndrome.
  - Sepsis.

Clinical Features

- Common presentations:
  - Asymptomatic
  - Palpitations
  - Lightheadedness
  - Malaise
  - Chest pressure
  - Shortness of breath
  - Syncope.

Diagnosis

- ECG – irregularly irregular with absence of P waves.
- Aberrant conduction (e.g., bundle branch blocks) results in wide complex AF.

Management

- Hemodynamically unstable AF or rapid AF with evidence of accessory pathway (e.g. WPW):
  - Direct current synchronized cardioversion (DCV):
    - 200 J biphasic is most efficacious.

- Can start anticoagulation simultaneously.
- Longer duration of AF is associated with decreased likelihood of successful cardioversion.
- Hemodynamically stable AF without evidence of accessory pathway:
  - Rate control:
    - Beta blockers (e.g. metoprolol, esmolol): advantageous in thyrotoxicosis.
    - Calcium channel blockers (e.g. diltiazem, verapamil):
      - Preferred in chronic obstructive pulmonary disease/asthma patient.
      - Amiodarone; can promote chemical cardioversion; should not be used in pregnancy.
- Elective ED Cardioversion of recent onset AF, defined as clear AF onset less than 48 hours:
  - DCV.
    - Pros:
      - Rapid conversion to NSR.
      - High success rate (with biphasic energy delivery).
    - Cons:
      - Contraindicated in digitalis toxicity or hypokalemia.
      - NPO time for procedural sedation may increase ED stay.
  - Pharmacologic cardioversion:
    - Pros:
      - Procedural sedation not required.
    - Cons:
      - Can potentiate additional arrhythmias.
      - Can take longer to cardiovert (one to six hours).
      - Slightly less successful than DCV, although if pharmacologic cardioversion fails, antiarrhythmic administration may facilitate subsequent DCV.
    - Medications most used (note: American Heart Association, AHA, recommendations are primarily from studies examining inpatient cardioversion/onset later than 48 hours):
      - Class I AHA recommendations: flecainide, ibutilide, propafenone.
      - Class IIb: amiodarone, propafenone, flecainide.
      - Class IIIb: procainamide:
        - Used most often in ED protocols with good success.
        - Described in the Ottawa Aggressive Protocol [1].
        - Can be used in WPW/preexcitation.
    - Contraindications to elective ED cardioversion:
      - Unknown onset of AF.
      - High embolic risk (CHA_2DS_2-VASc score).

- Other medical reason necessitates admission.
- Potential benefits:
  - Patient satisfaction;
  - Potential cost savings (patient is not admitted) [2];
  - Decreased length of stay [2];
- Risks:
  - Hypotension.
  - Thromboembolic event.
  - Recurrence rate of 3–17% [2].
  - Bradycardia.
  - Chest wall burn from defibrillator pads.
  - Atrioventricular block.
  - Non-sustained VT.

Debriefing Plan

Plan for approximately 30 minutes for discussion.

Potential Questions for Discussion

- What are the ECG findings in AF?
- What is the treatment of AF with RVR, with and without instability?
- What are common medical conditions associated with the development of AF?
- What are the indications/contraindications to performing ED cardioversion for stable AF?
- What are the risks/benefits of elective ED cardioversion to your patient?

REFERENCES FOR ATRIAL FIBRILLATION WITH RAPID VENTRICULAR RESPONSE

1. Oishi, M. and Xing, S. (2013). Atrial fibrillation: management strategies in the emergency department. *Emerg. Med. Pract.* 15 (2): 1–26.
2. Von Besser, K. and Mills, A.M. (2011). Is discharge home after emergency department cardioversion safe for the treatment of recent onset atrial fibrillation? *Ann. Emerg. Med.* 58: 517–520.

SELECTED READING FOR ATRIAL FIBRILLATION WITH RAPID VENTRICULAR RESPONSE

Chenoweth, J. and Diercks, D. (2012). Management of atrial fibrillation in the acute setting. *Curr. Opin. Crit. Care.* 18: 333–340.

PEDIATRIC PERICARDITIS

Educational Goals

Learning Objectives

1. Assess a pediatric patient with chest pain and formulate a differential diagnosis (MK, PBL, PC).
2. Select appropriate diagnostic studies, including labs, imaging, and ECG for a pediatric patient with chest pain (MK).
3. Formulate appropriate treatment, consultation, and disposition for a pediatric patient with pericarditis (MK, PBL, PC, ICS, P, SBP).
4. Recognize pericardial effusion on ultrasound and perform pericardiocentesis for hemodynamically unstable patient (optional for advanced learners) (PC, MK).
5. Demonstrate clear communication with the nurse, patient, family and consultants (ICS).

Critical Actions Checklist

☐ Perform a history and physical exam (PC).
☐ Obtain and interpret an ECG (MK).
☐ Recognize pericarditis on ECG (MK).
☐ Perform or order a bedside cardiac ultrasound to evaluate for pericardial effusion (MK, PC).
☐ Perform a bedside pericardiocentesis if indicated (MK, PC).

Critical actions can be changed to address the educational needs of the learner. For example, the patient can present with myopericarditis, or can become unstable from tamponade physiology.

Simulation Set-up

Environment: ED treatment room.

Mannequin: Pediatric simulator mannequin in a hospital gown.

Props: To be displayed on monitor or available via handouts in scenario room when asked for:
- Images (see online component for Pericarditis Scenario 2.3 at https://www.wiley.com/go/thoureen/simulation/workbook2e)
  - ECG which shows normal sinus rhythm with diffuse ST elevation (Figure 2.9).
  - Normal chest x-ray (Figure 2.10).

- Laboratory tests (see online component as above):
  - Basic metabolic panel (Table 2.17).
  - Complete blood count (Table 2.18).
  - Troponin (Table 2.19).
  - Lactate (Table 2.20).
  - D-dimer (Table 2.21).
  - Coagulation panel (Table 2.22).
  - Inflammatory markers (Table 2.23).
- Videos (see online component as above):
  - Normal cardiac ultrasound (Video 2.1).
  - Cardiac ultrasound demonstrating tamponade physiology (Video 2.2).

Available supplies:
- Basic airway and code cart including defibrillator

Medications:
- Pre-labeled bags:
  - Liter bags of 0.9% saline or lactated Ringer's solution (LR)
- Pre-labeled syringes:
  - Nonsteroidal anti-inflammatory drug (*NSAID*) (e.g., ketorolac).
  - Opioid analgesics (e.g., morphine, fentanyl)
- Pericardiocentesis kit, spinal or ultrasound needle with syringe, and/or pericardiocentesis task trainer (optional).
- Bedside ultrasound machine (optional).

Distractor: none

A low-cost pericardiocentesis task trainer can be made, if a formal task trainer is not available [1]. Alternatively, if a pericardiocentesis task trainer is unavailable, the learner can verbalize the steps of a pericardiocentesis.

Actors

- Patient with pediatric male voice. He can provide his own history throughout the scenario unless the facilitator makes the patient unstable and minimally conversant.
- Parent can provide additional history.
- Nurse can start IV lines, administer medications and fluids, provide any supplies and cue learners if needed.
- All consultants can be available by telephone consultation.

Case Narrative

Scenario Background

A seven-year-old boy presents with chest pain that started this morning and worsened throughout the day, so his mother picked him up from soccer practice. The patient reports pain in the middle of his chest, leaning forward improves his pain. He reports two days of malaise. He denies any fever, chills, cough, sore throat, shortness of breath, nausea, vomiting, abdominal pain, lightheadedness or syncope.

> Background can be presented by an EMS provider, nurse, parent or can be provided by a triage sheet.

Chief complaint: Chest pain.
Patient's medical history: None.
Medications: None.
Allergies: No known drug allergies.
Family history: Non-contributory.
Social history: Vaccinated, no tobacco, alcohol or drugs. No bullying, feels safe and supported at home and school. Makes As and Bs.

Initial scenario conditions

The patient is alert, oriented and provides full history.

Vital signs: Temp 98.6°F (37°C), HR 88, RR 22, BP 102/60, SpO_2 99% on room air.
Head: Normocephalic and atraumatic.
HEENT: No pharyngeal erythema or exudate.
Heart: Regular rate and rhythm, with no murmurs or gallops, + pericardial friction rub.
Lungs: Clear bilaterally.
Abdomen: Soft and nontender.
Extremities: No gross deformities, warm and well perfused.
Neurologic: Alert and oriented × 4, moves all extremities.
Skin: Normal, no rash.

> Physical exam findings not available on your mannequin can be reported verbally if asked for by learners (e.g., pericardial friction rub).

See flow diagram (Figure 2.11) for further scenario changes described.

Case Narrative, Continued

The learner should perform a history and physical exam and initiate appropriate work-up. ECG, labs, imaging, and an ultrasound can be provided to the learner as requested. If ECG is not ordered immediately, the patient will complain of more chest pain.

For novice and intermediate learners, the patient will continue to report pain until treated with NSAIDs. The bedside ultrasound will demonstrate no pericardial effusion (Video 2.1). After evaluation, the patient can ultimately be discharged home with appropriate treatment. The learner may choose to call the patient's primary care provider or pediatrician to ensure follow up.

For advanced learners, the patient can progressively worsen and become hypotensive from a pericardial effusion causing tamponade physiology. Bedside ultrasound can assist in diagnosis (Video 2.2) and emergent pericardiocentesis will be required.

The case can be altered to include an elevated troponin and/or fever and significant leukocytosis, warranting further evaluation and admission.

The case ends when pericarditis is diagnosed, the patient is appropriately treated, the diagnosis is communicated to the patient and his parent(s), and the patient is appropriately dispositioned.

Instructor Notes

Pathophysiology

- The pericardium is a double-walled sac that is made of a visceral and parietal layer.
- Pericarditis is an inflammation of the pericardial sac.
- Most common in male adolescents.
- Median age of 14.5 years.
- Etiology:
  - Most common: idiopathic.
  - Infectious:
    - Primarily viral (coxsackievirus, Epstein–Barr virus, influenza, echovirus, adenovirus, etc.).
    - Rarely bacterial or fungal.
  - Autoimmune (lupus, rheumatic fever, juvenile arthritis, etc.).
  - Neoplasm and paraneoplastic syndromes.
  - Drug-induced (isoniazid, procainamide, hydralazine, cyclosporine).
  - Trauma (blunt, penetrating, iatrogenic).
  - Post-radiotherapy.
  - Metabolic (uremia, hypothyroidism, etc.).
- Generally self-limited with resolution of symptoms in one week:
  - Infrequently chronic.
  - Recurrent in about 10% of cases.

Clinical Features

- Chest pain:
  - Retrosternal pain that is typically sharp.
  - Pleuritic and worse with coughing.
  - Improved by sitting up and leaning forward.
  - Onset is normally acute.
  - May radiate to neck, shoulders and back.
  - Atypical presentations of dull pain and unilateral arm pain do occur.
- Pericardial friction rub:
  - Heard best with the stethoscope diaphragm at left lateral sternal border, at end expiration, with the patient learning forward.
  - Usually intermittent and present in only one third of patients and is specific but with low sensitivity [2].
- Fever – only about half of pediatric patients present with fever [3].

Diagnosis

- Primarily clinical and supported by ECG findings.
- ECG findings:
  - Classically diffuse ST elevation.
  - Other findings: sinus tachycardia, ST depression, PR depression, reciprocal ST depression in lead aVR, T-wave flattening.
- Imaging studies:
  - Chest x-ray is normal unless a large pericardial effusion is present.
  - Cardiac ultrasound
    - If effusion is present, majority will be small, rare to have tamponade.
- Laboratory studies:
  - No definitive laboratory diagnosis of pericarditis.
  - Troponin elevation indicative of myopericarditis.
  - Inflammatory markers (white cell count, erythrocyte sedimentation rate, C-reactive protein) may be elevated; not sensitive or specific.
- Treatment:
  - Although rare, if pericardial tamponade is present, perform a pericardiocentesis.
  - Treat inflammation:
    - NSAIDs (ibuprofen, ketorolac) are first line.
    - Steroids are generally reserved for refractory cases or drug allergy to NSAIDs.
    - Colchicine has strong evidence to support its use in adults but is not yet fully supported in pediatric patients.
  - If bacterial etiology, administer antibiotics.

- Disposition
  - Majority of acute pericarditis is uncomplicated and can be discharged home with outpatient follow up.
  - Admit all high-risk patients:
    - Large effusion or pericardial tamponade.
    - Immunocompromised state.
    - History of anticoagulation.
    - Acute trauma.
    - Failure to respond to outpatient management.
    - Elevated troponin; myopericarditis.
    - Intractable pain.
    - Ill-appearing.

Debriefing Plan

Plan for approximately 30 minutes for discussion.

Potential Questions for Discussion

- How does acute pericarditis present?
- What are the causes of acute pericarditis in a pediatric patient?
- What are the typical ECG findings in pericarditis?
- What is the treatment for acute pericarditis in a pediatric patient?
- What is the role of ultrasound in the diagnosis of pericarditis?
- What are the indications for admission versus discharge in a patient with acute pericarditis?

REFERENCES FOR PEDIATRIC PERICARDITIS

1. Durani, Y., Giordano, K., and Goudie, B.W. (2010). Myocarditis and pericarditis in children. *Pediatr. Clin. North Am.* 57 (6): 1281–1303.
2. Imazio, M., Gaita, F., and LeWinter, M. (2015). Evaluation and treatment of pericarditis: a systematic review. *JAMA* 314 (14): 1498–1506.
3. Ratnapalan, S., Brown, K., and Benson, L. (2011). Children presenting with acute pericarditis to the emergency department. *Pediatr. Emerg. Care* 27 (7): 581–585.

SELECTED READING FOR PEDIATRIC PERICARDITIS

Sullivan, A., Khait, L., and Favot, M. (2018). A novel low-cost ultrasound-guided pericardiocentesis simulation model: demonstration of feasibility. *J. Ultrasound Med.* 37 (2): 493–500.

APPENDIX

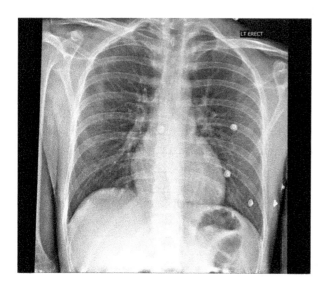

FIGURE 2.1   Normal chest x-ray.

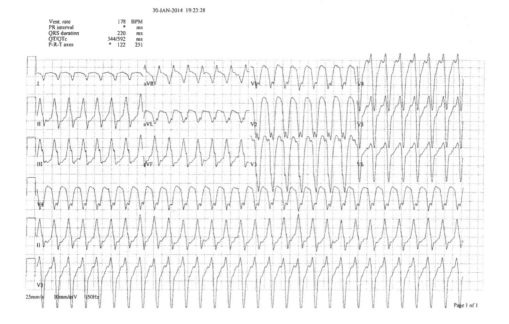

FIGURE 2.2   Sustained monomorphic ventricular tachycardia electrocardiogram.

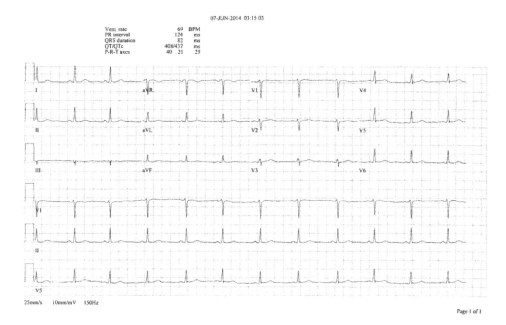

07-JUN-2014 03:15:03

Vent. rate	69	BPM
PR interval	124	ms
QRS duration	82	ms
QT/QTc	408/437	ms
P-R-T axes	40 21	29

25mm/s   10mm/mV   150Hz

Page 1 of 1

FIGURE 2.3   Previous electrocardiogram.

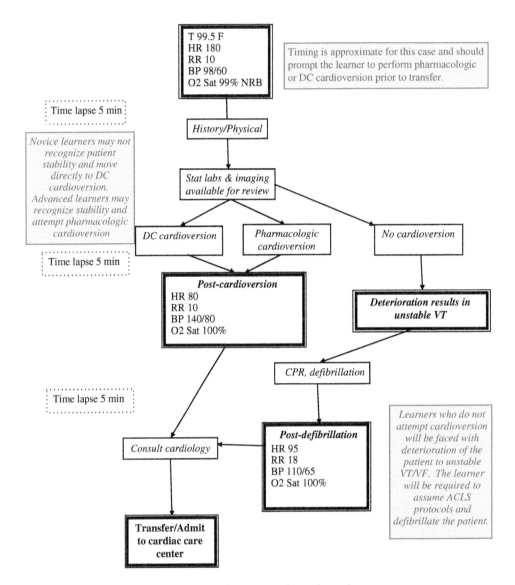

FIGURE 2.4   Flow diagram monomorphic ventricular tachycardia.

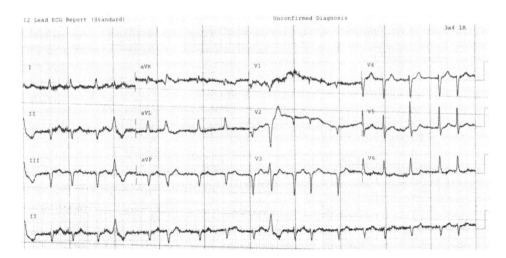

FIGURE 2.5 Electrocardiogram: atrial fibrillation with rapid ventricular rate.

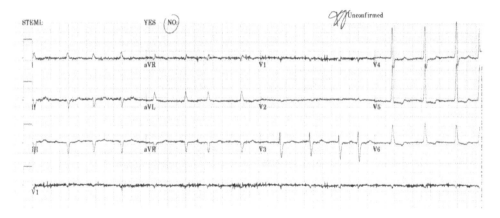

FIGURE 2.6 Electrocardiogram: atrial fibrillation, normal rate.

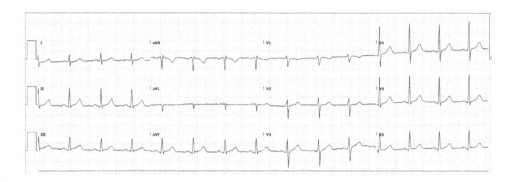

FIGURE 2.7 Electrocardiogram: normal sinus rhythm.

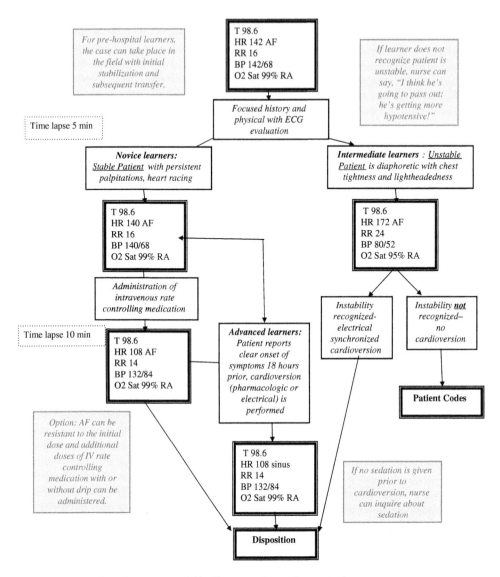

FIGURE 2.8   Flow diagram atrial fibrillation with rapid ventricular rate.

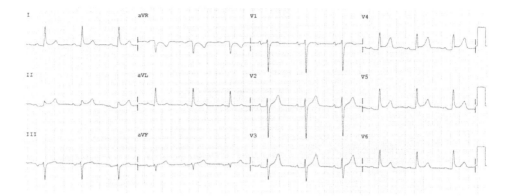

FIGURE 2.9   Electrocardiogram with diffuse ST elevation.

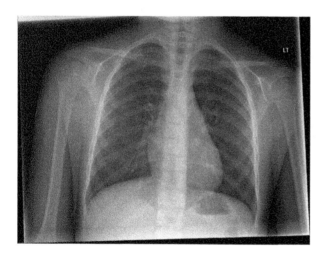

FIGURE 2.10   Normal chest x-ray.

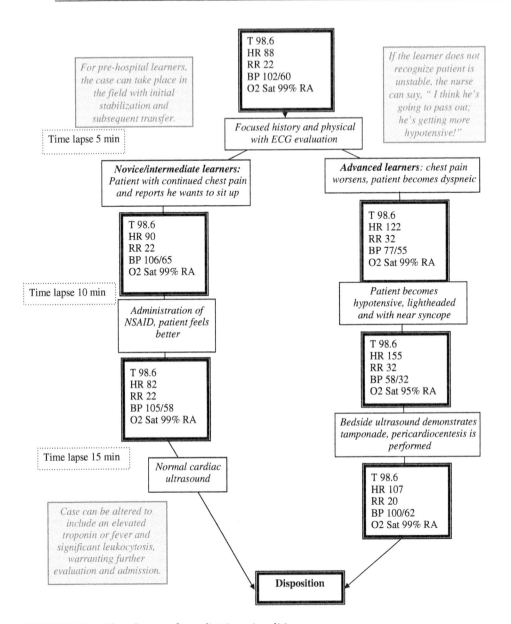

FIGURE 2.11   Flow diagram for pediatric pericarditis.

TABLE 2.1 Complete blood count.

Test	Value	Reference range
White blood cells (k/μl)	6.5	3.5–11.0
Hemoglobin (g/dl)	13.0	10.5–15.0
Hematocrit (%)	39	32–45
Mean corpuscular volume (fl)	92	81–100
Platelets (k/μl)	311	150–400

TABLE 2.2 Chemistry.

Test	Value	Reference range
Sodium (mmol/l)	138	135–145
Potassium (mmol/l)	3.3	3.6–5.1
Chloride (mmol/l)	108	98–110
CO_2 (mmol/l)	20	20–30
Blood urea nitrogen (mg/dl)	16	6–24
Creatinine (mg/dl)	0.7	0.4–1.3
Glucose (mg/dl)	118	67–109

TABLE 2.3 Magnesium level.

Test	Value	Reference range
Magnesium (mg/dl)	2.2	1.8–2.5

TABLE 2.4 Troponin.

Test	Value	Range
Troponin (ng/ml)	0.01	< 0.03 normal
		≥ 0.03–0.3 borderline
		> 0.2 abnormal

TABLE 2.5 Coagulation panel.

Test	Value	Reference range
Prothrombin time (seconds)	10.5	9.4–11.5
International normalized ratio	1.0	0.9–1.2
Partial thromboplastin time (seconds)	28.0	24.2–32.0

TABLE 2.6   Chemistry.

Test	Value	Reference range
Sodium (mmol/l)	138	135–145
Potassium (mmol/l)	3.8	3.6–5.1
Chloride (mmol/l)	108	98–110
CO_2 (mmol/l)	24	20–30
Blood urea nitrogen (mg/dl)	18	6–24
Creatinine (mg/dl)	0.9	0.4–1.3
Glucose (mg/dl)	118	67–109
Calcium (mg/dl)	9.7	8.6–10.3

TABLE 2.7   Complete blood count.

Test	Value	Reference range
White blood cells (k/µl)	8.4	3.5–11.0
Hemoglobin (g/dl)	13.4	10.5–15.0
Hematocrit (%)	39	32–45%
Mean corpuscular volume (fl)	92	81–100
Platelets (k/µl)	268	150–400

TABLE 2.8   Troponin.

Test	Value	Reference range
Troponin (ng/ml)	0.01	< 0.07

TABLE 2.9   Cardiac B-type natriuretic peptide.

Test	Value	Reference range
Cardiac B-type natriuretic peptide (pg/ml)	98	< 100

TABLE 2.10   Coagulation panel.

Test	Value	Reference range
Prothrombin time (seconds)	10.5	9.4–11.5
International normalized ratio	1.0	0.9–1.2
Partial thromboplastin time (seconds)	28.0	24.2–32.0

TABLE 2.11 Lactate.

Test	Value	Reference range
Lactate (mmol/l)	1.2	0.5–2.0

TABLE 2.12 D-dimer.

Test	Value	Reference range
D-dimer (µg/ml FEU)	0.47	< 0.50

FEU, fibrinogen-equivalent units.

TABLE 2.13 Liver function tests.

Test	Value	Reference range
Albumin (g/dl)	4.3	3.7–4.8
Total protein (g/dl)	8.0	6.3–8.3
Total bilirubin (mg/dl)	0.5	0.3–0.5
Direct bilirubin (mg/dl)	0.0	0.0–0.2
Alkaline phosphatase (iu/l)	67	38–120
Alanine aminotransferase (iu/l)	10	7–52
Aspartate aminotransferase (iu/l)	22	13–39

TABLE 2.14 Thyroid function test.

Test	Value	Reference range
Thyroid-stimulating hormone (iu/ml)	0.75	0.530–6.340
Free tetraiodothyronine (iu/ml)	1.11	0.6–1.60

TABLE 2.15 Fingerstick glucose.

Lab	Value	Reference range
Fingerstick glucose (mg/dl)	118	70–109

TABLE 2.16 Urinalysis.

Test	Value	Reference range
Color	Yellow	
Specific gravity	1.027	1.005–1.030
pH	7.0	5.0–8.0
Protein (mmol/l)	24	20–30
Glucose	18	Negative
Hemoglobin	Negative	Negative
Urobilinogen (mg/dl)	< 0.2	< 0.2
Red blood cells (/hpf)	0	0–3
White blood cells (/hpf)	0	0–5
Bacteria	None	None
Nitrites	Negative	Negative
Leukocyte esterase	Negative	Negative

hpf, high power factor.

TABLE 2.17 Chemistry.

Test	Value	Reference range
Sodium (mmol/l)	138	135–145
Potassium (mmol/l)	3.5	3.5–5.1
Chloride (mmol/l)	108	98–110
CO_2 (mmol/l)	23	20–30
Blood urea nitrogen (mg/dl)	7	6–24
Creatinine (mg/dl)	0.4	0.4–1.3
Glucose (mg/dl)	81	67–109
Calcium (mg/dl)	8.9	8.6–10.3

TABLE 2.18 Complete blood count.

Test	Value	Reference range
White blood cells (k/µl)	10.8	3.5–11.0
Hemoglobin (g/dl)	14.4	10.5–15.0
Hematocrit(%)	44	32–45
Mean corpuscular volume (fl)	98	81–100
Platelets (k/µl)	268	150–400

TABLE 2.19 Troponin.

Test	Value	Reference range
Troponin (ng/ml)	0.01	< 0.07

TABLE 2.20 Lactate.

Test	Value	Reference range
Lactate (mmol/l)	0.8	0.5–2.0

TABLE 2.21 D-dimer.

Test	Value	Reference range
D-dimer (µg/ml FEU)	0.280	< 0.50

FEU, fibrinogen-equivalent units.

TABLE 2.22 Coagulation panel.

Test	Value	Reference range
Prothrombin time (seconds)	10.5	9.4–11.5
International normalized ratio	1.0	0.9–1.2
Partial thromboplastin time (seconds)	28.0	24.2–32.0

TABLE 2.23 Inflammatory markers.

Test	Value	Reference range
C-reactive protein (mg/dl)	1.8	< 0.5
Erythrocyte sedimentation rate (mm/hour)	22	0–15

CHAPTER 3

Cutaneous Emergencies

Daa'iyah R. Cooper[1,2] and Afrah A. Ali[1,2]

[1] University of Maryland Medical Center, Baltimore, MD, USA
[2] Department of Emergency Medicine, University of Maryland School of Medicine, Baltimore, MD, USA

HENOCH–SCHÖNLEIN PURPURA

Educational Goals

Learning Objectives

1. Develop a differential diagnosis of a pediatric patient with purpuric rash (MK).
2. Recognize common presenting symptoms and clinical findings in Henoch–Schönlein purpura (*HSP*) (MK).
3. Demonstrate appropriate management of HSP, including HSP with multiple organ involvement (MK, PC).

Critical Actions Checklist

☐ Obtain a complete history from parent, including medications and vaccinations (PC, ICS).
☐ Undress patient and perform complete physical examination (PC).
☐ Order laboratory evaluations including urinalysis (MK).
☐ Consult pediatrics for admission (PC, ICS).

Emergency Medicine Simulation Workbook: A Tool for Bringing the Curriculum to Life,
Second Edition. Edited by Traci L. Thoureen and Sara B. Scott.
© 2022 John Wiley & Sons Ltd. Published 2022 by John Wiley & Sons Ltd.
Companion website: www.wiley.com/go/thoureen/simulation/workbook2e

Simulation Set-Up

Environment: Emergency Department treatment room.

Mannequin: Elementary school-age, pediatric simulator mannequin, with moulage to bilateral lower legs and hands to simulate purpura. Patient is dressed in regular clothing. Purpura can be moulaged with washable makeup in red and purple hues applied to extremities of simulator.

Props: To be displayed on a plasma screen/ computer screen and/or printed out on handouts in scenario room when asked for/return from lab:
- Images (see online component for HSP, Scenario 3.1 `https://www.wiley.com/go/thoureen/simulation/workbook2e`):
  - Chest x-ray (normal) (Figure 3.1).
  - Abdominal x-ray (normal) (Figure 3.2).
  - Abdominal ultrasound (Figure 3.3).
- Laboratory tests (see online component as above):
  - Complete blood count (Table 3.1).
  - Comprehensive metabolic panel (Table 3.2).
  - Lactate (Table 3.3).
  - Coagulation panel (Table 3.4).
  - Urinalysis (Table 3.5).
  - Erythrocyte sedimentation rate (Table 3.6).
  - C-reactive protein (*CRP*) (Table 3.7).

Available supplies:

- Intravenous (IV) start supplies, nasal cannula, cardiac monitor and leads, pulse oximetry
- Medications:
  - 250 ml bags of IV fluids such as 0.9% saline, Plasma-Lyte, and lactated Ringer's solution (*LR*).
  - Pre-labeled syringes:
    - Parenteral steroids.
    - Opioid analgesic medication.
  - Antipyretics/pain medications.
  - Oral steroids.

Distractor: Patient's parent can repeatedly ask, "Do you think he is having a side effect of the antibiotics the doctor gave him?"

Actors

- Patient's parent may be an actor/standardized patient or instructor/faculty member.
- Patient's voice is a youthful male. Patient should sound uncomfortable and low energy. He is able to follow commands and answer questions.
- Emergency department (ED) nurse can administer medications/fluids. The nurse does have some medical knowledge and may cue learners if needed.
- Pediatrician/additional consultants, such as dermatology will be available via "phone consultation."

Case Narrative

Scenario Background

A 10 year-old male is brought to the ED by his parent, who says the child has had an "upper respiratory infection" for over a week now and it is getting worse. His family doctor prescribed amoxicillin three days ago, after five days of sore throat, body aches, and some cough. He has a new rash that started two days ago, and he could not go to school today because of body pain. Patient is complaining of some pain in his legs (particularly knees and ankles). He also endorses some generalized abdominal discomfort, which gets worse with eating (only if asked).

Patient's medical history: None.
Medications: Multivitamin, Amoxicillin.
Allergies: No known drug allergies.
Family history: Maternal grandmother has hypertension.
Social history: Lives at home with parents, attends school (fifth grade).

Initial Scenario Conditions

Young boy brought from triage area accompanied by his parent.

Vital signs:	Temp 100.5°F (38.1°C), HR 118, RR 26, BP 115/61, SpO$_2$ 100% on room air.
General appearance:	alert, appears uncomfortable.
Head:	Head is atraumatic, normocephalic.
Eyes:	Pupils 4 mm and reactive to light.
Neck:	Supple, shotty submandibular lymphadenopathy.
Heart:	Tachycardic and regular, distal pulses intact.
Lungs:	Normal effort, lungs clear to auscultation throughout; no wheezing, rales, or rhonchi.

Abdomen:	Hypoactive bowel sounds, diffuse tenderness to palpation, no rebound, no guarding.
Genitourinary:	Mild scrotal edema; no scrotal tenderness.
Extremities:	1+ bilateral lower extremity edema to knees with skin findings noted below.
Skin:	Scattered palpable purpura noted to legs, knees, and hands, bilaterally.
Neurologic:	Alert and oriented × 3; no focal neurological deficits.

See flow diagram (Figure 3.4) for the case narrative.

Physical exam findings not available on your mannequin can be reported verbally if asked for by learners; for example, if your mannequin cannot simulate scrotal edema, this finding can be verbally reported when the structure is examined.

Case Narrative, Continued

Learners should begin by performing an initial assessment of the patient, including gaining IV access.

A complete history of present illness and past medical history, including medication and vaccine history, and a complete physical exam should be performed.

After taking the history and performing the physical, the learner should order laboratory and imaging tests that will help to narrow down their working diagnosis.

Novice learners can be prompted by the patient's parent or the nurse to report a potential list of diagnoses; for example, "Doctor, what could be causing this?" or "What do you think he has?"

The learner should recognize the patient's slightly increased heart rate and blood pressure for his age and attempt to correct this by providing pain control, antipyretics and/or IV fluids for the increased heart rate.

The patient will complain of abdominal pain that progressively worsens throughout the encounter. The severe abdominal pain in addition to other symptoms of HSP should prompt consideration of this diagnosis and the initiation of steroids.

After reviewing lab results and any available imaging ordered, learners should properly disposition the patient to pediatrics service. They should call and present the case and their working diagnosis to the admitting doctor.

Novice learners can be prompted about administering steroids by the admitting doctor; for example, "You mentioned he is complaining of rash, abdominal pain and nausea? What do you think the diagnosis may be? Did you start him on steroids?"

The case ends when the patient has been provided symptomatic treatment, initial laboratory/imaging evaluation has been completed, and learners have appropriately considered admission for uncontrolled abdominal and joint pain.

Instructor Notes

Pathophysiology of Henoch–Schönlein Purpura

- Also called immunoglobulin A (IgA) vasculitis.
- Self-limited, systemic, nongranulomatous, autoimmune complex disease.
- Multiorgan involvement.
- Nonthrombocytopenic small vessel vasculitis.
- Etiology is unclear, but is associated with:
  - Medications (quinolones, acetaminophen, codeine).
  - Vaccinations (measles, mumps and rubella, influenza, hepatitis).
  - Infections (streptococcus, staphylococcus, mycoplasma).
  - Neoplasms (prostate cancer, non-small-cell lung cancer).
  - Genetic disorders (alpha 1 antitrypsin deficiency, familial Mediterranean fever).

Clinical Features

- Classic tetrad:
  - Nonthrombocytopenic palpable purpura.
  - Arthralgias/arthritis.
  - Renal involvement.
  - Gastrointestinal involvement.
- Cutaneous involvement:
  - Rash most common presenting symptom:
    - Initially erythematous to urticarial macular wheels developing into distinct, symmetric, non-blanching, palpable purpura and petechiae with ecchymoses that coalesce
  - Dependent areas (legs/buttocks) most common distribution.
  - Can also be seen in upper extremities, face, and trunk.
- Gastrointestinal involvement:
  - Colicky abdominal pain that worsens with food.
  - ± nausea, vomiting, hematemesis, melena, hematochezia.
  - Rarely intussusception (ileoileal), ischemic necrosis of the bowel wall, intestinal perforation, massive gastrointestinal bleeding, acute acalculous cholecystitis, hemorrhagic ascites with serositis, pancreatitis, and biliary cirrhosis.

- Musculoskeletal involvement:
  - Approximately 15% of patients with HSP present with arthritis as the initial symptom, and overall arthralgia or arthritis occurs in 75% of children [1].
- Renal involvement:
  - Hematuria (microscopic or gross) most common.
  - Proteinuria is common with hematuria but rarely isolated.
  - Usually self-limiting.
  - Around 1% of cases of HSP nephritis progress to end- stage renal disease [2].

Diagnosis

- Clinical diagnosis:
  - American College of Rheumatology criteria: three or more of the following:
    - Age 20 years or less at disease onset.
    - Palpable purpura.
    - Acute abdominal pain with gastrointestinal bleeding.
    - Biopsy showing granulocytes in the walls of small arterioles or venules in superficial layers of skin.
  - Pediatric Rheumatology Society criteria: palpable purpura plus at least one of the following:
    - Diffuse abdominal pain.
    - IgA deposition in any biopsy.
    - Arthritis/arthralgias.
    - Renal involvement (hematuria and/or proteinuria).
- Tissue biopsy can be employed in atypical cases.

Management

- Nonsteroidal anti-inflammatory drugs (NSAIDs) and acetaminophen for arthralgias/arthritis.
- Avoid aspirin in children.
- Discontinue potentially causative medications.
- Oral steroid indications: severe rash, edema, severe colicky abdominal pain, renal, scrotal and/or testicular involvement:
  - IV steroids can be used if oral steroids are not tolerated.
  - High-dose, pulse IV steroids are indicated in patients with nephrotic range proteinuria.

Debriefing Plan

Plan for approximately 30 minutes for discussion.

Potential Questions for Discussion

- What is the general approach to a patient presenting with acute rash?
- What is the differential diagnosis for purpuric rash?
- When are steroids indicated in HSP? When are IV steroids used in HSP?
- What clinical findings in HSP predict a worse prognosis?

REFERENCES FOR HENOCH–SCHÖNLEIN PURPURA

1 Hetland, L.E., Susrud, K.S., Lindahl, K.H. et al. (2017). Henoch–Schönlein purpura: a literature review. *Acta Derm. Venereol.* 97 (10): 1160–1166.
2 Guo, D. and Lam, J.M. (2016). Henoch-Schönlein purpura. *CMAJ* 188 (15): E393.

SELECTED READING FOR HENOCH–SCHÖNLEIN PURPURA

Reid-Adam, J. (2014). Henoch–Schönlein purpura. *Pediatr. Rev.* 35 (10): 447–449.

NECROTIZING FASCIITIS

Educational Goals

Learning Objectives

1. Demonstrate appropriate fluid resuscitation and antimicrobial therapy in a patient with sepsis (MK, PC).
2. Interpret results and recognize limitations of imaging modalities in the initial evaluation of necrotizing fasciitis (MK, PC).
3. Demonstrate early surgical consultation in a rapidly progressive soft-tissue infection (SBP, MK, PC).

Critical Actions Checklist

☐ Obtain appropriate IV access (two large-bore IV cannulas) (PC).
☐ Undress patient and perform complete physical examination (PC).
☐ Order appropriate IV fluid resuscitation for a septic patient (MK, PC).
☐ Administer appropriate antibiotics (MK, PC).
☐ Consult appropriate surgeon and report concern for necrotizing fasciitis (ICS, P, SBP).

Simulation Set-Up

Environment: Emergency Department treatment room.

Mannequin: Adult male simulator mannequin, in hospital gown and covered by a sheet. Erythema/ecchymosis is moulaged on the right upper thigh/hip. Skin changes can be moulaged with washable makeup in red and purple hues applied to the proximal thigh of the right lower extremity.

Props: To be displayed on a plasma screen/computer screen or printed out on handouts and ready when asked for/ "resulted":

- Images (see online component for necrotizing fasciitis, Scenario 3.2, https://www.wiley.com/go/thoureen/simulation/workbook2e):
  - Right hip x-ray showing subcutaneous air (Figure 3.5).
  - Ultrasound of soft tissue showing diffuse thickening in the subcutaneous tissue and perifascial fluid (Figure 3.6).
  - Computed tomography (CT) slice from pelvis extending to upper thighs showing subcutaneous air on right (Figure 3.7).
- Laboratory tests (online component as above):
  - Complete blood count (Table 3.8)
  - Comprehensive metabolic panel(Table 3.9)
  - Lactate (Table 3.10)

- Coagulation panel (Table 3.11)
- Type and screen (Table 3.12)
- Urinalysis (Table 3.13)
- Arterial blood gas (Table 3.14)
- Serum ketones (Table 3.15)
- CRP (Table 3.16).

Available supplies:

- Basic airway supplies.
- Cardiac monitor, cardiac leads and pulse oximetry.
- Medications (labeled bags/syringes may be used in place of actual medicine syringes or bags):
  - Liter bags of 0.9% saline and LR.
  - Pre-labeled IV bags:
    - IV broad-spectrum antibiotics (e.g., piperacillin-tazobactam, meropenem, clindamycin, metronidazole, vancomycin).
    - IV vasopressor (e.g., epinephrine, norepinephrine, vasopressin).
  - Pre-labeled syringes:
    - Regular insulin.
    - Opioid analgesic.
Distractor: none

Actors

- Patient voice is male. The patient should express feelings of severe pain, which are out of proportion to history and exam findings. He should have low energy which progresses to lethargy and slight confusion with uncontrolled leg pain. He is able to follow commands and answer questions.
- ED nurse can administer medications/fluids. The nurse does have some medical knowledge and may cue learners if needed.
- Surgeon is available via telephone consultation.

Case Narrative

Scenario Background

Forty-one year-old man brought in by EMS due to worsening right leg pain after a fall out of the shower 1.5 days ago, hitting his right upper thigh on the bathtub causing a small abrasion. The patient is unable to bear weight on his right leg due to pain. Today, he noted redness/skin discoloration that was not there when he went to bed.

Over-the-counter medications have not helped. If asked, patient's sugar has been elevated above 300 mg/dl for the last 12 hours, although he has not eaten because of loss of appetite. He has not noted any fevers, but has not taken his temperature.

Patient's medical history: Hypertension, diabetes mellitus, diabetic neuropathy.
Medications: Insulin glargine, insulin aspart, hydrochlorothiazide.
Allergies: No known drug allergies.
Family history: Diabetes mellitus in both parents.
Social history: Former smoker; quit six months ago; drinks EtOH occasionally.

Initial scenario conditions

Patient brought in by EMS, moaning in pain.

Vital signs: Temp 100.4°F (38°C), HR 130, RR 30, BP 90/50, SpO$_2$ 99% on room air.
Head: Head is atraumatic, normocephalic.
Eyes: Pupils 4 mm and reactive to light; eyes open (eyes half closed as case progresses).
Neck: Supple.
Heart: Tachycardic and regular, distal pulses diminished.
Lungs: Tachypneic, shallow respirations, clear breath sounds.
Abdomen: Hyperactive bowel sounds, soft, nondistended, nontender, no masses.
Extremities: No gross deformities.
Skin: Approximately 6 cm diameter area of erythema to proximal, dorsal right thigh that surrounds a small healing abrasion. The abraded area is more of a dusky/purplish appearance compared with the surrounding erythema; some subcutaneous emphysema palpable.
Neurologic: Grossly intact, motor 5/5 throughout except motor in proximal right lower extremity limited due to pain; bilateral decreased sensation noted to plantar surface of feet symmetrically.

See Figure 3.8 for a flow diagram of the case narrative details.

Case Narrative, Continued

Learners of all levels should initially perform a primary trauma survey, obtain appropriate IV access, administer IV fluids and pain medication. Identification of cutaneous findings on the extremity with tenderness, as well as pain out of proportion to exam, should prompt concern for necrotizing fasciitis.

If the patient does not receive analgesia, the patient will continue to moan until given. The nurse can also prompt stating, "He looks so uncomfortable Doctor, can we give him something?"

Learners should order appropriate antibiotics and obtain surgical consultation. The patient should also be evaluated and treated for sepsis and hyperglycemia. Imaging should not delay surgical consultation, but the learners should evaluate the patient for acute traumatic injury with imaging.

After five minutes, failure to manage hemodynamic instability will lead to further decompensation and ultimately a lack of responsiveness of the patient. He will maintain his airway throughout the case. If appropriate hemodynamic and antimicrobial management is initiated, there will be a period of stabilization. During this time, any ordered imaging/labs return. For novice learners, the case may end here after consultation with surgery and admission.

For advanced learners, after approximately five minutes, the patient can begin to deteriorate significantly becoming asystolic and requiring cardiopulmonary resuscitation (*CPR*) then get return of spontaneous circulation (*ROSC*) after one round of CPR.

The case ends when the patient is stabilized and the surgeon has been made aware of the patient's need for emergent surgical evaluation for possible necrotizing fasciitis.

Instructor Notes

Pathophysiology

- Insult to the soft tissue which rapidly progresses to widespread systemic toxicity.
- Bacteria proliferate and invades subcutaneous tissue and deep space fascia, releasing exotoxins causing tissue ischemia [1, 2].
  - Typically polymicrobial: a combination of Gram-positive cocci, Gram-negative rods, and anaerobes.

Risk Factors

- Advanced age.
- Comorbidities:
  - Diabetes mellitus.
  - Alcoholism.
  - Peripheral vascular disease.
  - Heart disease, renal failure.
  - Chronic skin ulcers/infections.
  - Immunosuppression:
    - Human immunodeficiency virus, cancer, immune system impairment.
- Drugs: use of NSAIDs, IV drug abuse [3].

Clinical Features

- Severe pain that is out of proportion to physical findings.
- Involved area may be erythematous and tender with marked edema and crepitus.
- Vitals signs may show tachycardia, fever and hypotension.

Diagnosis

- Primarily a clinical diagnosis based on history and physical examination [4]
- Laboratory risk indicator for necrotizing fasciitis (*LRINEC*) score can be used as an aid to differentiate between cellulitis with abscess and necrotizing fasciitis [5]:
  - CRP
  - White blood cell count
  - Hemoglobin
  - Sodium
  - Creatinine
  - Glucose
- Imaging may help to facilitate diagnosis:
  - Plain radiographs: poor sensitivity, may show subcutaneous gas.
  - Ultrasound: may show fluid collection along the fascial plane, fascial irregularity, and subcutaneous air.
  - CT with IV contrast: usually shows fascial thickening of deep facial planes and non-enhancing deep fascia on contrast imaging suggesting necrosis [6].
- Surgical exploration is the only way to confirm the diagnosis.

Management

- Aggressive fluid resuscitation.
- Broad-spectrum antibiotics. Coverage should also include methicillin-resistant *Staphylococcus aureus* coverage and clindamycin for antitoxin effects.
- Consult surgical service for emergent surgical debridement.
- Provide tetanus prophylaxis as indicated [7, 8].

Debriefing Plan

Plan for approximately 30 minutes of discussion.

Potential Questions for Discussion

- What are the pertinent clinical findings in necrotizing fasciitis?
- What are the risk factors for necrotizing fasciitis?
- What is the LRINEC score and how is it used in the diagnosis of necrotizing fasciitis?
- What is the management for necrotizing fasciitis?

REFERENCES FOR NECROTIZING FASCIITIS

1. Sarani, B., Strong, M., Pascual, J. et al. (2009). Necrotizing fasciitis: current concepts and review of the literature. *J. Am. Coll. Surg.* 208 (2): 279–288.
2. Maltezou, H.C. and Giamarellou, H. (2006). Community-acquired methicillin-resistant *Staphylococcus aureus* infections. *Int. J. Antimicrob. Agents.* 27 (2): 87–96.
3. Cainzos, M. and Gonzalez-Rodriguez, F.J. (2007). Necrotizing soft tissue infections. *Curr. Opin. Crit. Care.* 13 (4): 433–439.
4. Swain, R.A., Hatcher, J.C., Azadian, B.S. et al. (2013). A five-year review of necrotizing fasciitis in a tertiary referral unit. *Ann. R. Coll. Surg. Engl.* 95 (1): 57–60.
5. Gönüllü, D., Ilgun, A.S., Demiray, O. et al. (2019). The potential prognostic significance of the laboratory risk indicator for the necrotizing fasciitis (LRINEC) score in necrotizing fasciitis. *Chirurgia (Bucur)* 114 (3): 376–383.
6. Zacharias, N., Velmahos, G.C., Salama, A. et al. (2010). Diagnosis of necrotizing soft tissue infections by computed tomography. *Arch. Surg.* 145 (5): 452–455.
7. Nordqvist, G., Walldén, A., Brorson, H. et al. (2015). Ten years of treating necrotizing fasciitis. *Infect. Dis. (Lond).* 47 (5): 319–325.
8. Bucca, K., Spencer, R., Orford, N. et al. (2013). Early diagnosis and treatment of necrotizing fasciitis can improve survival: an observational intensive care unit cohort study. *A. N. Z. J. Surg.* 83 (5): 365–370.

TOXIC EPIDERMAL NECROLYSIS

Educational Goals

Learning Objectives

1. Develop a differential diagnosis for a febrile patient with widespread rash (MK).
2. Recognize the clinical signs and symptoms of toxic epidermal necrolysis (*TEN*) (PC, MK).
3. Demonstrate appropriate treatment for TEN (PC, MK).
4. Demonstrate appropriate disposition and consultation (ICS, SBP, P).

Critical Actions Checklist

- ☐ Assess airway, breathing and circulation (PC, MK).
- ☐ Obtain two large-bore IV cannulas (PC, MK).
- ☐ Calculate total body surface area involved (PC, MK).
- ☐ Initiate IV fluid resuscitation (MK).
- ☐ Order pain medications (PC, MK).
- ☐ Start broad-spectrum antibiotics to cover potential sepsis (PC, MK).
- ☐ Cover the wounds with non-adherent dressing or saline soaked gauze (PC, MK, SBP).
- ☐ Disposition to a burn unit (ICS, SBP, P).
- ☐ Communicate the diagnosis and plan with the patient (ICS, P).

Simulation Set-Up

Environment: ED treatment area.

Mannequin: Adult female simulator mannequin. Patient is dressed in a hospital gown, lying on the bed. Skin on the neck, upper thorax, and abdomen moulaged to illustrate bullae and desquamation. The lips can be covered with red dried out paint to have an appearance of cracked skin.

Simulated desquamated skin can be made using tinted tissue paper that has been dried out and placed on the mannequin with red paint underneath.

Props: To be displayed on a plasma screen/computer screen or printed on handouts to be distributed when participants request test results:
- Images (see online component for TEN, Scenario 3.3 at https://www.wiley.com/go/thoureen/simulation/workbook2e).
  - Chest x-ray showing right lower lobe infiltrate (Figure 3.9).
- Laboratory tests:
  - Complete blood count (Table 3.17).
  - Comprehensive metabolic panel (Table 3.18).
  - Lactate (Table 3.19).
  - Urinalysis (Table 3.20).
  - Pregnancy test (Table 3.21).

Available supplies:

- Basic airway and code cart.
- Medications (labeled bags/syringes may be used in place of actual medicine syringes or bags):
  - Liter bags of 0.9% saline and LR
  - Pre-labeled IV bags:
    - Broad-spectrum antibiotics (e.g. piperacillin-tazobactam, cefepime).
    - Vasopressor (e.g. epinephrine, norepinephrine, vasopressin).
  - Pre-labeled syringes:
    - Opioid analgesics.
  - Wound dressing:
    - Non-adhesive dressing/gauze.
    - Sterile gauze.
    - Bottle of 0.9% saline.

Distractor: (optional) patient will keep repeating that her symptoms are secondary to infection in her bloodstream. Patient can state, "My urinary infection has gotten into my blood, I have read it on Google; it's called sepsis, it's dangerous if missed."

Actors

- Patient's voice is female, soft spoken, in pain.
- The nurse can help with placing the patient on the monitor, starting IV access and giving medication. The nurse does have medical knowledge and can cue learners to expose the patient and examine the rash/lesions.
- The burn/intensive care consultant can be present via "phone consultation."

Case Narrative

Scenario Background

A 25-year-old woman presents to the ED via EMS complaining of feeling weak and fatigued for the past two days, as well as having increased urinary frequency for one week. She was seen by her primary care physician and diagnosed with a urinary tract infection. She was started on an antibiotic, which she is taking as prescribed. Dryness and cracking of her lips started two days ago with mouth sores and subjective fevers at home. She also complains of decreased appetite, red and itchy eyes, and a dry, non-productive cough. She has not been able to eat or drink much due to painful swallowing and a sore throat. There is a painful rash with blisters over her chest and right arm that started yesterday evening and spread to the abdomen and back this morning. She has been taking ibuprofen for two to three days with minimal relief.

> For advanced learners, the information about the rash can be withheld until the patient is exposed and examined.

Patient's medical history:	Asthma.
Medications:	Sulfamethoxazole/trimethoprim, albuterol as needed, ibuprofen as needed.
Allergies:	None.
Patient's surgical history:	None.
Family history:	None.
Social history:	Non-smoker, Drinks one to two glasses of wine on weekends, denies recreational drugs.

Initial scenario conditions

Patient is lying on the stretcher, moaning in pain.

Vital signs:	Temp 101.1°F (38.4°C), HR 120, RR 28, BP 104/64, SpO$_2$ 91 on room air.
Weight:	65 kg.
General:	Alert, oriented × 3, uncomfortable, in pain.
Head:	Normocephalic, atraumatic.
Eyes:	Pupils equal and reactive to light, extraocular movement intact, bilateral conjunctival hyperemia.
HEENT:	Normal tympanic membranes, normal nose. Lips crusted and erythematous with desquamation around the corners of the mouth. Tongue without edema. Oropharynx with an erosive, deep ulcer anterior.

Neck:	Full range of motion, mild erythema noted, no blisters.
Heart:	Tachycardic, regularly regular rhythm, no murmur, no gallops, no rubs.
Lungs:	Tachypnea, mild respiratory distress, no wheezes, no rales, no stridor, crackles to right base.
Abdomen:	Soft, non-tender, no organomegaly, Bowel sounds normal.
Genitourinary:	Erosive ulcers noted on the vaginal wall.
Neurologic:	Cranial nerves II–XII intact, motor strength intact, sensation intact.
Extremities:	Right upper extremity: bullae and erythematous lesion with desquamation and sloughing of skin.
Skin:	Erythematous macules with purpuric center on the neck, upper thorax, abdomen, mixed with areas of desquamation and sloughing, with intermittent blisters and vesicles. If asked, there is a positive Nikolsky sign.

Physical exam findings not available on your mannequin (e.g., vaginal ulcers) can be reported verbally by the nurse when requested by the learner.

See Figure 3.10 for a flow diagram of the case narrative described.

Case Narrative, Continued

Learners of all levels should place the patient on a cardiac monitor and a pulse oximeter, and should obtain vital signs. Patient should be placed on supplemental oxygen. The learner should recognize that the symptoms are likely caused by TEN secondary to her antibiotic. Two IV lines should be placed for initiation of appropriate fluid resuscitation, antipyretics and broad-spectrum antibiotics will improve the patient's vital signs. Learners should obtain laboratory studies and chest radiograph. The learner will have to appropriately consult burn center for case to end. If the learner calls dermatology consult, they will advise wound care, treatment of the underlying sepsis, and transfer.

Failure to appropriately resuscitate the patient with IV fluids and antibiotics will lead to decompensation of the condition. The patient will become hypotensive and obtunded with worsening respiratory distress. The learner should recognize the impending airway failure and appropriately intubate the patient. The patient should be resuscitated with fluids prior to intubation. If an attempt is made to intubate a hypotensive patient, the patient will go into pulseless electrical activity and the earners will need to initiate advanced cardiac life support (Advanced Cardiovascular Life Support). They will get ROSC after one round of ACLS. The scenario ends when the patient is stabilized and admitted to a burns unit.

For advanced learners, the patient can become increasingly obtunded, with worsening respiratory distress, regardless of initial interventions, and require intubation for airway protection and mechanical ventilation.

Instructor Notes

Pathophysiology of Toxic Epidermal Necrolysis

- Delayed mucocutaneous hypersensitivity reaction.
- Extensive necrosis and detachment of the epidermis.
- Involves more than 30% total body surface area [1].

Risk Factors

- Most common cause is medication:
  - High-risk drugs include nevirapine, lamotrigine, carbamazepine, phenytoin, phenobarbital, cotrimoxazole and other sulfonamides, sulfasalazine, allopurinol, oxicams.
  - Low-risk drugs include sertraline, acetic acid, NSAIDs, macrolides, quinolones, cephalosporins, aminopenicillins [2].
- Infection: HIV, mycoplasma pneumonia, tuberculosis.
- Collagen vascular disorders: systemic lupus erythematosus.
- Cancers: bone, ovarian, hematological.

Clinical Features

- Initially nonspecific prodrome of flu-like symptoms.
- ± fever, nasal congestion, sore throat, cough, odynophagia, fatigue and malaise.
- Cutaneous lesions → painful, ill defined, erythematous macules with purpuric center which progress to vesicles and bullae.
  - Start on the trunk and extend to the extremities in a symmetrical fashion.
  - Mucosal involvement of oral, vaginal and perineal lesions is common [3].
- Positive Nikolsky sign → the ability to extend the area of superficial sloughing by applying gentle lateral pressure on the surface of the skin.
- Electrolyte imbalances and dehydration due to massive fluid losses.
- Septicemia is the main cause of morbidity and mortality [4].
- Pneumonia is a common pulmonary complication, which can progress to acute respiratory distress syndrome requiring mechanical ventilation [5].

Diagnosis

- Primarily clinical.

Management

- Assess airway, breathing and circulation.
- Discontinue offending agent.

- Aggressive fluid resuscitation.
- Pain control.
- Prophylactic antibiotics are not recommended.
- Broad-spectrum antibiotics can be used for suspected sepsis.
- Corticosteroid use is controversial.
- IV immunoglobulin in conjunction with dermatology consult.
- Calculate *SCORTEN* (SCORe of toxic epidermal necrolysis)
  - Prognostic score for mortality based on seven clinical and laboratory values:
    1. Age ≥ 40 years.
    2. Heart rate ≥ 120 beats per min
    3. Cancer/hematologic malignancy.
    4. Body surface area detachment $\geq 10\%$ (at day 1).
    5. Serum blood urea nitrogen (*BUN*) > 28 mg/dl.
    6. Serum bicarbonate level < 20 mEq/l.
    7. Serum glucose level > 252 mg/dl.
  - Can be used to help identify appropriate level of care for a patient with TEN [6].
- Admission to a burn unit [7, 8].
- Patients with severe disease (skin detachment $> 30\%$ of the body surface area) or a SCORTEN score ≥ 2 should be transferred to a specialist burn unit.

Debriefing Plan

Plan for approximately 30 minutes of discussion.

Potential Questions for Discussion

- What are the risk factors associated with TEN?
- What is the management of TEN?
- What are the indications of antibiotics in TEN?
- What factors can help to determine the appropriate disposition for TEN?
- What are the complications of TEN?

REFERENCES FOR TOXIC EPIDERMAL NECROLYSIS

1. Downey, A., Jackson, C., Harun, N., and Cooper, A. (2012). Toxic epidermal necrolysis: review of pathogenesis and management. *J. Am. Acad. Dermatol.* 66 (6): 995–1003.
2. Mockenhaupt, M., Viboud, C., Dunant, A. et al. (2008). Stevens–Johnson syndrome and toxic epidermal necrolysis: assessment of medication risks with emphasis on recently marketed drugs: the EuroSCAR-study. *J. Invest. Dermatol.* 128 (1): 35–44.

3. Papp, A., Sikora, S., Evans, M. et al. (2018). Treatment of toxic epidermal necrolysis by a multidisciplinary team: a review of literature and treatment results. *Burns* 44 (4): 807–815.

4. Lerch, M., Mainetti, C., Terziroli Beretta-Piccoli, B. et al. (2018). Current perspectives on Stevens–Johnson syndrome and toxic epidermal necrolysis. *Clin. Rev. Allergy Immunol.* 54 (1): 147–176.

5. de Prost, N., Mekontso-Dessap, A., Valeyrie-Allanore, L. et al. (2014). B. Acute respiratory failure in patients with toxic epidermal necrolysis: clinical features and factors associated with mechanical ventilation. *Crit. Care Med.* 42 (1): 118–128.

6. Bastuji-Garin, S., Fouchard, N., Bertocchi, M. et al. (2000). SCORTEN: a severity-of-illness score for toxic epidermal necrolysis. *J. Invest. Dermatol.* 115 (2): 149–153.

7. Palmieri, T.L., Greenhalgh, D.G., Saffle, J.R. et al. (2002). A multicenter review of toxic epidermal necrolysis treated in U.S. burn centers at the end of the twentieth century. *J. Burn Care Rehabil.* 23 (2): 87–96.

8. McGee, T. and Munster, A. (1998). Toxic epidermal necrolysis syndrome: mortality rate reduced with early referral to regional burn center. *Plast. Reconstr. Surg.* 102 (4): 1018–1022.

APPENDIX

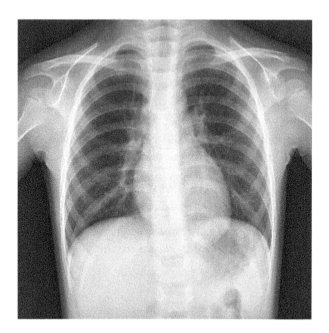

FIGURE 3.1   Pediatric chest x-ray (normal).

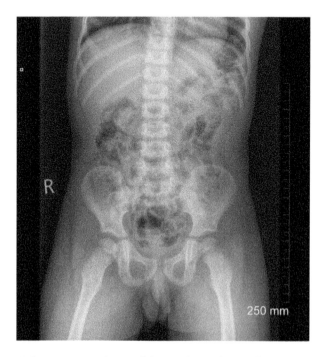

FIGURE 3.2   Pediatric abdominal x-ray (normal).

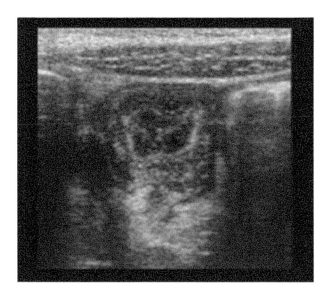

FIGURE 3.3 Abdominal ultrasound showing small-bowel wall thickening.

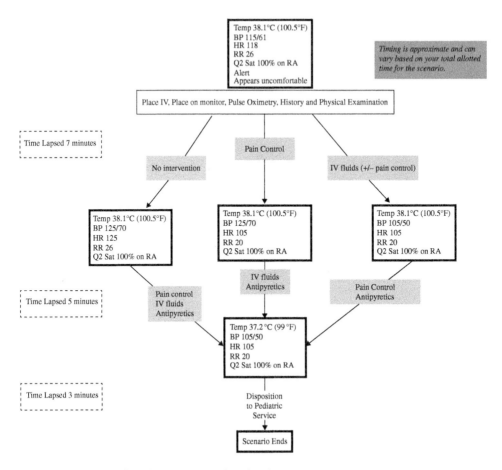

FIGURE 3.4   Case flow diagram, Henoch–Schönlein purpura.

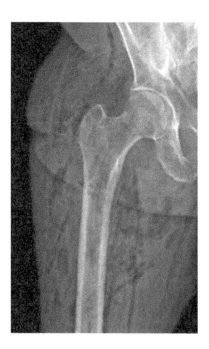

FIGURE 3.5 Femur x-ray showing subcutaneous air without fracture.

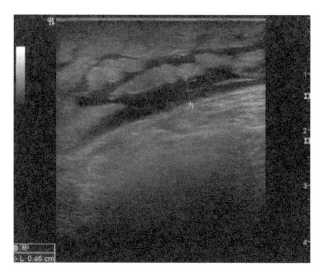

FIGURE 3.6 Soft-tissue ultrasound showing emphysema along the deep fascia, and increased echogenicity of the overlying fatty tissue with interlacing fluid collections.

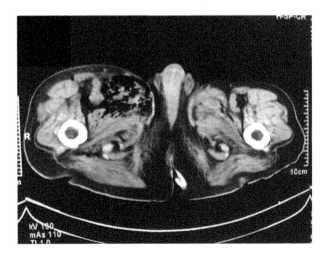

FIGURE 3.7   Computed tomography of the thigh showing the presence of gas in the tissues, with necrosis and asymmetric fascial thickening.

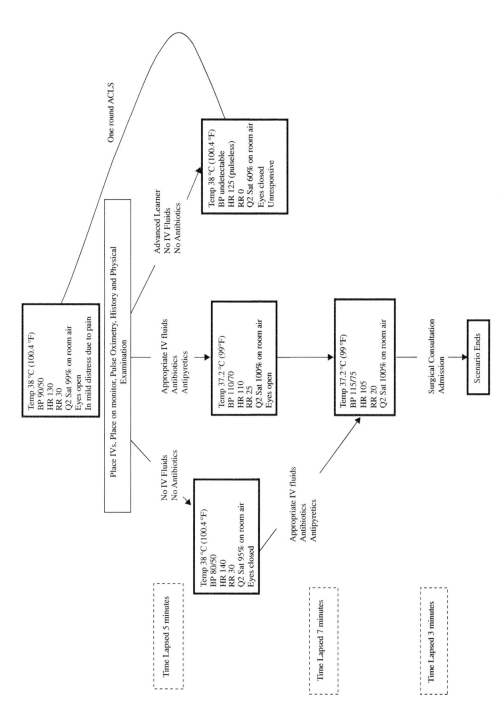

FIGURE 3.8 Case flow diagram for necrotizing fasciitis.

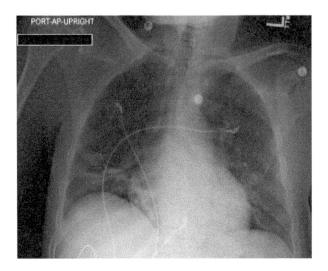

FIGURE 3.9   Chest x-ray showing right lower lobe infiltrate.

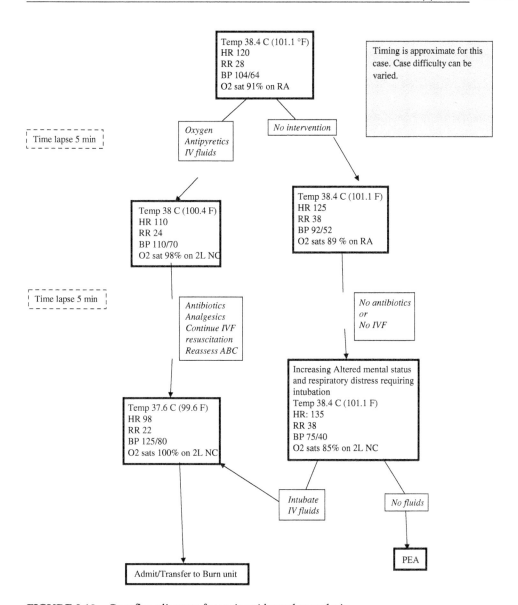

FIGURE 3.10   Case flow diagram for toxic epidermal necrolysis.

TABLE 3.1   Complete blood count.

Test	Value	Reference range
White blood cell count ($\times 10^3/\mu l$)	15.1	4.5–13.5
Red blood cell count ($\times 10^6/\mu l$)	5.3	4.00–5.20
Hemoglobin (g/dl)	15.6	11.5–15.5
Hematocrit (%)	46.8	35–45
Platelet count ($\times 10^3/\mu l$)	550	150–450
Mean corpuscular volume (fl)	93	77–95
Mean corpuscular hemoglobin (pg)	33	25–33
Mean corpuscular hemoglobin concentration (%)	36.3	32–36
Neutrophils (%)	65	33–61
Lymphocytes (%)	27	28–48
Eosinophils (%)	6	0–3
Basophils (%)	0	0–1
Monocytes (%)	2	2–6

TABLE 3.2   Comprehensive metabolic panel.

Test	Value	Reference range
Sodium (mEq/l)	147	130–147
Potassium (mEq/l)	5.0	3.5–5.1
Chloride (mEq/l)	105	95–108
Carbon dioxide (mEq/l)	25	20–30
Blood urea nitrogen (mg/dl)	20	2–20
Creatinine (mg/dl)	1.1	0.5–1
Glucose (mg/dl)	90	60–100
Calcium (mg/dl)	9	8.8–10.8
Aspartate aminotransferase (iu/l)	35	10–40
Alanine aminotransferase (iu/l)	35	10–40
Alkaline phosphatase (iu/l)	525	140–560
Total protein (g/dl)	7	5.7–8
Total bilirubin (mg/dl)	1.3	< 1.5

TABLE 3.3   Lactate.

Test	Value	Reference range
Lactate (mEq/l)	1.1	0.5–2

TABLE 3.4   Coagulation studies.

Test	Value	Reference range
Partial thromboplastin time (seconds)	60	60–70
International normalized ratio	1	0.8–1.1

TABLE 3.5   Urinalysis.

Test	Value	Reference range
Appearance	Clear; amber	Clear to hazy; light yellow to amber
Blood	Positive	Negative
Bilirubin	Negative	Negative
Glucose	Negative	Negative
Ketones	Negative	Negative
Leukocyte esterase	Negative	Negative
Nitrites	Negative	Negative
pH	6.5	5–8
Protein	Negative	Negative
Specific gravity	1.025	1.001–1.030
Red blood cells (/hpf)	8	0–3
White blood cells(/hpf)	0	0–5
Squamous epithelial cells(/hpf)	2	≤15–20
Hyaline casts(/lpf)	0	0–2
Mucous	None	None to slight
Bacteria	None	None

TABLE 3.6 Erythrocyte sedimentation rate.

Test	Value	Reference range
Erythrocyte sedimentation rate (mm/hour)	15	< 10

TABLE 3.7 C-reactive protein.

Test	Value	Reference range
C-reactive protein (mg/l)	12	0–10

TABLE 3.8 Complete blood count.

Test	Value	Reference range
White blood cell count ($\times 10^3$/µl)	15.3	4.3–13.8
Red blood cell count ($\times 10^6$/µl)	4.3	4.2–5.9
Hemoglobin (g/dl)	15.0	13.5–17.5
Hematocrit (%)	45	38.8–50
Platelet count ($\times 10^3$/µl)	162	150–450

TABLE 3.9 Comprehensive metabolic panel.

Test	Value	Reference range
Sodium (mEq/l)	133	135–147
Potassium (mEq/l)	5.1	3.7–5.2 mEq/l
Chloride (mEq/l)	108	96–106 mEq/l
Carbon dioxide (mEq/l)	21	23–29 mEq/l
Blood urea nitrogen (mg/dl)	22	10–20
Creatinine (mg/dl)	1.5	0.6–1.3
Glucose (mg/dl)	498	70–100
Calcium (mg/dl)	9	8.5–10.2

TABLE 3.10   Lactate level.

Test	Value	Reference range
Lactate (mEq/l)	2.4	0.5–2

TABLE 3.11   Coagulation panel.

Test	Value	Reference range
Partial thromboplastin time (seconds)	65	60–70
International normalized ratio	1	0.8–1.1

TABLE 3.12   Type and screen.

Test	Value	Reference range
Blood type	B positive	Not applicable

TABLE 3.13   Urinalysis.

Test	Value	Reference range
Appearance	Hazy; amber	Clear to hazy; light yellow to amber
Blood	Negative	Negative
Bilirubin	Negative	Negative
Glucose	3+	Negative
Ketones	Negative	Negative
Leukocyte esterase	1+	Negative
Nitrites	Negative	Negative
PH	6.5	5–8
Protein	Negative	Negative
Specific gravity	1.035	1.001–1.030

TABLE 3.14 Arterial blood gas.

Test	Value	Reference range
pH	7.35	7.38–7.44
Partial pressure of carbon dioxide (mmHg)	29	38–42
Bicarbonate (mEq/l)	21	23–28
Sodium (mEq/l)	133	136–145
Chloride (mEq/l)	108	98–106
Albumin (g/dl)	4.0	3.5–5.5

TABLE 3.15 Serum ketones.

Test	Value	Reference range
Ketone bodies (mg/dl)	< 1	< 1

TABLE 3.16 C-reactive protein.

Test	Value	Reference range
C reactive protein (mg/l)	14	0–10

TABLE 3.17 Complete blood count.

Test	Result	Reference range
White blood cells ($\times 10^3/\mu l$)	14.7	4.3–13.8
Hemoglobin (g/dl)	8.3	13.5–17.5
Hematocrit (%)	26.1	38.8–50
Platelets ($\times 10^3/\mu l$)	419	150–450

TABLE 3.18 Comprehensive metabolic panel.

Test	Result	Reference range
Sodium (mEq/l)	141	135–147
Potassium (mEq/l)	4.3	3.7–5.2
Chloride (mEq/l)	103	96–106
Bicarbonate (mEq/l)	27	23–29
Blood urea nitrogen (mEq/l)	40	10–20
Creatinine (mg/dl)	1.7	0.6–1.3
Glucose (mg/dl)	123	70–100
Calcium (mg/dl)	8.5	8.5–10.2
Magnesium (mg/dl)	2.4	1.6–2.3
Phosphate (mg/dl)	5.2	2.5–4.5
Alkaline phosphatase (iu/l)	70	140–560
Alanine aminotransferase (iu/l)	40	10–40
Aspartate aminotransferase (iu/l)	32	10–40
Albumin (g/dl)	3.1	3.5–5

TABLE 3.19 Lactate level.

Test	Result	Reference range
Lactate (mmol/l)	4.6	0.7–2

TABLE 3.20   Urinalysis.

Test	Value	Reference range
Appearance	Yellow	Clear to hazy; light yellow to amber
Blood	Negative	Negative
Bilirubin	Negative	Negative
Glucose	Negative	Negative
Ketones	Negative	Negative
Leukocyte esterase	+3	Negative
Nitrites	Positive	Negative
PH	6.0	5–8
Protein	Negative	Negative
Specific gravity	1.035	1.001–1.030
White blood cells (/hpf)	30–40	0–5
Red blood cells (/hpf)	2–4	0–2

TABLE 3.21   Pregnancy test.

Test	Result	Reference range
Pregnancy test	Negative	Negative

CHAPTER 4

Environmental Emergencies

Moira Davenport[1,2] and Brittany N. Muller[2]

[1] Temple University School of Medicine, Philadelphia, PA, USA
[2] Emergency Medicine Residency, Allegheny General Hospital, Pittsburgh, PA, USA

HEAT INJURY

Educational Goals

Learning Objectives

1. Recognize a patient with heat injury (MK, PC, ICS).
2. Demonstrate appropriate management for heat injury (MK, PC).
3. Develop a differential diagnosis for altered mental status (MK, PC).
4. Demonstrate appropriate management of fluids and electrolytes in a patient with hyponatremia (MK, PC).

Critical Actions Checklist

☐ Check vital signs, including core temperature (PC).
☐ Obtain electrocardiogram (ECG) (PC).
☐ Establish intravenous (IV) access (PC).
☐ Check electrolytes before administering IV fluids (MK).
☐ Initiate continuous core temperature monitoring (PC).

Emergency Medicine Simulation Workbook: A Tool for Bringing the Curriculum to Life,
Second Edition. Edited by Traci L. Thoureen and Sara B. Scott.
© 2022 John Wiley & Sons Ltd. Published 2022 by John Wiley & Sons Ltd.
Companion website: www.wiley.com/go/thoureen/simulation/workbook2e

- ☐ Initiate cooling (MK, PC).
- ☐ Stop cooling when temperature reaches 102°F (39°C) (MK, PC).
- ☐ Administer benzodiazepines as needed for shivering (MK, PC).
- ☐ Appropriately correct hyponatremia (MK).

Simulation Set-Up

Environment: Standard simulation room mocked up as a medical tent for a marathon. A multiple bed simulation room may also be used to recreate a medical tent setting.

Mannequin: The mannequin should be wearing running shorts and a sports (wicking material) shirt and sneakers. The patient should be male. No oxygen or IVs should be in place to start the scenario.

Props: To be displayed on screen or printed out in scenario room and available for distribution when requested by the learner:

- Images (see online component for Heat Injury Scenario 4.1 at https://www. wiley.com/go/thoureen/simulation/workbook2e):
  - ECG demonstrating sinus tachycardia at 125 beats/minute. Normal axis, normal intervals. No acute ST-T wave changes (Figure 4.1).
- Laboratory tests (see online component as above):
  - Point-of-care chemistry panel (Table 4.1).
  - Point-of-care hemoglobin/hematocrit (Table 4.2).

Available supplies:

- Automated external defibrillator.
- Basic airway supplies (bag valve mask, oxygen tank).
- Medications:
  - IV fluids (liter bags) of 0.9% saline, lactated Ringer's solution (*LR*) and 5% dextrose in water (D5W).
  - 100 ml bags of 3% saline.
  - Pre-labeled syringes:
    - IV benzodiazepine (e.g., midazolam).
- Cooling equipment (e.g., ice bath: kids swimming pool filled with water/ice, cooling blankets, ice bags or other commercially available cooling device).

Distractor: None

Actors

- Patient voice is male.
- Nurse can perform point-of-care testing and administer IV fluids.

Case Narrative

Scenario Background

Scenario takes place at the finish line medical tent at a regional marathon. A participant collapsed 50 meters after the finish line and was brought to the medical tent for further evaluation.

Chief complaint: Found down
Patient medical history: Unknown
Medications: Unknown
Allergies: Unknown
Family history: Unknown
Social history: Unknown

Initial Scenario Conditions

A 25-year-old man is brought to the finish line medical tent. He is awake but is not answering questions appropriately.

Vital signs: Temp 37.4°C (99°) tympanic, HR 128, RR 22, BP 158/92, 98% SpO$_2$ on room air (core temperature 106°F, 41.1°C, if specifically requested).
HEENT: Normocephalic, atraumatic. Posterior pharynx clear, mucous membranes dry.
Eyes: Pupils 4 mm and equally reactive to light.
Neck: No lymphadenopathy.
Heart: Tachycardic, regular. 1+ pulses distally.
Lungs: Tachypneic, no rales, rhonchi, or wheezes.
Abdomen: Soft, non-tender, non-distended. Bowel sounds decreased.
Extremities: No clubbing, cyanosis, or edema.
Skin: Warm without diaphoresis.
Neurologic: Moves all extremities equally and spontaneously. Does not answer questions appropriately. Does not follow commands.

See flow diagram (Figure 4.2) for further scenario changes described.

Case Narrative, Continued

All learners should specifically request a rectal temperature, obtain an ECG, establish IV access, and check electrolytes prior to starting IV fluids. If a core temperature is requested, it is 106°F (41.1°C).

Continuous core temperature monitoring and active cooling procedures should be initiated. For student learners, the case could end here.

More advanced learners are expected to administer benzodiazepines if the patient starts shivering during the cooling process, and should stop cooling procedures once the core temperature reaches 102°F (39°C). This can be achieved by having the patient state "I'm cold" or by having the nurse mention that the patient's teeth are chattering and he is shivering.

Learners should recognize hyponatremia. Advanced learners should calculate the appropriate rate of sodium correction. Learners may administer hypertonic saline (100 cc of 3% solution) for hyponatremia.

If the learners provide fluid resuscitation without consideration of appropriate sodium correction (e.g., if they administer D5W, or if more than 500 ml of LR or 0.9% saline is administered) the patient starts to seize. At this point, benzodiazepines should be administered, but without effect, and the patient goes into cardiac arrest.

The case ends when the patient is transferred to a tertiary care facility or when five minutes have lapsed without the core temperature being measured.

Instructor Notes

Pathophysiology

- Heat injury occurs when the body generates more heat than it can dissipate:
  - Causes ischemia and oxidative and nitrosative stress (main cause for morbidity and mortality).
- Heat is dissipated through four primary mechanisms:
  1. Convection: electromagnetic waves move heat from a warmer object to a cooler one.
  2. Evaporation: vaporization of water removes heat from an object.
  3. Radiation: air/liquid moving across an object removes heat from an object.
  4. Conduction: direct transfer of heat from a warmer object to a cooler one.
- Athletes primarily lose heat through radiation and evaporation:
  - The ambient temperature during an endurance event can affect an athlete's ability to cool.

Clinical Features

- Spectrum of disease with signs and symptoms that vary and help determine the category of exertional heat illness:
  - Heat exhaustion
    - Core temperature typically 101–104°F (38.3–40°C).
    - Cannot continue with exercise.
    - No central nervous system (*CNS*) dysfunction.
  - Heat injury:
    - Core temperature > 104°F (> 40°C)
    - End-organ dysfunction:
      - Kidney, liver, muscle (rhabdomyolysis)

- No CNS dysfunction
- Heat stroke
- Core temperature > 104 °F (>40 °C)
- Defined by CNS dysfunction
  - Disorientation
  - Headache
  - Behavior changes
  - Altered mental status
  - Coma
  - Seizure
- All types of heat illness may include:
  - Vital sign changes
  - Tachycardia
  - Hypotension
  - Generalized weakness
  - Presyncope/syncope:
    - Profuse sweating or no sweating
    - Gastrointestinal symptoms: abdominal cramps, nausea, vomiting, diarrhea
    - Muscle cramps

Diagnosis

- Primarily clinical, based on elevated temperature and symptoms:
  - Core temperature should be used to evaluate for hyperthermia
  - Rectal
  - Bladder
  - Esophageal
- Laboratory abnormalities may include:
  - Low serum bicarbonate
  - Elevated creatinine kinase
  - Elevated creatine
  - Transaminitis

Management

- Airway/breathing:
- Supplemental oxygen as needed.
- Circulation:
  - IV fluids:
    - At a rate that ensures urinary output at 1 ml/kg/hour.

- If there is clinical consideration of hyponatremia, electrolytes should be checked prior to starting fluid administration. Calculate the appropriate rate of fluid replacement to avoid the complications of rapidly correcting sodium.
  - Consider ECG to evaluate for cardiac conduction abnormalities.
- Active cooling:
  - Ice packs to the axilla, groin, and head.
  - Immersion in an ice bath.
  - Administer cold IV fluids.
  - Urinary catheter lavage with cold fluids.
  - Stopped once the patient's temperature reaches 102°F (39°C).
  - Antipyretics have not been shown to decrease cooling times.

Debriefing Plan

Plan for around 20 minutes for discussion.

Potential Questions for Discussion

- What are the different types of heat-related injuries?
- What is the differential diagnosis for the collapsed athlete?
- What are the risks associated with rapid correction of hyponatremia?
- How is heat stroke managed?

SELECTED READINGS FOR HEAT INJURY

Asplund, C.A., O'Connor, F.G., and Noaks, T.D. (2011). Exercise-associated collapse: an evidence based review and primer for clinicians. *Br. J. Sports Med.* 45 (14): 1157–1162.

Casa, D.J., Armstrong, L.E., Ganio, M.S. et al. (2005). Exertional heat stroke in competitive athletes. *Curr. Sports Med. Rep.* 4 (6): 309–317.

Luning, H., Mangelus, C., Carlstrom, E. et al. (2019). Incidence and characteristics of severe exercise-associated collapse at the world's largest half-marathon. *PLoS One* 14 (6): e0217465.

JELLYFISH ENVENOMATION

Educational Goals

Learning Objectives

1. Recognize symptoms of a jellyfish envenomation (MK).
2. Demonstrate appropriate, geographically relevant management of jellyfish envenomation (MK, PC).
3. Recognize Irukandji syndrome (MK).
4. Develop a differential diagnosis for the patient's presentation (MK, PC).
5. Recognize indications for transfer to a higher level of care (MK, PC, SBP).
6. Demonstrate appropriate consultation with a medical toxicologist or the poison control center (PC, ICS, SBP).

Critical Actions Checklist

- ☐ Check vital signs, including temperature (PC).
- ☐ Expose the patient (PC).
- ☐ Establish IV access and start IV fluids (PC).
- ☐ Initiate transfer to higher level of care (PC).
- ☐ Deactivate nematocyst (PC).
- ☐ Administer opioids for early Irukandji syndrome(PC).
- ☐ Consult poison control or medical toxicologist (PC, SBP, ICS).

Simulation Set-Up

Environment: Free-standing emergency department (ED) near a popular beach in Northern Australia; case occurs on New Year's Day.

Alternatively, for prehospital providers, this case could take place in a lifeguard or first-aid station at the beach.

Mannequin: Pediatric male mannequin, elementary-aged size, dressed in swim shorts. The clothes should be wet. An optional wig can be used to show wet hair. Moulage with additional silicone skin on the left lower extremity to represent edema along the lateral aspect of the leg from the middle third of the tibia to the syndesmosis. Use washable make-up to demonstrate erythema in the area with a central area of induration with multiple small puncture wounds located in the center.

Props: None.

Available supplies:

- Standard first aid equipment (gauze squares, antibiotic ointment, tweezers, irrigation bins, antibiotic ointment, gauze bandage roll, elastic bandages)
- Adhesive tape
- Ice bag or cold pack
- IV fluids (liter bags) of 0.9% saline, LR and D5W
- Bottle labeled as 5% acetic acid

Distractor: Parent is initially yelling at the child to hold still and stop crying, which is making the child cry more.

Actors

- Patient has a male child's voice and he is crying. Once the parent is no longer yelling at the child, he becomes more cooperative.
- Nurse can obtain requested supplies and administer IV fluids and medications.
- Parent is yelling at the child to cooperate but calmed when given an explanation of the diagnosis and care.

Case Narrative

Scenario Background

You are providing medical coverage at a free-standing emergency department near a popular public beach in Northern Australia. A seven-year-old boy is brought in by parents for evaluation of left lower leg pain that started while swimming. His parent brought him to the ED because he continued to cry in pain after exiting the water.

Chief complaint:	Leg pain
Patient medical history:	Mild asthma
Medications:	Albuterol MDI
Allergies:	Penicillin
Family history:	Multiple family members with mild asthma
Social history:	third-grade student

Initial Scenario Conditions

A seven-year-old boy, awake, alert and oriented×3 in no respiratory distress but moaning in pain.

Case may start with EMS on scene evaluating stability, initiating treatment, and transporting according to local EMS protocols. EMS may then hand the patient over to the ED care team.

Vital signs: Temp 98.1°F (36.7°C) oral, HR 128, RR 32, BP 110/74, SpO$_2$ 98% on room air.

Weight: 23 kg.

HEENT: Normocephalic, atraumatic. Pupils equal, round, and reactive to light and accommodation. Extraocular movement intact. Posterior pharynx clear, mucous membranes moist.

Neck: No lymphadenopathy. No midline tenderness.

Heart: Tachycardic, regular. No murmurs, rubs or gallops. 2+ pulses throughout.

Lungs: Tachypneic, no rales, rhonchi or wheezes.

Abdomen: Soft, non-tender, non-distended.

Extremities: No clubbing, cyanosis or edema of the bilateral upper and right lower extremities. Left lower extremity has edema along the lateral aspect of the leg from the middle third of the tibia to the syndesmosis. There is erythema in the area with a central area of induration. There are multiple small puncture wounds in the central area of induration.

Skin: Findings as described above.

Neurologic: No focal deficits.

See flow diagram (Figure 4.3) for further scenario changes described.

Case Narrative, Continued

The patient should be placed on a cardiac monitor and vitals signs should be continually assessed. An IV line should be placed and weight-based fluid resuscitation should be started. The learner should ask about possible mechanisms of injury, including trauma, potential bites and envenomations. All learners should examine the left lower extremity. If the learner does not ask about possible jellyfish envenomation, the case ends within five minutes.

The left lower extremity should be elevated. Analgesics should be given in appropriate doses. The learner should recommend nematocyst deactivation with seawater, 0.9% saline or vinegar (typically 5% acetic acid). If tap water or another hypotonic solution is used for deactivation the patient starts to decompensate. Once the nematocyst is deactivated, it may be removed by adhesive tape. Use of other methods (tweezers) results in patient decompensation. Alternatively, the deactivated nematocyst may be left in place during transport.

After approximately 10 minutes, the patient starts to complain of increasing pain to all extremities as well as abdominal pain. The learner should give IV opiates for pain control. Once the patient starts to show evidence of cardiovascular instability, box jellyfish antivenom should be considered and a call for transfer should be initiated.

The case ends when the patient is transferred to a tertiary care facility or when five minutes have lapsed without EMS being called

Instructor Notes

Background

- Jellyfish are marine invertebrates.
- Subdivided into five classes
  - Cubozoa:
    - Contains the deadliest species, the Australian box jellyfish (Chironex fleckeri) and the Irukandji jellyfish (Carukia barnesi), which can cause Irukandji syndrome.
    - Found in tropical Australia and other areas of the Indo-Pacific.
    - Most Australian jellyfish envenomations occur from November to April.
  - Hydrozoa:
    - Not actually true jellyfish.
    - Portugese man of war (Physalia species) is in this class.
    - Found in nontropical waters of the Atlantic, Pacific, and Indian Oceans, as well as the Caribbean and Sargasso Seas [1].
  - Scyphozoa.
  - Anthozoa.
  - Staurozoa:
    - Geographic location should be taken into consideration to assess potential severity of envenomation.
- Jellyfish stings are from tentacles covered in cells containing stinging barbed threads or tubules [1].
  - Mechanical or chemical stimulation induces an osmotic gradient causing the threads or barbs to expel venom.
  - Venom composition depends on the species of jellyfish.

Clinical Features

- Localized reaction is typically seen:
  - Classically, lesions are linear, painful, erythematous and/or urticarial.
- Systemic symptoms:
  - Rare in Physalia envenomations.
  - C. fleckeri envenomations can cause sudden cardiac arrest, cardiogenic shock.

- C. barnesi envenomations can cause delayed symptoms of abdominal/back pain, accompanied by symptoms similar to sympathomimetic toxicity (Irukandji syndrome).
  - Cardiomyopathy with pulmonary edema and cardiogenic shock can occur in severe cases.

Diagnosis

- Primarily clinical and from history of seawater immersion.

Management

- Deactivation of undischarged nematocysts.
  - Immerse the affected area in sea water or 0.9% saline.
  - Use of vinegar (4–6% acetic acid) for at least 30 seconds is no longer recommended for **all** jellyfish envenomations.
    - Vinegar is still recommended for C. barnesi, C. alata, and Pelagia noctiluca. (C. fleckeri is controversial but recommended in the Australian Resuscitation Council Guidelines [2])
- Removal of tentacles:
  - Rinse off site with seawater to remove tentacles.
  - Manual removal is recommended.
    - Adhesive tape should be applied to the area and quickly removed.
    - Skin scraping with a sharp object (potentially harmful and should be used if tape is not available or not successful).
- Symptomatic treatment:
  - Analgesics:
    - Immerse stung area in hot water for 20 minutes unless C. fleckeri or non-tropical regions.
    - Consider cold packs (especially C. fleckeri).
    - Topical lidocaine.
  - Antihistamines.
  - Topical steroids.
  - Antibiotics:
    - Topical after minor sting.
    - Secondary infection very rare.
- Antivenom:
  - Available for C. fleckeri.
  - Should only be used once nematocyst removal has occurred.
  - Should be given within one hour of sting for symptoms of severe cardiotoxicity.

- Adult and pediatric dose is the same (20 000 units IV per vial) and can be administered multiple times.

Debriefing Plan

Plan for 20–30 minutes for discussion.

Potential Questions for Discussion

- Why is geographic location important in determining the potential severity of a jellyfish envenomation?
- In what parts of the world might you see severe systemic symptoms from jellyfish envenomation?
- What is Irukandji syndrome? In what geographic location might this occur following a jellyfish envenomation?
- What can be done to reduce pain from a jellyfish envenomation?

REFERENCES FOR JELLYFISH ENVENOMATION

1. Lakkis, N.A., Maalouf, G.J., and Mahmassani, D.M. (2015). Jellyfish stings: a practical approach. *Wilderness Environ. Med.* 26: 422–429.
2. Australian Resuscitation Council. (2010). *Envenomation: Jellyfish Stings.*Guideline 9.4.5. East Melbourne, Victoria: ARC. https://resus.org.au/guidelines (accessed 1 September 2021).

SELECTED READING FOR JELLYFISH ENVENOMATION

Honeycutt, J.D., Jonas, C.E., and Smith, R.F. (2014). Treatment of jellyfish envenomation. *Am. Fam. Phys.* 89 (10): 823A–823C.

HIGH-ALTITUDE PULMONARY EDEMA

Educational Goals

Learning Objectives

1. Diagnose high-altitude pulmonary edema (*HAPE*) (MK, PC).
2. Initiate management for HAPE (MK, PC).
3. Develop differential diagnosis of dyspnea (MK).
4. Formulate a treatment plan that includes altitude descent and transfer to higher level of care (MK, PC, SBP).

Critical Actions Checklist

- ☐ Obtain vital signs, including temperature and oxygen saturation (PC).
- ☐ Obtain EKG (PC).
- ☐ Initiate cardiac monitoring (PC).
- ☐ Establish IV access (PC).
- ☐ Perform a complete physical exam (PC).
- ☐ Initiate oxygen therapy (PC).
- ☐ Arrange for descent and transfer to a tertiary care facility (PC, SBP).
- ☐ Administer nifedipine for HAPE (optional for advanced learners)

Simulation Set-Up

Environment: A multiple bed simulation room may be used to recreate a slopeside medical clinic.

Mannequin: Adult female mannequin should be placed in a base layer of tight-fitting long underwear, multiple layers of wicking material shirts, ski pants including a bib and shoulder straps, a ski jacket, helmet, goggles, and ski boots. No oxygen or IV should be in place to start the scenario. Moulage should include red cheeks from being outdoors.

Props: To be displayed on screen or printed out in scenario room and available for distribution when requested by the learner:

- Laboratory tests (see online component for HAPE, Scenario 4.3 at https://www.wiley.com/go/thoureen/simulation/workbook2e):
  - Point-of-care:
    - Basic metabolic panel (Table 4.3).
    - Troponin (Table 4.4).

- Hemoglobin (Table 4.5).
- Pregnancy test (Table 4.6).

Available supplies:

- Airway supplies, code cart, and defibrillator.
- Medications:
  - IV fluids (liter bags) of 0.9% saline, LR and D5W.
  - Pre-labeled syringes:
    - Benzodiazepine of choice.
    - Furosemide.
    - Acetazolamide.
  - Pre-labeled IV bags:
    - 100 ml bags of 3% saline.
- Optional: bottle labeled as oral nifedipine.

Distractor: None.

Actors

- Patient's voice is female.
- Nurse can perform point-of-care testing and can administer IV fluids and/or medications. The nurse can cue learners if needed to progress the case.
- Ski patrol officer can be available by phone consultation to facilitate rapid descent from the slopeside clinic site.
- Hyperbaric medical specialist available by telephone consultation.

Case Narrative

Scenario Background

A 33 year old woman is brought into a slopeside medical clinic (at 11 000 ft) after being assisted off the slope by ski patrol. The skier initially flagged down the ski patrol to ask for help as she was feeling short of breath after getting off the chair lift. On further discussion, the patient states that she arrived at the resort approximately 24 hours ago. She had been skiing this morning, but had to stop due to progressive dyspnea. She was able to wave down the ski patrol and ask for assistance. She reports that she also had felt short of breath and light-headed while riding up the chair lift, which she has never experienced.

Chief complaint:	"I'm . . . short . . . of . . . breath."
Patient medical history:	Asthma.
Medications:	Albuterol as needed.
Allergies:	None.

Family history:	Non-contributory.
Social history:	No tobacco or drug use. Social alcohol use. Patient is an avid climber that lives in Chicago, Illinois but travels frequently for hikes/climbs.

Initial Scenario Conditions

Patient is in mild distress due to dyspnea.

Vital signs:	99.7°F (37.6°C), HR 119, RR 28, BP 142/87, 88% SpO$_2$ on room air.
HEENT:	Normocephalic, atraumatic. Posterior pharynx clear, mucous membranes moist.
Eyes:	Pupils 4 mm reactive to light; extraocular movements intact.
Neck:	No lymphadenopathy.
Heart:	Tachycardic, regular. 2+ pulses throughout. No murmur. No jugular vein distension.
Lungs:	Tachypneic with rales bilaterally.
Abdomen:	Soft, non-tender, non-distended.
Extremities:	Cyanotic nail beds. No peripheral edema.
Skin:	Warm and dry.
Neurologic:	Alert and oriented × 3. No focal deficits. Moves all extremities equally and spontaneously.

Physical exam findings not available on your mannequin (e.g., cyanotic nail beds) can be reported verbally, if asked for by learners. Visual findings could also be presented via projected images.

See the flow diagram (Figure 4.4) for further scenario changes described.

Case Narrative, Continued

All learners should initiate continuous pulse oximetry and establish IV access, provide supplemental oxygen, and complete a thorough history and physical. Radiography is unavailable at the slopeside clinic.

All learners should arrange for descent upon recognizing edema on lung exam. For advanced learners, descent is not immediately available, and they should initiate medical therapy with nifedipine.

If supplemental oxygen is not administered or if there is aggressive IV fluid administration, the patient will begin to decompensate. If corrective measures are not taken, the patient will have a pulseless electrical activity arrest over the course of 10 minutes.

The case ends when the patient has been stabilized on oxygen and descent has been initiated or when there is a delay of more than 5 minutes in initiating altitude descent or treatment for HAPE.

Instructor Notes

Pathophysiology

- Hypoxia secondary to high altitude induces pulmonary hypertension:
  - Leads to fluid leakage from pulmonary capillaries causing pulmonary edema.
- HAPE typically starts to develop at 3000 m (10 000 ft) above sea level:
  - Most common fatal manifestation of severe high-altitude illness.

Clinical Features

- Symptoms begin gradually two to four days after arrival at high altitude
  - Initial symptoms include dyspnea on exertion, generalized fatigue, and dry cough
  - Progresses to dyspnea with rest and productive cough with watery sputum
- Exam often reveals scattered rales without jugular vein distension or peripheral edema.

Diagnosis

- Primarily clinical:
  - Based on the patient's history of rapid ascent with progressive dyspnea and evidence of pulmonary edema.
- Chest x-ray and/or bedside ultrasound can demonstrate pulmonary edema.

Management

- Supplemental oxygen:
  - Consider positive pressure oxygen delivery when available.
- Rapid descent after stabilization:
  - Descend until symptoms resolve; 3000 ft is generally adequate.
- If descent is unavailable:
  - Rest.
  - Supplemental oxygen.
  - Nifedipine: 30 mg orally twice daily (reduces pulmonary arterial pressure).
  - Hyperbaric therapy, if available (simulates descent).

- Fluid management:
  - IV fluids should be given judiciously in the setting of pulmonary edema.

Debriefing Plan

This discussion should take 20–30 minutes.

Potential Questions for Discussion

- What is the differential diagnosis for progressive dyspnea in high-altitude settings?
- What are classic symptoms, exam findings, and imaging abnormalities associated with HAPE?
- What is the appropriate management for HAPE?
- What treatments are used for HAPE if descent is unavailable?

SELECTED READINGS FOR HIGH-ALTITUDE PULMONARY EDEMA

Pennardt, A. (2013). High-altitude pulmonary edema: diagnosis, prevention and treatment. *Curr. Sports Med. Rep.* 12 (2): 115–119.

Wilkins, M.R., Ghofrani, H.A., Weissmann, N. et al. (2015). Pathophysiology and treatment of high-altitude pulmonary vascular disease. *Circulation* 131: 582–590.

Paralikar, S.J. (2012). High altitude pulmonary edema-clinical features, pathophysiology, prevention and treatment. *Indian J. Occup. Environ. Med.* 16 (2): 59–62.

APPENDIX

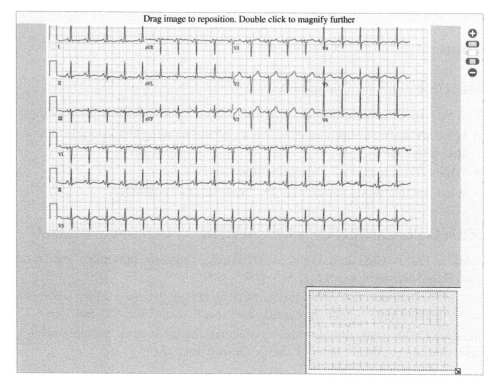

Drag image to reposition. Double click to magnify further

FIGURE 4.1   Electrocardiogram with sinus tachycardia.

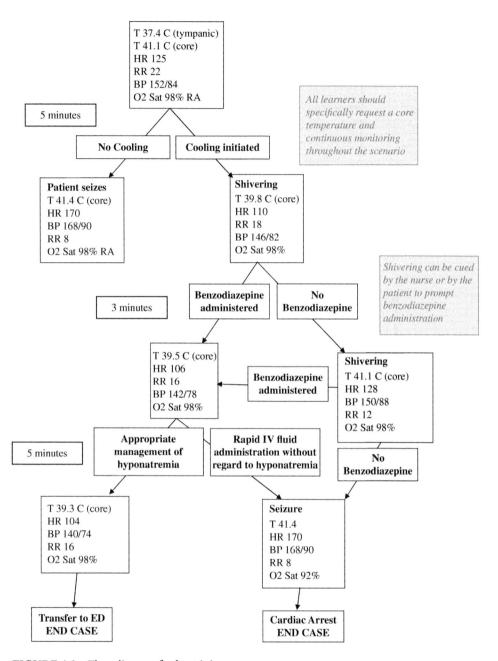

FIGURE 4.2 Flow diagram for heat injury.

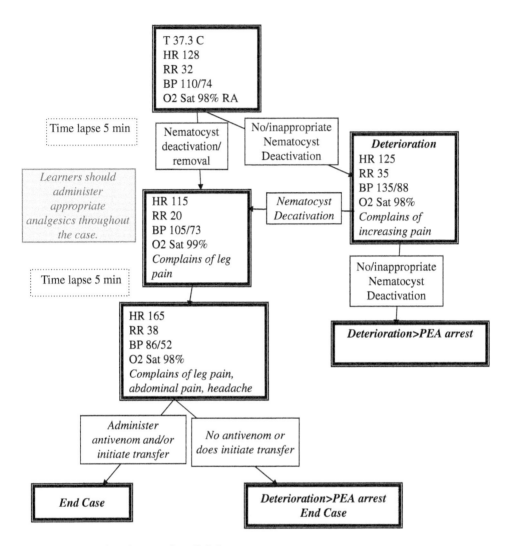

FIGURE 4.3   Flow diagram for jellyfish envenomation.

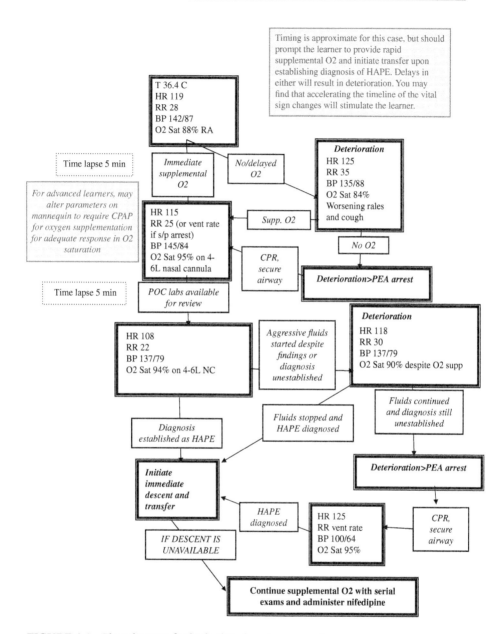

Timing is approximate for this case, but should prompt the learner to provide rapid supplemental O2 and initiate transfer upon establishing diagnosis of HAPE. Delays in either will result in deterioration. You may find that accelerating the timeline of the vital sign changes will stimulate the learner.

T 36.4 C
HR 119
RR 28
BP 142/87
O2 Sat 88% RA

Time lapse 5 min

Immediate supplemental O2

No/delayed O2

Deterioration
HR 125
RR 35
BP 135/88
O2 Sat 84%
Worsening rales and cough

For advanced learners, may alter parameters on mannequin to require CPAP for oxygen supplementation for adequate response in O2 saturation

HR 115
RR 25 (or vent rate if s/p arrest)
BP 145/84
O2 Sat 95% on 4-6L nasal cannula

Supp. O2

CPR, secure airway

No O2

Deterioration>PEA arrest

Time lapse 5 min

POC labs available for review

HR 108
RR 22
BP 137/79
O2 Sat 94% on 4-6L NC

Aggressive fluids started despite findings or diagnosis unestablished

Deterioration
HR 118
RR 30
BP 137/79
O2 Sat 90% despite O2 supp

Fluids continued and diagnosis still unestablished

Diagnosis established as HAPE

Fluids stopped and HAPE diagnosed

Deterioration>PEA arrest

Initiate immediate descent and transfer

HAPE diagnosed

HR 125
RR vent rate
BP 100/64
O2 Sat 95%

CPR, secure airway

IF DESCENT IS UNAVAILABLE

Continue supplemental O2 with serial exams and administer nifedipine

FIGURE 4.4   Flow diagram for high-altitude pulmonary edema.

TABLE 4.1   Point-of-care chem 7 blood panel.

Test	Value	Reference range
Glucose (mg/dl)	92	70–115
Sodium (mmol/l)	118	135–145
Chloride (mmol/l)	98	96–106
Potassium (mEq/l)	4.1	3.5–4.5
CO_2 (mEq/l)	26	23–29
Blood urea nitrogen (mg/dl)	13	11–23
Creatinine (mg/dl)	0.98	0.7–1.5

TABLE 4.2   Point-of-care hemoglobin and hematocrit.

Test	Value	Reference range
Hemoglobin (g/dl)	16.1	13–17
Hematocrit(%)	47.6	38–48

TABLE 4.3   Point-of-care chem 8 basic metabolic panel.

Test	Value	Reference range
Glucose (mg/dl)	117	70–115
Sodium (mmol/l)	142	135–145
Chloride (mmol/l)	102	96–106
Potassium (mEq/l)	4.1	3.5–4.5
Bicarbonate (mEq/l)	18	23–29
Blood urea nitrogen (mg/dl)	18	11–23
Creatinine (mg/dl)	0.84	0.7–1.5
Calcium (mg/dl)	10.1	9–11

TABLE 4.4   Point-of-care troponin.

Test	Value	Reference range
Troponin (ng/ml)	< 0.01	< 0.03

TABLE 4.5   Point-of-care hemoglobin.

Test	Value	Reference range
Hemoglobin (g/dl)	14.5	13–17

TABLE 4.6   Point-of-care pregnancy test.

Test	Value	Reference range
Pregnancy (urine)	Negative	Negative

CHAPTER 5

Hematologic and Oncologic Emergencies

Ashley Pickering and Sarah B. Dubbs

Department of Emergency Medicine, University of Maryland School of Medicine, Baltimore, MD, USA

INTRACRANIAL HEMORRHAGE IN A PATIENT WITH HEMOPHILIA

Educational Goals

Learning Objectives

1. Recognize common congenital bleeding disorders (MK).
2. Identify and properly manage major bleeding in a patient with hemophilia (MK, PC).
3. Identify and manage intracranial hemorrhage (*ICH*) in a patient with hemophilia (MK, PC).
4. Demonstrate proper administration of clotting factor (MK, PC).
5. Recognize signs of decompensation and need for airway management in a pediatric patient with ICH (MK, PC).
6. Perform rapid sequence intubation (*RSI*) in a pediatric patient (MK, PC).
7. Initiate appropriate consultations with hematology, pediatric intensive care and neurologic surgery (SBP, ICS).
8. Communicate with the parents of a critically ill child (ICS).

Emergency Medicine Simulation Workbook: A Tool for Bringing the Curriculum to Life,
Second Edition. Edited by Traci L. Thoureen and Sara B. Scott.
© 2022 John Wiley & Sons Ltd. Published 2022 by John Wiley & Sons Ltd.
Companion website: www.wiley.com/go/thoureen/simulation/workbook2e

Critical Actions Checklist

- ☐ Obtain history of hemophilia (MK, PC, ICS).
- ☐ Administer appropriate factor replacement immediately prior to obtaining imaging (MK, PC).
- ☐ Order computed tomography (CT) of the head (MK, PC).
- ☐ Perform pediatric RSI (PC).
- ☐ Communicate with patient's parents (ICS, P).
- ☐ Consult hematology, pediatric intensivist, and neurosurgery (ICS, P, SBP).

Simulation Set-up

Environment: Emergency department (ED) trauma resuscitation bay. This may also start "on scene" and transition to a hospital setting.

Mannequin: Male pediatric elementary-aged simulator mannequin in street clothes, seated in bed. The mannequin has a 3 cm diameter hematoma on the left parieto-occipital scalp. This can be moulaged with makeup and clay/putty.

Props: To be displayed on plasma screen/computer screen or printed out on handouts in scenario room when asked for/return from lab:

- Images (see online component for Hemophilia, Scenario 5.1 at https://www.wiley.com/go/thoureen/simulation/workbook2e):
  - Pediatric CT head representative slice showing subdural hematoma with skull fracture and midline shift (Figure 5.1).
  - Factor replacement (Figure 5.2).
- Laboratory tests (see online component as above):
  - Complete blood count (Table 5.1).
  - Complete metabolic panel (Table 5.2).
  - Coagulation panel (Table 5.3).

Available supplies:

- Basic pediatric airway and code cart.
- Pediatric emergency measuring tape.
- Medications:
  - Liter bags of 0.9% saline and lactated ringer's solution (*LR*).
  - Pre-labeled syringes:
    - RSI medications.
    - Analgesic medication (e.g., fentanyl, morphine).

- Factor VIII replacement.
- Pre-labeled IV bags:
  - Sedative medication (e.g., midazolam, propofol).
- Video-assisted laryngoscope (optional).

Distractor: Parent not physically present in the ED and history cannot be fully obtained without calling the parent.

Actors

- Patient voice is male. Patient is initially crying softly and complaining of a headache. Initially awake and responsive. He automatically volunteers that he has a "bleeding problem," but does not know the specific name of the disease.
- Emergency medical services (EMS) may be an actor or another learner. They are able to give the history of patient's fall on the playground at school.
- Patient's parent can be reached by phone. When told why the child is in the ED they will become upset and immediately provide the history of hemophilia. Depending on the level of learner, they can suggest factor replacement, give instructions on administration and even provide basic hemophilia education.
- ED nurse can administer medications/fluids. The nurse does have some medical knowledge and may cue learners if needed.
- Hematology, pediatric intensive care and neurosurgery consultants available via phone.

Case Narrative

Scenario Background

A six-year-old boy fell in the playground, striking his head on the ground, which was dirt/grass. He did not lose consciousness, got up immediately and was crying. He has been complaining of a headache, and the school reports he has a history of a "bleeding problem," so they sent him to the hospital for further evaluation.

Chief complaint:	fall.
Patient's medical history:	Hemophilia A (patient says he has a "bleeding problem." Specific disease name can only be obtained from the parent).
Medications:	Factor VIII replacement (child unaware of this, only obtained if learner asks parent).
Allergies:	None.
Family history:	Non-contributory.
Social history:	Lives with his parents, attends elementary school.

Initial scenario conditions

Male pediatric patient in street clothes, seated in bed.

> Case may start with EMS receiving this case on scene as presented, and performing their objectives to initiate treatment and transport, including recognizing the need for transport despite low mechanism of injury and possible immobilization of the patient. Alternatively, case background may be presented prior to case.

Vital signs:	Temp 37.1, HR 103, RR 24, BP 101/65, SpO$_2$ 99 on room air (normal for age).
Weight:	19 kg.
Head:	Head with 3 cm diameter hematoma on the left parieto-occipital scalp.
Eyes:	Pupils 4 mm and reactive to light bilaterally.
Neck:	Non-tender to palpation.
Heart:	Regular rhythm, no murmurs.
Chest:	No tenderness, no deformity.
Lungs:	Clear bilaterally.
Abdomen:	Soft, non-tender, no distension, no bruising.
Extremities:	Non-tender, no deformities, full range of motion.
Skin:	Scalp hematoma as above, otherwise normal.
Neurologic:	Glasgow Coma Scale score of 15, interacts appropriately, normal strength/sensation.

> *Physical exam findings not available on your mannequin can be reported verbally if asked for by learners; e.g., if the mannequin does not have reactive pupils you can verbally report the pupillary exam when it is requested.*

See flow diagram (Figure 5.3) for further scenario changes described.

Case Narrative, Continued

Learners of all levels should initially perform a primary trauma survey, obtain a history of a "bleeding problem" and contact the parent by phone for more information and consent to treat. For all learners, the history of hemophilia A can be provided by the patient's parent. For novice learners, the parent can also provide education on factor administration.

Learners should appropriately administer factor VIII before obtaining imaging. A hematology consultant or pharmacist can be available for phone consultation for learners of all levels regarding factor replacement dosing.

If the learners do not call the patient's parent for specific details of the past medical history, or if the factor administration is delayed for head CT or lab results, the patient will begin to decompensate but can be temporarily stabilized with appropriate factor administration.

For all learners, an intracerebral hemorrhage (ICH) will be present on head CT. The case can end here for novice learners after consultation with hematology, pediatric intensive care and neurosurgery.

For advanced learners, despite factor replacement, the patient will begin to decompensate and require intubation for airway protection.

All learners should have a critical conversation with the patient's parent (via phone) regarding the patient's condition at this point. The case ends when the patient is stabilized and transferred to the pediatric intensive care unit.

Instructor Notes

Pathophysiology

- Hemophilias are X-linked recessive disorders of clotting factors:
  - Hemophilia A
    - Factor VIII deficiency
    - Approximately 80% of cases
  - Hemophilia B
    - Christmas disease
    - Factor IX deficiency
- Both affect the intrinsic pathway of coagulation

Clinical Features

- Dependent on disease severity:
  - Factor activity <1%
    - Severe post-traumatic or post-surgical bleeding.
    - Spontaneous and traumatic hemarthroses.
    - Deep tissue bleeding.
    - Recurrent mucocutaneus bleeding.
  - Factor activity 1–5%:
    - Post-traumatic or post-surgical bleeding.
  - Factor activity 6–40%:
    - Mild disease.
    - Female carriers of the hemophilia gene may have excessive bleeding, especially with menstruation.

Diagnosis

- Primarily historical in ED setting:
  - Factor activity less than 40% normal.
- Lab findings:

- Prolonged activated partial thromboplastin time (PTT).
- Normal prothrombin time/international normalized ratio (INR), platelet counts and bleeding time.

Management

- Assess and manage airway, breathing, circulation.
- Factor replacement:
  - Do not delay for imaging or lab results.
  - Use the patient's own factor if it is available.
  - Dependent on factor activity and bleed severity.
- Factor activity:
  - Patients typically know their baseline factor activity.
  - If unknown, assume 0% activity.
  - Factor VIII: 1 iu/kg raises factor level by 2%.
  - Factor IX: 1 iu/kg raises factor level by 1%.
- Bleed severity:
  - Major bleed: raise factor level to 100%; empiric dosing: factor VIII 40–50 iu/kg, factor IX 80–100 iu/kg:
    - Hemarthrosis
    - Deep muscle hematoma
    - Compartment syndrome
    - ICH
    - Spinal cord hemorrhage
    - Gastrointestinal
    - Airway/neck/throat
    - Ophthalmic
  - Minor bleed: raise factor level to 40–50%; empiric dosing: factor VIII 20–25 iu/kg, factor IX 40–50 iu/kg:
  - Superficial muscle hematoma
  - Oral bleeding
  - Epistaxis
  - Renal hematoma
  - Skin and soft-tissue bleeding
  - If specific factor replacement is unavailable:
    - Desmopression: causes release of von Willebrand factor and allows extra factor VIII to be carried in plasma.

- Cryoprecipitate: small amount of factor VIII.
- Fresh frozen plasma (FFP): small amounts of factors VIII and IX. Watch for volume overload.
- Considerations for patient disposition:
  - Admission:
    - Patients receiving multiple factor replacement doses.
    - Any bleeding in the head, neck, pharynx, retropharynx, or retroperitoneum.
    - Bleeding in areas with potential for compartment syndrome.
    - Head injuries without ICH, with any of the following:
      - Severe mechanism of injury
      - Neurologic symptoms
        - Headache with increased severity
        - Irritability
        - Vomiting
        - Seizures
        - Vision problems
        - Focal neurologic deficits
        - Stiff neck
        - Altered level of consciousness
      - Past ICH (increased risk of recurrence)
  - Discharge:
    - Follow-up should be coordinated with the patient's hematologist or primary care provider.

Debriefing Plan

Plan for approximately 30 minutes for discussion.

Potential Questions for Discussion

- What is the approach to a patient with hemophilia presenting with bleeding?
- What drugs or medications can be given if specific factor replacement is not available?
- What are examples of major bleeding in patients with hemophilia?
- What lab work is needed to initiate treatment of bleeding in the hemophilic patient?
- If this patient had not had ICH what would be the appropriate disposition and follow up?

SELECTED READINGS FOR INTRACRANIAL HEMORRHAGE IN A PATIENT WITH HEMOPHILIA

Butler, R., Raffini, L., Witmer, C. et al. (2019). *Emergency Department Clinical Pathway for Evaluation/Treatment of Children with Hemophilia and Closed Head Injury (CHI)*. Philadelphia, PA: Children's Hospital of Philadelphia https://www.chop.edu/clinical-pathway/hemophilia-with-head-trauma-clinical-pathway (accessed 1 September 2021).

García Sánchez, P., Molina Gutiérrez, M., Martín Sánchez, J. et al. (2018). Head trauma in the haemophilic child and management in a paediatric emergency department: descriptive study. *Haemophilia*. 24 (4): e187–e193.

Lee, L.K., Dayan, P.S., Gerardi, M.J. et al. (2011). Intracranial hemorrhage after blunt head trauma in children with bleeding disorders. *J. Pediatr.* 158 (6): 1003–1008.e1-2.

National Hemophilia Foundation (2019). *Guidelines for Emergency Department Management of Individuals with Hemophilia and Other Bleeding Disorders*. New York, NY: National Hemophilia Foundation.

Woods, G.M., Dunn, M.W., and Dunn, A.L. (2018). Emergencies in hemophilia. *Clin. Pediatr. Emerg. Med.* 19 (2): 110–121.

THROMBOTIC THROMBOCYTOPENIC PURPURA

Educational Goals

Learning Objectives

1. Recall the causes of microangiopathic hemolytic anemia (*MAHA*) and thrombocytopenia (MK).
2. Identify thrombotic thrombocytopenic purpura (*TTP*) (MK, PC, ICS).
3. Differentiate TTP from sepsis with disseminated intravascular coagulation (*DIC*) (MK, PC).
4. Demonstrate appropriate management of TTP with plasma exchange/plasmapheresis (MK, PC).
5. Identify alternative treatments if plasma exchange/plasmapheresis is not immediately available (MK, PC).
6. Initiate appropriate consultations (hematology, nephrology, critical care) (SBP, ICS).
7. Demonstrate good communication skills in discussions of care with a family member of a critically ill patient (ICS).
8. Perform percutaneous sheath introducer (*PSI*) or multilumen access catheter (*MAC*) placement for initiation of plasma exchange(MK, PC).

Critical Actions Checklist

- ☐ List TTP and sepsis with DIC in the differential diagnosis (MK, PC).
- ☐ Obtain laboratory studies to help differentiate between TTP and other causes of MAHA (MK, PC).
- ☐ Consult with hematology, nephrology and critical care (PC, ICS).
- ☐ Appropriately communicate with patient's boyfriend and/or family member (ICS, P).
- ☐ Perform PSI or MAC placement (PC).
- ☐ Initiate plasma exchange/plasmapheresis (MK, PC).

Simulation Set-up

Environment: ED resuscitation room. This may also start on scene and transition to a hospital setting.

Mannequin: Female adult simulator mannequin in hospital gown. Petechiae on arms and legs moulaged with make-up. Icteric sclera can be moulaged with yellow erasable marker or make-up. If you are unable to place central lines with your mannequin, you will also need a separate central line task trainer.

Props: To be displayed on plasma screen/ computer screen or printed out on handouts in scenario room when asked for/return from lab:

- Images (see online component for TTP, Scenario 5.2 at https://www.wiley. com/go/thoureen/simulation/workbook2e).
  - ECG showing sinus tachycardia (Figure 5.4).
  - Chest X-Ray which is normal (Figure 5.5).
  - CT Head which is normal (Figure 5.6).
- Laboratory tests (see online component as above):
  - Complete blood count (Table 5.4).
  - Complete metabolic panel (Table 5.5).
  - Lactate (Table 5.6).
  - Lactate dehydrogenase (*LDH*) (Table 5.7).
  - Coagulation panel (Table 5.8).
  - Manual differential/peripheral smear (Table 5.9).

Any imaging or lab work not provided can be verbally reported as normal or pending.

Available supplies:

- Basic airway and code cart.
- Medications:
  - Blood products (red blood cells, fresh frozen plasma, platelets).
  - Liter bags of 0.9% saline and LR.
    - PSI or MAC kit.
    - Central line trainer.

Distractor: None.

Actors

- Patient voice is an adult female. Patient appears tired, but oriented and able to provide medical history.
- EMS may be an actor or another learner.
- ED nurse can administer medications/fluids. The nurse does have medical knowledge and may cue learners if needed.
- Boyfriend is available by phone and can provide a history of confusion and poor intake of food and drink, increasing over two to three days.
- Hematology, nephrology, and critical care consult available for telephone consultation.

See flow diagram (Figure 5.7) for further scenario changes described.

CASE NARRATIVE

Scenario Background

A 33 year-old woman arrives via EMS for "flu-like" symptoms. Her co-workers called EMS because she had not been acting herself all day, saying that she was "tired." The patient thinks she is fine and does not need medical care, but will get checked out to make everyone feel better.

Chief complaint:	Flu-like symptoms.
Patient's medical history:	Lupus.
Medications:	None; patient has not seen a doctor in three years.
Allergies:	None.
Family history:	Diabetes.
Social history:	Lives with her boyfriend, who is available by telephone.

Initial Scenario Conditions

Young adult female in a gown, lying in bed, who appears tired and is mildly confused.

> Case may start with EMS receiving this case on scene as presented and performing their objectives to initiate treatment and transport, including recognizing the need for transport, based on lethargy and mild confusion, despite the patient stating that she is "OK." Alternatively, case background may be presented by EMS on arrival in ED.

Vital signs:	Temp 101.3°F (38.5°C), HR 141, RR 27, BP 110/65, SpO$_2$ 95 on room air.
Head:	Atraumatic.
EENT:	Scleral icterus, pupils symmetric and reactive, otherwise normal.
Neck:	No meningismus.
Heart:	Tachycardic, regular rhythm, + systolic murmur.
Lungs:	Tachypnea, clear to auscultation bilaterally.
Abdomen:	Soft, non-tender, no organomegaly.
Extremities:	No deformities, no edema.
Skin:	Scattered petechiae on arms and legs.
Neurologic:	Drowsy, but oriented × 3. Normal strength and sensation.

> *Physical exam findings not available on your mannequin, such as scleral icterus, can be reported verbally if asked for by learners.*

See flow diagram (Figure 5.7) for further scenario changes described.

Case Narrative, Continued

Learners of all levels should initially perform a primary survey and fingerstick blood glucose. They should recognize vital sign abnormalities as concerning for sepsis. They should also identify petechiae on exam. Lab and imaging studies should be ordered for further evaluation of findings.

If learners want to perform a diagnostic lumbar puncture, the nurse should ask about the results of lab studies, and should particularly comment on the platelet count.

All learners should consult critical care and/hematology. Consultants can cue learners, if needed, by asking questions regarding etiology of thrombocytopenia and suggesting lab work to help with diagnosis and management. If they do not consult hematology, then the patient's state worsens. If learners do not consult critical care or hematology, the hospitalist can refuse the admission and prompt consideration for notifying these consultants.

For advanced learners who diagnose TTP and initiate consultation for plasma exchange/plasmapheresis, there should be a delay in availability of the consultant. If this occurs, learners need to transfuse FFP as a temporizing measure and recall that transfusing platelets should be avoided. They should place a PSI or MAC so that plasma exchange/plasmapheresis can be started as soon as available. If learners do not place the line or give FFP, the patient's state worsens and the case ends prompting discussion.

All learners should have a critical conversation with the patient's significant other (via phone).

The case ends when the patient is transferred to intensive care or to another hospital for plasma exchange/plasmapheresis.

Instructor Notes

Pathophysiology

- Microvascular thrombosis involving capillaries and arterioles of multiple organs leading to:
  - Thrombocytopenia.
  - MAHA.
  - Thrombi are mainly comprised of platelets and von Willebrand's factor.
  - May be inherited, acquired through an autoimmune mechanism, or idiopathic.

Clinical Features

- Symptoms of TTP are related to:
  - Thrombocytopenia due to platelet dysfunction.
  - MAHA.

- Classic pentad (rarely observed in clinical practice):
  - Neurologic dysfunction (headache, seizures, coma).
  - MAHA.
  - Thrombocytopenia with purpura.
  - Fever (usually late symptom).
  - Acute renal failure.
- May also include:
  - Cardiac failure.
  - Splenomegaly.
  - Jaundice.

Diagnosis

- Should be considered in any patient with MAHA and thrombocytopenia.
- Laboratory findings:
  - Schistocytes on peripheral smear.
  - Low hemoglobin.
  - Low platelets; may not be severe (average 25 000/µl).
  - Elevated LDH.
  - Elevated indirect bilirubin.
  - Acute kidney injury and/or electrolyte abnormalities.
  - Urinalysis showing proteinuria, hematuria, and/or casts.
- Differentiating from other causes of MAHA or thrombocytopenia:
  - DIC:
    - Elevated INR, PTT and D-dimer.
    - Significant bleeding.
- Hemolytic uremic syndrome (*HUS*):
  - More renal involvement and fewer neurologic symptoms than TTP.
  - Often history of diarrhea.
  - Common in pediatrics.
- Immune thrombocytopenic purpura (*ITP*):
  - Thrombocytopenia without schistocytes.
  - Typically not acutely ill.
- Hemolysis, elevated liver enzymes, low platelet count (HELLP: hemolysis, elevated liver enzymes and low platelets syndrome):
  - Pregnant/postpartum state.
  - More significant transaminitis.

Management

- Plasma exchange/plasmapheresis:
  - Definitive treatment
  - Filters circulating antibodies against ADAMTS13 and ADAMTS13 multimers.
- FFP:
  - Temporizing measure if plasmapheresis is not immediately available.
- Steroids:
  - Administer with plasmapheresis.
- Intravenous immune globulin:
  - For failed plasmapheresis.
- Splenectomy:
  - Refractory cases.
- Transfusing platelets should be avoided:
  - Increased morbidity due to arterial thrombosis.

Debriefing Plan

Plan for approximately 30 minutes for discussion.

Potential Questions for Discussion

- What is the classic pentad of TTP and how commonly does it present?
- What two lab findings should make you consider TTP in your differential diagnosis?
- How do you differentiate between TTP and other causes of MAHA or thrombocytopenia (DIC, HUS, HELLP, ITP)?
- What is the definitive treatment for TTP?
- Which blood products may be used in TTP and which should be avoided?

SELECTED READINGS FOR THROMBOTIC THROMBOCYTOPENIC PURPURA

Coppo, P. and Veyradier, A. (2012). Current management and therapeutical perspectives in thrombotic thrombocytopenic purpura. *Presse. Med.* 41: 163–176.

Kessler, C.S., Khan, B.A., and Lai-Miller, K. (2012). Thrombotic thrombocytopenic purpura: a hematological emergency. *J. Emerg. Med.* 43: 538–544.

Scully, M., Hunt, B.J., Benjamin, S. et al. (2012). Guidelines on the diagnosis and management of thrombotic thrombocytopenic purpura and other thrombotic microangiopathies. *Br. J. Hematol.* 158: 323–335.

TUMOR LYSIS SYNDROME

Educational Goals

Learning Objectives

1. Recognize tumor lysis syndrome (*TLS*) (MK).
2. Identify metabolic abnormalities associated with TLS (MK, PC).
3. Manage hyperkalemia in the setting of TLS (MK, PC).
4. Demonstrate appropriate fluid resuscitation in a patient with TLS (MK, PC).
5. Plan disposition to an appropriate level of care (PC).
6. Demonstrate appropriate use of rasburicase in TLS (MK, PC).

Critical Actions Checklist

☐ Obtain ECG (PC).
☐ Recognize signs of hyperkalemia on ECG (MK, PC).
☐ Treat hyperkalemia (MK, PC).
☐ Recognize TLS (MK).
☐ Administer IV fluids (MK, PC).
☐ Consult oncology (ICS, P).
☐ Admit to intensive care unit (ICS, P).

Simulation Set-up

Environment: ED patient room.

> For prehospital providers, the case may also start on scene and transition to a hospital setting.

Mannequin: Male simulator mannequin, in hospital gown. Scattered petechiae can be moulaged on lower legs with make-up. Baldness can be moulaged using a skin-tone skull cap.

Props: To be displayed on plasma screen/computer screen or printed out on handouts in scenario room when asked for/return from lab:

- Images (see online component for TLS, Scenario 5.3 at URL to follow)
  - ECG showing peaked T waves (Figure 5.8).

- Chest x-ray which is normal (Figure 5.9).
- Laboratory tests (see online component as above):
  - Complete blood count (Table 5.10).
  - Complete metabolic panel (Table 5.11).
  - Lactate (Table 5.12).
  - Magnesium (Table 5.13).
  - Phosphate (Table 5.14).
  - Uric acid (Table 5.15).
  - LDH (Table 5.16).

Available supplies:

- Basic airway and code cart.
- Medications:
  - Liter bags of 0.9% saline and LR or PlasmaLyte.
  - Pre-labeled syringes:
    - Benzodiazepines.
    - RSI medications commonly used in your institution.
    - Calcium gluconate.
    - Regular insulin.
    - 50% dextrose.
    - Sodium bicarbonate.
  - Nebulizer mask.

Distractor: None.

Actors

- Patient voice is male. Patient should sound fatigued and generally weak.
- EMS may be an actor or another learner.
- ED nurse can administer medications/fluids. The nurse does have medical knowledge and my cue learners if needed.
- Oncologist and critical care physician available via telephone consultation.

Case Narrative

Scenario Background

A 25 year old man with B-cell lymphoma presents with complaining of dehydration. He complains of fatigue and weakness. Denies fever. He received intravenous chemotherapy four days prior.

Chief complaint:	Dehydration.
Patient's medical history:	None.
Medications:	None.
Allergies:	Penicillin.
Family history:	Hypertension, diabetes.
Social history:	No tobacco, alcohol or drug use.

Initial Scenario Conditions

Young man lying on stretcher, appears fatigued, but in no distress.

Vital signs:	Temp 99.3°F (37.4°C), HR 106, RR 22, BP 105/56, SpO$_2$ 99% on room air.
Head:	Head is atraumatic, bald.
Eyes:	Pupils 4 mm and reactive to light, conjunctiva pale.
Mouth:	Mucous membranes dry.
Neck:	No meningismus.
Heart:	Tachycardic and regular. No murmurs/rubs/gallops.
Lungs:	Normal.
Abdomen:	Normal.
Extremities:	No gross deformities, pulses 2+ and equal.
Skin:	Petechiae scattered on lower extremities.
Neurologic:	Alert and oriented. Moves all extremities with equal strength.

See flow diagram (Figure 5.10) for further scenario changes described.

Case Narrative, Continued

Learners of all levels (EMS, students and postgraduate learners) should perform a primary survey, history, and physical. They should be expected to initiate a broad workup based on the recent chemotherapy and generalized symptoms. Some will go down a path toward sepsis management, which would be very reasonable to begin with; however, they should recognize the constellation of metabolic abnormalities that indicate TLS.

An ECG will show signs of hyperkalemia. If hyperkalemia is not treated appropriately, the patient will decompensate into pulseless electrical activity arrest.

After review of all the initial studies, learners may request additional lab studies, including phosphorus, uric acid, and/or LDH, if not previously ordered. If they do not order additional studies, they may be prompted to do so.

If TLS is still not recognized, and learners attempt to admit the patient without further therapy or oncology consultation, the admitting physician can prompt consideration of the diagnosis of TLS. The patient should be admitted to intensive care after oncology consultation.

For advanced learners, aggressive IV fluid hydration should be initiated and administration of rasburicase should be considered or initiated. If both interventions are not made, the patient will decompensate and begin to have a seizure. Once stabilized, the patient should be admitted to the intensive care.

Instructor Notes

Pathophysiology

- Autolysis in hematologic malignancies or solid tumors with very high cell turnover may cause TLS:
  - Triggered by cytotoxic chemotherapy and other cancer treatments.
  - Releases intracellular contents into the bloodstream:
    - Potassium poses the most immediate threat.
    - Phosphate precipitates with calcium (leading to hypocalcemia).
    - The calcium–phosphate crystals further exacerbate renal injury.
  - Cellular DNA is metabolized to uric acid:
    - Accumulates in the renal tubules exacerbating renal injury
- TLS most common after cytotoxic chemotherapy:
  - Can also occur as the initial presentation of cancer.

Clinical Features

- Patients may be asymptomatic, or present with vague symptoms:
  - Generalized weakness.
  - Fatigue.
  - Nausea and vomiting.
- The metabolic derangements can manifest as:
  - Renal failure.
  - Cardiac dysrhythmias.
  - Seizures.
  - Altered mental status.

Diagnosis

- Laboratory abnormalities:
  - Hyperkalemia.
  - Hypocalcemia.
  - Elevated creatinine.
  - Hyperphosphatemia.
  - Hyperuricemia.
  - Elevated LDH.
- The Cairo and Bishop definition of TLS provides criteria for laboratory and clinical TLS (Table 5.17).

Management

- Fluid administration:
  - Fluid boluses and maintenance fluids with a goal urine output of 2 ml/kg/hour.
    - Use caution with significant renal failure or heart failure.
- Evaluation and treatment of hyperkalemia:
  - Obtain ECG to evaluate for cardiotoxicity.
  - Cardiac membrane stabilization:
    - Calcium.
    - NOTE: Calcium should be reserved for patients with signs of cardiotoxicity as excess calcium can worsen renal failure by fueling precipitation of phosphate.
  - Shift potassium intracellularly:
    - Insulin/dextrose.
    - Albuterol.
    - Sodium bicarbonate.
  - Elimination of potassium:
    - Loop diuretics or dialysis.
- Management of hyperuricemia:
  - Allopurinol:
    - Inhibits metabolism of DNA protein to uric acid.
    - Does NOT affect uric acid that has already been made.
    - Takes 48–72 hours to affect uric acid levels.
  - Rasburicase:
    - Recombinant urate oxidase (uricase).
    - Converts uric acid to allantoin.
    - Urine soluble and able to be excreted through the urinary system.
    - Immediate decrease in uric acid levels.
    - Often requires approval from oncology or pharmacy representatives.
      - Extremely high financial cost.
      - Potential for hypersensitivity reactions with repeated doses.
  - Urine alkalinization is no longer recommended.
- Management of hyperphosphatemia:
  - Moderate hyperphosphatemia (5.5–6 mg/dl):
    - Fluid hydration.
    - Oral phosphate binders.
    - Reduction of dietary phosphate intake.
  - Severe hyperphosphatemia ($\geq$ 6 mg/dl)

- May require dialysis for definitive treatment.
- Management of hypocalcemia:
  - Treatment of hyperphosphatemia will improve hypocalcemia.
  - Intravenous calcium repletion only for cases with severe symptoms such as cardiac conduction abnormalities, muscle spasm or tetany, paresthesias, altered mental status, or seizures.
- Seizure:
  - Addressed and managed as any other seizure.
  - Consider calcium infusion, if refractory to benzodiazepines or antiepileptics.
  - May be secondary to severe hypocalcemia.
  - Admit to intensive care:
    - Continuous cardiac and hemodynamic monitoring.
    - Frequent lab analysis and clinical reevaluation.

Debriefing Plan

Plan for approximately 20 minutes for discussion.

Potential Questions for Discussion

- What patient population is at highest risk of developing TLS?
- What lab abnormality in TLS is most acutely life threatening?
- What special considerations should be given to treating hyperkalemia in TLS?
- What ECG findings suggest hyperkalemia?
- What is rasburicase and what are the indications for its use?

SELECTED READINGS FOR TUMOR LYSIS SYNDROME

Cairo, M.S. and Bishop, M. (2004). Tumour lysis syndrome: new therapeutic strategies and classification. *Br. J. Haematol.* 127 (1): 3–11.

Coiffier, B., Altman, A., Pui, C.-H. et al. (2008). Guidelines for the Management of Pediatric and Adult Tumor Lysis Syndrome: an evidence-based review. *J. Clin. Oncol.* 26 (16): 2767–2778.

Dubbs, S.B. (2018). Rapid fire: tumor lysis syndrome. *Emerg. Med. Clin. North Am.* 36 (3): 517–525.

Klemencic, S. and Perkins, J. (2019). Diagnosis and management of oncologic emergencies. *West J. Emerg. Med.* 20 (2): 316–322.

APPENDIX

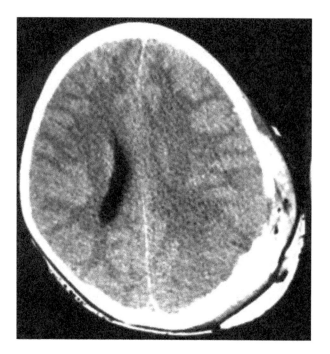

FIGURE 5.1   Pediatric computed tomography head slice showing intracerebral hemorrhage and midline shift.

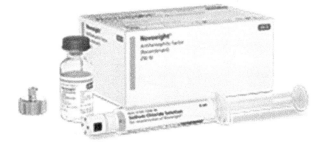

FIGURE 5.2   Factor replacement.

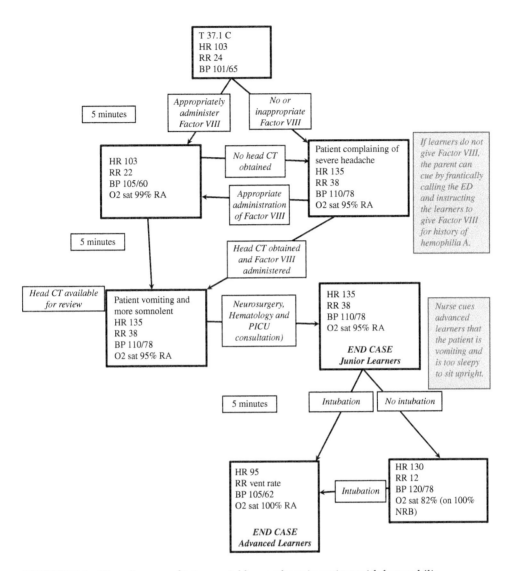

FIGURE 5.3 Flow diagram of intracranial hemorrhage in patient with hemophilia.

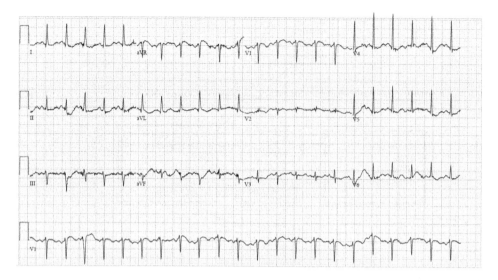

FIGURE 5.4   Electrocardiogram showing sinus tachycardia.

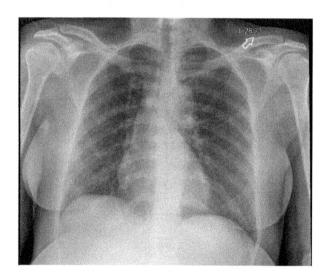

FIGURE 5.5   Chest x-ray (normal).

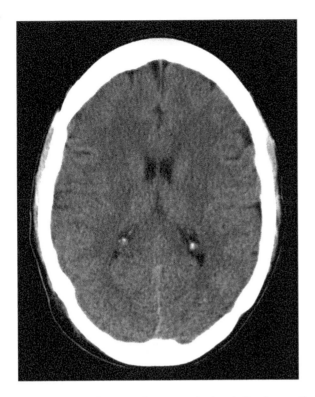

FIGURE 5.6   Computed tomography head slice (normal).

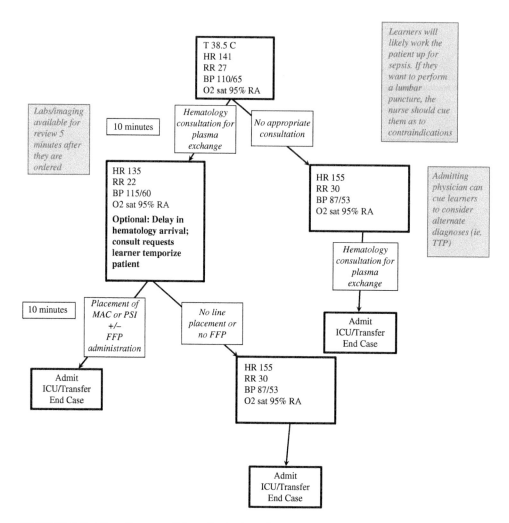

FIGURE 5.7   Flow diagram of thrombotic thrombocytopenic purpura.

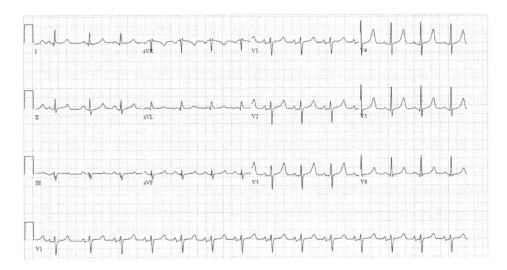

FIGURE 5.8   Electrocardiogram showing peaked T waves.

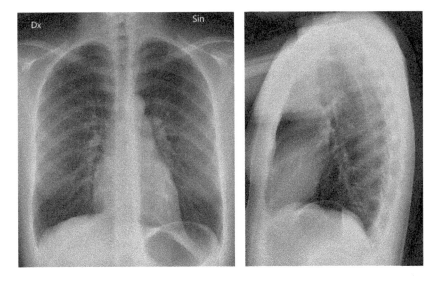

FIGURE 5.9   Chest x-ray (normal).

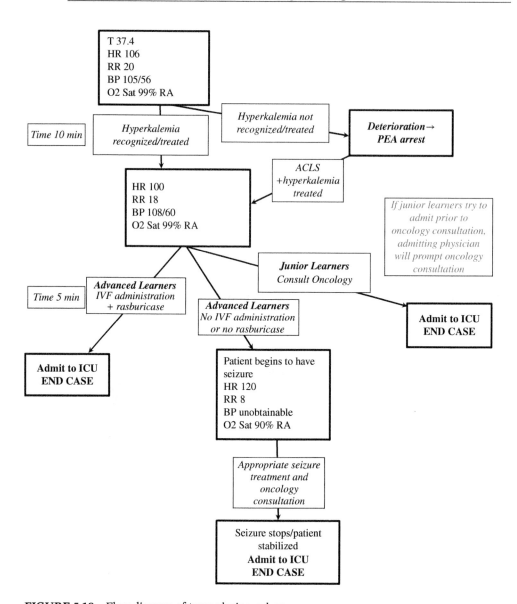

FIGURE 5.10   Flow diagram of tumor lysis syndrome.

TABLE 5.1   Complete blood count.

Test	Result	Reference range
White blood cell count (cells/mm³)	9300	4000–15 500
Hemoglobin (g/dl)	11.2	11.5–14.5
Hematocrit (%)	29.3	33–43
Platelet count(× 10³/µl)	152	150–450

TABLE 5.2   Complete metabolic panel.

Test	Value	Reference range
Sodium (mEql/l)	141	130–147
Potassium (mEql/l)	4.5	3.5–5.1
Chloride (mEql/l)	100	95–108
Carbon dioxide (mEql/l)	21	20–30
Glucose (mg/dl)	99	60–100
Blood urea nitrogen (mg/dl)	19	2–20
Creatinine (mg/dl)	0.5	0.3–0.7
Albumin (g/dl)	3.9	3.5–5.5
Alanine aminotransferase (iu/l)	24	15–50
Aspartate aminotransferase (iu/l)	13	5–55
Total bilirubin (mg/dl)	1.3	< 1.5
Alkaline phosphatase (iu/l)	184	100–420
Lactate dehydrogenase (iu/l)	225	100–500

TABLE 5.3   Coagulation panel.

Test	Value	Reference range
Prothrombin time (seconds)	12.1	11–13
International normalized ratio	1.1	< 2.0
Activated partial prothromboplastin time (seconds)	43.8	25–35

TABLE 5.4 Complete blood count.

Test	Value	Reference range
White blood cells (k/μl)	13.5	4000–15 500
Hemoglobin (g/dl)	6.9	11.5–14.5
Hematocrit (%)	23.4	33–43
Platelets (k/μl)	11	150–450

TABLE 5.5 Complete metabolic panel.

Test	Value	Reference range
Sodium (mEql/l)	141	130–147
Potassium (mEql/l)	4.5	3.5–5.1
Chloride (mEql/l)	100	95–108
Carbon dioxide (mEql/l)	21	20–30
Glucose (mg/dl)	99	60–100
Blood urea nitrogen (mg/dl)	19	6–21
Creatinine (mg/dl)	2.1	0.7–1.3
Albumin (g/dl)	3.9	3.5–5.5
Aspartate aminotransferase (iu/l)	24	0–35
Alanine aminotransferase (iu/l)	13	0–35
Total bilirubin (mg/dl)	2.5	0.3–1.2
Alkaline phosphatase (iu/l)	84	36–92

TABLE 5.6 Lactate.

Test	Value	Reference range
Lactate (mmol/l)	3.2	0.5–2.2

TABLE 5.7 Lactate dehydrogenase.

Test	Value	Reference range
Lactate dehydrogenase (iu/l)	2336	60–160

TABLE 5.8 Coagulation panel.

Test	Value	Reference range
Prothrombin time (seconds)	15.7	11–13
International normalized ratio	1.2	< 2.0
Activated partial prothromboplastin time (seconds)	24.8	25–35

TABLE 5.9 Manual differential/peripheral smear.

Test	Value	Reference range
Red blood cell morphology	Abnormal	Normal
Schistocytes	2+	None
Macrocytes	Slight	None
Microcytes	1+	None

TABLE 5.10 Complete blood count.

Test	Value	Reference range
White blood cells (cells/mm³)	18 400	4000–15 500
Hemoglobin (g/dl)	6.6	12–16
Hematocrit (%)	22.7	36–47
Platelets (× 10^3/µl)	56	150–350

TABLE 5.11 Complete metabolic panel.

Test	Value	Reference range
Sodium (mEql/l)	133	130–147
Potassium (mEql/l)	7.2	3.5–5.1
Chloride (mEql/l)	101	95–108
Carbon dioxide (mEql/l)	21	20–30
Glucose (mg/dl)	98	60–100
Blood urea nitrogen (mg/dl)	23	6–21
Creatinine (mg/dl)	2.8	0.7–1.3
Albumin (g/dl)	3.9	3.5–5.5
Aspartate aminotransferase (iu/l)	20	0–35
Alanine aminotransferase (iu/l)	18	0–35
Total bilirubin (mg/dl)	0.6	0.3–1.2
Alkaline phosphatase (iu/l)	61	36–92
Calcium (mg/dl)	5.2	8.6–10.3

TABLE 5.12   Lactate.

Test	Value	Reference range
Lactate (mmol/l)	2.2	0.5–2.2

TABLE 5.13   Magnesium.

Test	Value	Reference range
Magnesium (mg/dl)	0.9	1.5–2.4

TABLE 5.14   Phosphate.

Test	Value	Reference range
Phosphate (mg/dl)	4.9	3.0–4.5

TABLE 5.15   Uric acid.

Lab	Value	Reference range
Uric acid (mg/dl)	10.4	2.5–8

TABLE 5.16   Lactate dehydrogenase.

Test	Value	Reference range
Lactate dehydrogenase (iu/l)	851	60–160

TABLE 5.17   Cairo and bishop definition of tumor lysis syndrome.

Laboratory	Clinical
Abnormality in ≥ 2 of:	Laboratory + at least 1 of:
• Potassium ≥6 mEq/l or 25% above baseline	• Creatinine ≥1.5x upper limit of normal
• Uric acid ≥8 mg/dl or 25% above baseline	• Cardiac dysrhythmia
• Phosphate ≥4.5 mg/dl or 25% above baseline	• Seizure
• Calcium ≤7.0 mg/dl or 25% below baseline	

Source: Adapted from Cairo, M.S., Bishop, M. Tumor lysis syndrome: new therapeutic strategies and classification. Br. J. Haematol. 2004; 127 (1): 3–11.

CHAPTER 6

Immune System Emergencies

Ashley C. Crimmins

Department of Emergency Medicine, University of Maryland School of Medicine, Baltimore, MD, USA

ANGIOEDEMA

Educational Goals

Learning Objectives

1. Identify and properly manage impending airway compromise in a patient with angioedema (MK, PC, SBP).
2. Obtain a focused history from a patient with angioedema (MK, PC, ICS, P).
3. Demonstrate appropriate use of medications for management of a patient with angiotensin-converting enzyme (*ACE*) inhibitor angioedema (MK, PC, SBP).

Critical Actions Checklist

☐ Assess airway, breathing, circulation (PC, MK).
☐ Obtain intravenous (IV) access, place patient on continuous cardiac monitoring and pulse oximetry (PC).
☐ Obtain history of possible inciting exposures (PC, MK, ICS).
☐ Perform awake or delayed sequence intubation for impending airway compromise (MK, PC).
☐ Admit patient to an intensive care unit (*ICU*) (MK, PC, SBP, ICS).

Emergency Medicine Simulation Workbook: A Tool for Bringing the Curriculum to Life,
Second Edition. Edited by Traci L. Thoureen and Sara B. Scott.
© 2022 John Wiley & Sons Ltd. Published 2022 by John Wiley & Sons Ltd.
Companion website: www.wiley.com/go/thoureen/simulation/workbook2e

☐ Counsel patient (or family) on the importance of avoiding ACE inhibitors and angiotensin receptor antagonists in the future (MK, PC, ICS).

Simulation Set-Up

Environment: Emergency department (ED) resuscitation room.

Mannequin: Adult female simulator mannequin in street clothes, sitting straight up on the stretcher. She has tongue edema and has secretions dribbling down her chin. If a high-fidelity mannequin is available, the mannequin can be programmed to have tongue edema and to simulate a difficult airway necessitating a fiberoptic or video-assisted approach or even cricothyroidotomy. Glycerin may be used to simulate secretions from the mouth.

Props:

- Images (see online component for angioedema, Scenario 6.1 at https://www.wiley.com/go/thoureen/simulation/workbook2e):
  - Post-intubation chest x-ray (Figure 6.1).
  - Patient photograph (Figure 6.2).
- Laboratory tests (see online component for angioedema, Scenario 6.1 at https://www.wiley.com/go/thoureen/simulation/workbook2e):
  - Complete blood count (Table 6.1).
  - Basic metabolic panel (Table 6.2).

> Any imaging or lab work not provided can be verbally reported as normal if the learners order the study.

Available supplies:

- Adult code cart and basic airway supplies.
- Oral mucosal atomizer.
- Medications:
  - Liter bags of 0.9% saline and/or lactated Ringer's solution (*LR*).
  - Pre-labeled syringes:
    - 4% lidocaine.
    - Epinephrine (1 : 1000 and 1 : 10 000 concentration).
    - Diphenhydramine.
    - Parenteral steroid of choice at your institution.
    - Histamine type 2 (*H2*) receptor antagonist of choice at your institution.

- Icatibant (depending on institutional availability).
- Rapid sequence intubation (*RSI*) medications (paralytic and induction medication of choice at your institution).
- Sedative of choice at your institution.
- Fiberoptic scope, video-assisted laryngoscope, transtracheal jet ventilation set-up, cricothyrotomy tray (optional).

Actors

- Patient voice is female. Patient is alert and oriented but has a muffled "hot potato" voice.
- ED nurse can administer medications/fluids. The nurse does have some medical knowledge base and my cue learners if needed.
- Family member has no medical knowledge but is appropriately concerned/ inquisitive (optional).
- Otolaryngology is available by telephone consultation.

Case Narrative

Scenario Background

A 55-year-old woman with a history of hypertension presents with several hours of tongue edema. She woke up with it several hours earlier. The patient tried to wait and see if it would improve, but it seems to be getting worse. She took some diphenhydramine prior to coming to the emergency department.

Chief complaint:	Throat swelling.
Patient's medical history:	Hypertension, diabetes mellitus.
Medications:	Lisinopril, metformin.
Allergies:	Penicillin.
Family history:	Non-contributory.
Social history:	Half pack of cigarettes daily for the past 30 years, drinks two beers weekly, no illicit drug use.

Initial Scenario Conditions

Middle-aged woman sitting straight up in bed and drooling. She asks for something to spit in.

Vital signs:	Temp 37 °C (98.6 °F), HR 105, RR 24, BP 143/81, O2 sat 99% RA
General:	Awake, alert, sitting up in bed, appears anxious
HEENT:	Normocephalic, atraumatic. Significant lip swelling. Phonation is muffled with a "hot potato" voice. If nasopharyngeal scope is used, the patient has swelling of the base of the tongue, the epiglottis and the aryepiglottic folds.

Neck: Supple, no lymphadenopathy, no stridor.
Lungs: Clear to auscultation bilaterally, no wheezes, rales or rhonchi.
Heart: Regular rate and rhythm, no murmurs.
Abdomen: Soft, non-tender, non-distended, active bowel sounds.
Extremities: Warm, dry, 2+ pulses, no peripheral edema.

Physical exam findings not available on your mannequin can be reported verbally if asked for by learners; e.g., if your mannequin does not simulate tongue/airway angioedema you can verbally report the tongue and airway when they are requested.

See flow diagram (Figure 6.3) for further scenario changes described.

Case narrative, continued

Learners should perform an initial assessment targeting airway and breathing and obtain appropriate IV access. They should consider administering epinephrine, antihistamines, and corticosteroids. The patient's angioedema will not respond to any of these measures and will worsen to the point of needing intubation. If learners request icatibant, the pharmacy may refuse to release it due to lack of indication for use in ACE inhibitor-related angioedema. Alternatively, icatibant may be given without any immediate change in the patient's condition. If otolaryngology is contacted prior to securing the patient's airway, they are in the operating room and unable to come to the patient's bedside.

Identification of impending airway compromise should be managed with intubation. For more novice learners, the airway can be secured with RSI and a small endotracheal tube (6.5 or 6.0 mm).

For more advanced learners, awake intubation or delayed-sequence intubation should be performed, which will result in patient stabilization. Attempts at RSI result in a "can't intubate-can't ventilate" scenario. Cricothyroidotomy or transtracheal jet ventilation within two minutes is required or the patient will become bradycardic, and will ultimately have an asystolic cardiac arrest. With cardiopulmonary resuscitation (*CPR*) and a surgical airway, the patient has return of spontaneous circulation and the patient's condition improves but the patient is hypotensive and tachycardic and will require further resuscitation.

Once the patient's airway is secured, the case may end with consultation/admission to the ICU.

Instructor Notes

Pathophysiology

- ACE inhibitors cause bradykinin accumulation by inhibiting conversion of bradykinin to inactive peptides [1].

- Hereditary angioedema is also bradykinin mediated:
  - Hereditary angioedema and ACE inhibitor-associated angioedema share a common pathway in the accumulation of bradykinin.

Clinical Features

- Angioedema most often involves the head, neck, face, lips, tongue, and larynx:
  - Typically asymmetric.
  - Occurs in 0.7% of patients treated with ACE inhibitors [1].
- Life-threatening edema of the upper airway occurs in 25–39% of cases of ACE inhibitor angioedema [2].

Diagnosis

- Primary a clinical diagnosis.

Management

- Primarily focused on airway management:
  - Awake intubation [3]:
    - Airway preparation (desiccation, topical anesthesia).
    - Consider midazolam (1–2 mg IV) for anxiolysis or ketamine (0.3–0.5 mg/kg IV) for sedation with preserved airway reflexes.
    - Can use a rigid endoscope or a flexible endoscope to evaluate the glottis and can proceed with intubation if needed.
  - Delayed sequence intubation [4]:
    - Can be considered if patient is too anxious or agitated to tolerate preoxygenation for intubation.
    - Ketamine 1–1.5 mg/kg is given by a slow IV push to produce a dissociative state.
    - Patient is subsequently preoxygenated until SpO_2 reaches 100% and for an additional two or three minutes.
    - Once a patient is adequately oxygenated and sedated, this may allow for topical anesthesia of the airway and fiberoptic assessment prior to intubation.
  - Medications:
    - Fresh frozen plasma (*FFP*):
      - Multiple case reports [5, 6].
      - No randomized controlled trials.
      - One published case report of worsening angioedema temporally associated with administration of FFP [7].
      - Risk of transfusion reaction and potential infectious exposure.

- Tranexamic acid (*TXA*):
  - May act on the bradykinin pathway.
  - Single case series suggests it is a promising treatment [8].
  - Low cost, easily available.
  - Theoretical risk of thrombosis, but a recent meta-analysis showed no increased risk of venous or arterial thrombosis [9].
- C1 esterase inhibitors:
  - Food and Drug Administration (FDA) approved for hereditary angioedema.
  - There are case reports that suggest an improvement in ACE inhibitor angioedema when C1 esterase inhibitors are administered [10, 11].
  - Case series suggests very little benefit [12].
  - No high-quality studies on use of C1 esterase inhibitors for ACE inhibitor angioedema.
- Icatibant:
  - Bradykinin B2 receptor antagonist that is FDA-approved for use in hereditary angioedema.
  - Trials have shown that it is not better than placebo for ACE inhibitor-related angioedema [13, 14].
- No recommendation due to no effect on symptoms [9]:
  - Epinephrine.
  - Antihistamines.
  - Corticosteroids.
- Identify potential inciting medications.
- Counsel patient to discontinue ACE inhibitors and ARBs.

Debriefing Plan

Plan for approximately 30 minutes for discussion.

Potential Questions for Discussion

- What is the management for angioedema?
- What medications should be considered and/or administered? What is the evidence behind these medications?
- What preparation should be taken prior to intubating patients with angioedema?
- What advanced airway techniques are useful in this situation? Which are available in your particular practice environment?
- When can a patient with angioedema safely be discharged?

REFERENCES FOR ANGIOEDEMA

1. Baş, M., Greve, J., Stelter, K. et al. (2015). A randomized trial of icatibant in ACE-inhibitor-induced angioedema. *N. Engl. J. Med.* 372 (5): 418–425.
2. Sánchez-Borges, M. and González-Aveledo, L.A. (2010). Angiotensin-converting enzyme inhibitors and angioedema. *Allergy Asthma Immunol. Res.* 2 (3): 195–198.
3. Tonna, J.E. and DeBlieux, P.M. (2017). Awake laryngoscopy in the emergency department. *J. Emerg. Med.* 52 (3): 324–331.
4. Weingart, S.D. (2011). Preoxygenation, reoxygenation, and delayed sequence intubation in the emergency department. *J. Emerg. Med.* 40 (6): 661–667.
5. Hassen, G.W., Kalantari, H., Parraga, M. et al. (2013). Fresh frozen plasma for progressive and refractory angiotensin-converting enzyme inhibitor-induced angioedema. *J. Emerg. Med.* 44 (4): 764–772.
6. Saeb, A., Hagglund, K.H., and Cigolle, C.T. (2016). Using fresh frozen plasma for acute airway angioedema to prevent intubation in the emergency department: a retrospective cohort study. *Emerg. Med. Int.* 2016: 6091510.
7. Adebayo, O. and Wilkerson, R.G. (2017). Angiotensin-converting enzyme inhibitor-induced angioedema worsened with fresh frozen plasma. *Am. J. Emerg. Med.* 35 (1): 192.e1–e2.
8. Beauchêne, C., Martins-Héricher, J., Denis, D. et al. (2018). Tranexamic acid as first-line emergency treatment for episodes of bradykinin-mediated angioedema induced by ACE inhibitors. *Rev. Med. Interne.* 39 (10): 772–776.
9. Zuraw, B.L., Bernstein, J.A., Lang, D.M. et al. (2013). A focused parameter update: hereditary angioedema, acquired C1 inhibitor deficiency, and angiotensin-converting enzyme inhibitor-associated angioedema. *J. Allergy Clin. Immunol.* 131 (6): 1491–1493.
10. Erickson, D.L. and Coop, C.A. (2016). Angiotensin-converting enzyme inhibitor-associated angioedema treated with c1-esterase inhibitor: a case report and review of the literature. *Allergy Rhinol. (Providence).* 7 (3): 168–171.
11. Hermanrud, T., Duus, N., Bygum, A., and Rasmussen, E.R. (2016). The use of plasma-derived complement C1-esterase inhibitor concentrate (Berinert®) in the treatment of angiotensin converting enzyme-inhibitor related angioedema. *Case Rep. Emerg. Med.* 2016: 3930923.
12. Perza, M., Koczirka, S., and Nomura, J.T. (2020). C1 esterase inhibitor for ace-inhibitor angioedema: a case series and literature review. *J. Emerg. Med.* 58 (3): e121–e127.
13. Sinert, R., Levy, P., Bernstein, J.A. et al. (2017). Randomized trial of icatibant for angiotensin-converting enzyme inhibitor-induced upper airway angioedema. *J. Allergy Clin. Immunol. Pract.* 5 (5): 1402–1409.e3.
14. Straka, B.T., Ramirez, C.E., Byrd, J.B. et al. (2017). Effect of bradykinin receptor antagonism on ACE inhibitor-associated angioedema. *J. Allergy Clin. Immunol.* 140 (1): 242–248.e2.

SELECTED READINGS FOR ANGIOEDEMA

Braun, J., Kingsley, G., van der Heijde, D. et al. (2000). On the difficulties of establishing a consensus on the definition of and diagnostic investigations for reactive arthritis. Results and discussion of a questionnaire prepared for the 4th international workshop on reactive arthritis, Berlin, Germany, July 3–6, 1999. *J. Rheumatol.* 27 (9): 2185–2192.

Chornenki, N.L.J., Um, K.J., Mendoza, P.A. et al. (2019). Risk of venous and arterial thrombosis in non-surgical patients receiving systemic tranexamic acid: a systematic review and meta-analysis. *Thromb. Res.* 179: 81–86.

PEDIATRIC ANAPHYLAXIS

Educational Goals

Learning Objectives

1. Recognize anaphylaxis (MK, PC).
2. Demonstrate standard treatment of anaphylaxis with appropriate first- and second-line medications delivered via appropriate routes (MK, PC).
3. Formulate a safe transfer of care/discharge plan anticipating a possible biphasic reaction (MK, PC, ICS).
4. Demonstrate communication skills by counseling the patient's parent on anaphylaxis identification and management (MK, PC, ICS).

Critical Actions Checklist

☐ Assess airway, breathing, circulation (PC, MK).
☐ Administer a weight-based dose of intramuscular (IM) epinephrine (PC, MK).
☐ Place patient on continuous cardiac monitoring and pulse oximetry (PC).
☐ Obtain venous access rapidly or move to alternate access methods such as intraosseous (IO) access (PC).
☐ Obtain history of potential inciting factors (PC, MK, ICS).
☐ Administer weight-based doses of antihistamine, corticosteroids, and IV fluid (PC, MK).
☐ Educate family on potential causes, signs and symptoms of anaphylaxis (PC, MK, ICS).

Simulation Set-Up

Environment: ED resuscitation room.

Mannequin: Female infant simulation mannequin in onesie. The patient has generalized erythroderma and periorbital edema. A red/pink washable marker can be used to simulate erythroderma/hives on mannequin skin. Latex or silicone can be used to create periorbital edema.

Props: None.

Available supplies:

- Length-based resuscitation tape (e.g., Broselow tape).
- Pediatric code cart and basic airway supplies.
- Medications:

- Liter bags of 0.9% saline and LR.
- Pre-labeled syringes:
  - Pediatric epinephrine auto-injector (or vial of epinephrine to be drawn up and administered).
  - Steroid of choice.
  - Diphenhydramine.
  - Histamine-H2 receptor antagonist of choice for your institution.
- IO needle/placement device (optional).

Distractor: None.

Actors

- EMS may be an actor or another learner.
- Patient is female. Moans and cries.
- ED nurse can administer medications/fluids. The nurse does have some medical knowledge base and my cue learners if needed.
- Parent has no medical knowledge but is appropriately concerned and inquisitive about the diagnosis. If asked, the parent states this has never happened before.

Case Narrative

Scenario Background

EMS was called to a local daycare for an allergic reaction. When they arrive, they find a nine-month-old girl with facial swelling and hives as well as two episodes of vomiting. Symptoms began while eating lunch. EMS administered IM epinephrine en route. They attempted IV access but were unsuccessful.

> Case may start with EMS receiving this case on scene as presented and performing their objectives to initiate treatment and transport, including administering epinephrine. Alternatively, case background may be presented prior to case as an EMS medical consult or by EMS on arrival.

Chief complaint:	Allergic reaction.
Patient's medical history:	Eczema.
Medications:	Crisaborole (topical)
Allergies:	No known drug allergies.
Family history:	Asthma and eczema in mom
Social history:	Lives at home with mom, dad, and four-year-old sister. No pets. Fully vaccinated and has her regular well-child checks.

Initial Scenario Conditions

Vital signs: (EMS arrival on scene): HR 150, RR 38, BP 65/palp, SpO$_2$ 98% on room air.
Weight: 8 kg, length: 27 in.
Vital signs: (ED arrival): Temp 98.6°F (37.0°C) HR 200, RR 40, BP 60/palp, SpO$_2$ 99% on non-rebreather mask.
General: Awake, alert, crying.
HEENT: Tongue edema, midline uvula, rhinorrhea.
Eyes: Periorbital edema.
Lungs: Diffuse expiratory wheezes, no rales.
Heart: Tachycardic, regular, no murmurs.
Abdomen: Soft, non-tender, non-distended, active bowel sounds.
Extremities: Warm, dry, well-perfused.
Skin: Diffuse erythroderma, some discrete hives.

Physical exam findings not available on your mannequin can be reported verbally if asked for by learners; e.g., if your mannequin cannot simulate periorbital edema, it can be verbally reported when the exam is performed/requested.

See flow diagram (Figure 6.4) for further scenario changes described.

Case Narrative, continued

Learners of all levels (EMS, students, and postgraduate learners) should perform a rapid evaluation of the patient, administer IM epinephrine, obtain appropriate IV access (for more novice learners this can be IV, for more advanced learners the patient may require IO), appropriately administer IV fluids, antihistamine(s), and corticosteroids. Failure to administer epinephrine within two minutes will lead to decompensation. If epinephrine is not provided within two minutes of decompensation, it leads to respiratory arrest and subsequent cardiac arrest.

If the patient goes into cardiac arrest, pulses should return and vitals should return to the initial emergency department state after two minutes of CPR and administration of IV (or IO) epinephrine.

Following appropriate anaphylaxis management, there is an initial period of stabilization, which allows for the parent to ask questions and the learner to educate the parent. The case may end here for students.

For post-graduate learners, the case can continue with a return to the initial state once epinephrine wears off and the requirement for additional epinephrine dosing and an epinephrine drip. The case ends when the patient is stabilized and a plan for admission to the intensive care unit has been communicated to the parent and an admitting team.

Instructor Notes

Pathophysiology

- Two types: immunologic mediated (immunoglobulin-mediated) and non-immunologic (results from mast cell and basophil degranulation without immunoglobulin involvement):
  - Immunoglobulin-mediated causes activation of antibodies on mast cells and basophils resulting in release of histamine, leukotrienes, prostaglandins, serotonin, proteases, and heparin [1]. These result in:
    - Vasodilation.
    - Increased vascular permeability.
    - Increased mucous secretion.
    - Increased bronchial smooth muscle tone.

Clinical Features

- The majority (80%) of cases involve skin symptoms [2]:
  - Typically, urticaria, pruritus, and/or diffuse erythroderma.
  - Cutaneous symptoms are more likely to be absent in children with food allergen or precipitating insect sting.
- Gastrointestinal symptoms:
  - Abdominal pain, nausea, vomiting, or diarrhea.
  - Have been associated with more severe outcomes [2].
- Pulmonary symptoms:
  - Dyspnea, wheezing, stridor, and reduced peak flow.
- Cardiovascular symptoms:
  - Tachycardia, hypotension, and syncope.
- Biphasic reaction → recurrence of symptoms after complete resolution:
  - Generally occurs within 8 hours, but can occur up to 72 hours [3].
  - Occurs in 6–11% of children.

Diagnosis

- Criteria for diagnosis include any of the following three definitions [2]:
  1. Acute onset of an illness (minutes to several hours) with involvement of the skin, mucosal tissue, or both, and at least one of:
     - Respiratory compromise.
     - Reduced blood pressure or associated symptoms of end-organ dysfunction.

2. Two of more of the following, which occur rapidly after exposure to a likely allergen for that patient:
   - Involvement of the skin-mucosal tissue.
   - Respiratory compromise.
   - Reduced blood pressure or associated symptoms.
   - Persistent gastrointestinal symptoms.
3. Reduced blood pressure after exposure to known allergen for that patient.

Management

- Medications:
  - Epinephrine
    - First priority.
    - Delays in administration are associated with increased morbidity, mortality, and biphasic reaction.
    - IM epinephrine (1 : 1000 concentration); dose 0.01 mg/kg to a maximum of 0.5 mg:
      - Infants weighing < 10 kg should be given exact weight-based dose whenever possible.
      - Use 0.15 mg dose for children 10–25 kg, and 0.30 mg dose for children >25 kg [3].
      - Epinephrine auto-injectors may be available in 0.1, 0.15, and 0.30 mg doses.
    - Continuous IV epinephrine infusion:
      - Consider for patients who are refractory to IM epinephrine or who require repeat doses.
      - Starting dose is 0.1 µg/kg/minute for both children and adults.
  - Antihistamines:
    - No evidence for utility in managing anaphylaxis but useful in treating urticaria and rhinorrhea.
    - Diphenhydramine:
      - Most widely available.
      - Available in oral and IV formulation.
      - IV administration preferred for anaphylaxis.
    - Dosing:
      - Pediatric: 1–2 mg/kg/dose.
      - Adult: 25–50 mg.
    - H2 blockers:
      - No evidence for relief of airway obstruction or shock [4, 5].
      - Option include IV famotidine

- Dosing:
  - Pediatric 20 mg/kg, maximum dose of 20 mg.
  - Adult 20 mg.
- Corticosteroids:
  - Slow onset, no role for treatment of acute anaphylaxis.
  - Thought to potentially prevent a biphasic reaction.
- Beta 2-agonist bronchodilators (e.g., albuterol):
  - May help treat respiratory symptoms of anaphylaxis.
- Discharge planning
  - Anaphylaxis emergency action plan should include:
    - Signs and symptoms of anaphylaxis.
    - Actions to be taken in the event of anaphylaxis.
    - Information on obtaining a medical alert bracelet.
  - Epinephrine auto-injectors:
    - Patients should receive a prescription for at least two doses.
    - Doses should be kept together and always with the patient, so that the patient has adequate treatment in the event of a protracted reaction prior to EMS arrival.
    - Parents and/or the patient should have education provided on how to use the specific auto-injector prescribed.

Debriefing Plan

Plan for approximately 30 minutes for discussion'

Potential Questions for Discussion

- What is the approach to a patient with anaphylaxis?
- How should vascular access be established? What are the options for access if a peripheral IV fails? What are the indications for moving on from attempts at peripheral access?
- If this patient were in respiratory distress, are there any special considerations for intubation?
- What patient education is important when discharging a patient with anaphylaxis?

REFERENCES FOR PEDIATRIC ANAPHYLAXIS

1. Reber, L.L., Hernandez, J.D., and Galli, S.J. (2017). The pathophysiology of anaphylaxis. *J. Allergy Clin. Immunol.* 140 (2): 335–348.

2. Sampson, H.A., Muñoz-Furlong, A., Campbell, R.L. et al. (2006). Second symposium on the definition and management of anaphylaxis: summary report: second National Institute of allergy and infectious disease/Food Allergy and Anaphylaxis Network symposium. *J. Allergy Clin. Immunol.* 117 (2): 391–397.

3. Chipps, B.E. (2013). Update in pediatric anaphylaxis: a systematic review. *Clin. Pediatr. (Phila).* 52 (5): 451–461.

4. Nurmatov, U.B., Rhatigan, E., Simons, F.E., and Sheikh, A. (2014). H2-antihistamines for the treatment of anaphylaxis with and without shock: a systematic review. *Ann. Allergy Asthma Immunol.* 112: 126.

5. Fedorowicz, Z., van Zuuren, E.J., and Histamine, H.N. (2012). H2-receptor antagonists for urticaria. *Cochrane Database Syst. Rev.* (3): CD008596.

REACTIVE ARTHRITIS

Educational Goals

Learning Objectives

1. List reactive arthritis as part of the differential diagnosis of a painful knee effusion (MK, PC).
2. Recognize association of reactive arthritis with urethritis and obtain relevant history (MK, PC, ICS).
3. Perform arthrocentesis of the knee (PC).
4. Differentiate inflammatory (reactive) arthritis from infectious arthritis with respect to arthrocentesis results (MK).
5. Demonstrate appropriate treatment of urethritis-associated reactive arthritis (MK, PC).

Critical Actions Checklist

☐ Perform a thorough musculoskeletal exam of a knee with a joint effusion (PC, MK).
☐ Perform a knee arthrocentesis (PC, MK).
☐ Correctly interpret knee arthrocentesis results (PC, MK).
☐ Obtain history of preceding urethritis (MK, PC).
☐ Order relevant testing for urethritis (MK, PC).
☐ Treat urethritis caused by common sexually transmitted infections (MK, PC).
☐ Discuss partner notification/treatment of suspected urethritis (MK, PC, ICS).

Simulation Set-Up

Environment: ED treatment room.

Standardized patient: Male, dressed in hospital gown, with swollen right knee and conjunctivitis. Can be moulaged with latex to mimic swelling around patella and use eye drops to simulate conjunctivitis.

Props: To be displayed on plasma screen/computer screen or printed out on handouts in scenario room when asked for/return from lab.

Images (see online component for reactive arthritis, Scenario 6.3 at https://www.wiley.com/go/thoureen/simulation/workbook2e):
 • Knee x-ray showing effusion (Figures 6.5 and 6.6).
 Laboratory tests (see online component as above):

- Urinalysis (Table 6.3).
- Complete blood count (Table 6.4).
- Basic metabolic panel (Table 6.5).
- Inflammatory markers (Table 6.6).
- Arthrocentesis panel (Table 6.7).
- Gonorrhea/chlamydia nucleic acid amplification test (*NAAT*) (Table 6.8).

Available supplies:

- Supplies for arthrocentesis:
  - Syringes, needles, sterile drape, chlorhexidine swabs.
  - Medications: local anesthetic agent of choice.
- Arthrocentesis task trainer or a trainer created using a three-dimensional printer [1] (optional).

Distractor: None.

Actors

- Patient is male. He provides relevant history and complains of pain with manipulation of the left knee. Patient notes on review of systems that his eyes have been irritated and he's been using drops for them.
- ED nurse can administer medications/fluids. The nurse does have some medical knowledge base and my cue learners if needed.
- Orthopedics and/or rheumatology can be available for telephone consultation.

Case Narrative

Scenario Background

A 23-year-old man presents with right knee pain. It began approximately a week ago. He does not remember hurting his knee, but plays basketball several times a week. He went to an urgent care two days ago, was told it was sprained, was started on around-the-clock ibuprofen and given a knee brace. However, the pain is getting worse, and the knee seems more swollen now. Over the past few days, he has had intermittent chills and sweats.

If asked specifically, his wrists and ankles feel stiff in the morning but that abates after 20 minutes. Also, if specifically asked, he is sexually active without barrier protection. He has been having dysuria for about two weeks but has not sought medical attention.

Chief complaint:	Knee pain
Patient's medical history:	Asthma
Meds:	Ibuprofen as needed
Allergies:	None

Family history:	Non-contributory
Social history:	No tobacco, occasional marijuana, no other drugs, no alcohol

Initial scenario conditions

Patient resting comfortably on hospital stretcher in no acute distress.

Vital signs:	Temp 100.2°F (37.8°C), HR 84, RR 18, BP 123/65, SpO$_2$ 99% on room air.
General:	Awake, alert, no acute distress but appears uncomfortable
Eyes:	Mild conjunctivitis.
Neck:	Supple, without lymphadenopathy.
Lungs:	Clear to auscultation bilaterally without wheezes, rales, or rhonchi.
Heart:	Regular rate and rhythm, no murmur, intact distal pulses.
Abdomen:	Soft, non-tender, non-distended, active bowel sounds.
Genitals:	Clear penile discharge, normal testicular exam, cremasteric reflex intact.
Musculoskeletal:	Right knee is swollen with joint effusion, warm, non-erythematous and painful with ROM. Negative anterior and posterior drawer test, negative Apley grind test. Remainder of joints demonstrate full active and passive ROM without swelling.

> Physical exam findings should be reported verbally when the learner demonstrates a thorough exam of that organ system. Sensitive organ systems (e.g., genitourinary exam) can be reported verbally when requested.

See flow diagram (Figure 6.7) or further scenario changes described.

Case narrative, continued

All learners should perform a thorough musculoskeletal exam, start an IV, obtain relevant lab work, and treat the patient's pain.

For student learners, the case can end once the results of the arthrocentesis have been returned and interpreted. If orthopedics is consulted, the orthopedic consultant can ask if the learners have also considered inflammatory causes.

A knee arthrocentesis skills session can be incorporated into the debriefing to allow for hands-on practice.

For more advanced learners, arthrocentesis should be performed using a task trainer (alternatively, in the absence of a task trainer, learners can recite the steps of performing a knee arthrocentesis). The case should not end until investigation into the cause of the inflammatory arthritis has been initiated in the form of a more thorough history, and potentially additional lab work. If advanced learners consult orthopedics for a suspected septic arthritis, the consultant can suggest they consider other causes.

Instructor Notes

Pathophysiology

- Immune-mediated arthritis associated with recent enteric, respiratory or uro-genital infection from the following organisms [2]:
  - *Salmonella.*
  - *Shigella* species.
  - *Yersinia.*
  - *Campylobacter.*
  - *Clostridium difficile.*
  - *Escherichia coli* (diarrheagenic strains).
  - *Chlamydia trachomatis, Chlamydia pneumoniae.*
  - *Ureaplasma urealyticum.*
  - *Mycoplasma genitalium.*
  - Group A beta-hemolytic *Streptococcus.*
    - 80% of patients are human leukocyte antigen-B27 positive, indicating some genetic predisposition to reactive arthritis [3].

Clinical Features

- Oligoarthritis or monoarthritis:
  - Develops one to four weeks after exposure to preceding infectious organism.
- Conjunctivitis, uveitis.
- Urethritis:
  - More common in men than women by a ratio of 5–10 : 1.
- Classic triad of eye symptoms, joint symptoms, and urethritis is only present in approximately one third of patients [3].

Diagnosis

- Criteria proposed by Braun et al. [4]:
  - Two major criteria and one minor criteria are suggested to be diagnostic.
  - A patient with either (i) both major criteria or (ii) one major criteria and one minor criteria are thought to have probable reactive arthritis.
  - Major criteria:
    - Arthritis with two of the following three characteristics:
    - Asymmetric
    - Mono- or oligoarticular

- Lower limbs predominantly affected.
- Preceding symptomatic infection:
  - Enteritis: diarrhea for at least one day, three days to six weeks before onset of infection.
  - Urethritis: dysuria or discharge for at least one day, three days to six weeks before onset of infection.
- Minor criteria:
  - Evidence of triggering infection
    - Positive NAAT in morning urine or urethral/cervical swab for *Chlamydia trachomatis*.
    - Positive stool culture for enteric pathogens associated with reactive arthritis.
  - Evidence of persistent synovial infection (positive immunohistology or polymerase chain reaction for *Chlamydia*).
  - Joint fluid leukocytes are 2000–64 000/ml [2].
  - Erythrocyte sedimentation rate and C-reactive protein typically elevated.

Management

- The mainstay of treatment is non-steroidal anti-inflammatory drugs.
- Initiation of antibiotic therapy is dependent on preceding causative organism.
  - Chlamydia urethritis should be treated with appropriate antibiotics.
  - Enteral infections generally do not persist beyond the symptomatic stage and do not require antibiotic treatment.
- Acute reactive arthritis generally lasts three to five months:
  - Can develop a chronic reactive arthritis.
  - Rheumatology may consider treating patients with disease-modifying antirheumatic drugs.
    - Sulfasalazine has been shown to induce clinical remission more rapidly than placebo if started during the first three months [2].

Debriefing Plan

Plan for approximately 30 minutes for discussion.

Potential Questions for Discussion

- What is in your differential diagnosis for an atraumatic swollen knee?
- What are the most common associated bacterial infections in reactive arthritis?
- What diagnostic testing is necessary to confirm the diagnosis?
- Which inciting bacterial infections require treatment?
- What is the prognosis for reactive arthritis?

REFERENCES FOR REACTIVE ARTHRITIS

1. Day, A.L., Barger, J.B., and Resuehr, D. (2019). A versatile, low-cost, three-dimensional-printed ultrasound procedural training phantom of the knee. *Eur. Med. J.* 4 (3): 68–72.

2. Hannu, T. (2011). Reactive arthritis. *Best Pract. Res. Clin. Rheumatol.* 25 (3): 347–357.

3. Stavropoulos, P.G., Soura, E., Kanelleas, A. et al. (2015). Reactive arthritis. *J. Eur. Acad. Dermatol. Venereol.* 29 (3): 415–424.

4. Braun, J., Kingsley, G., van der Heijde, D., and Sieper, J. (2000). On the difficulties of establishing a consensus on the definition of and diagnostic investigations for reactive arthritis. Results and discussion of a questionnaire prepared for the 4th international workshop on reactive arthritis, Berlin, Germany, July 3–6, 1999. *J. Rheumatol* 27 (9): 2185–2192.

APPENDIX

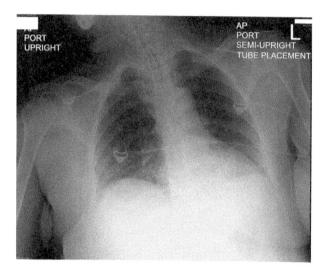

FIGURE 6.1 X-ray chest post-intubation.

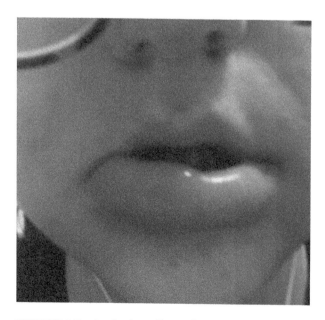

FIGURE 6.2 Angioedema lip swelling.

Scenario Flow Diagram: Angioedema

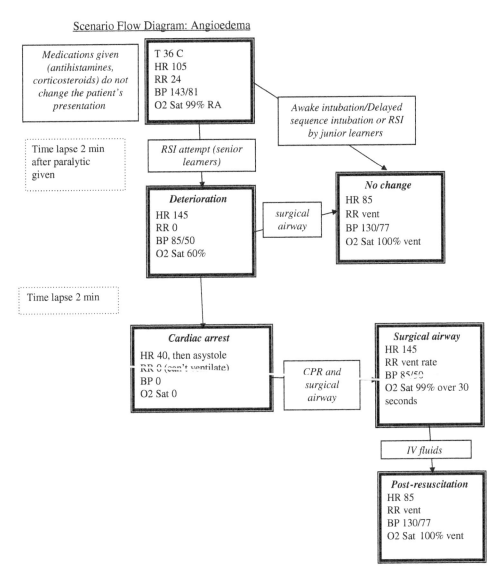

FIGURE 6.3 Flow diagram for angioedema.

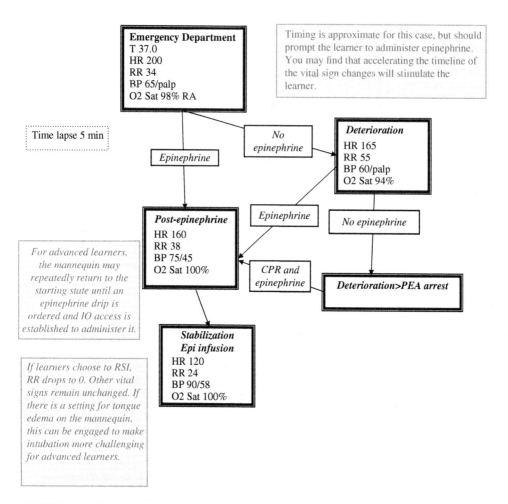

FIGURE 6.4   Flow diagram for pediatric anaphylaxis.

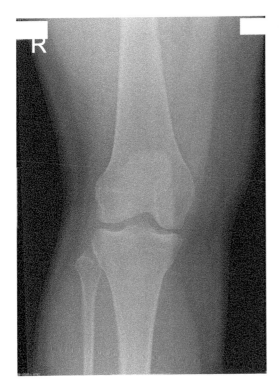

FIGURE 6.5   X-ray anteroposterior knee.

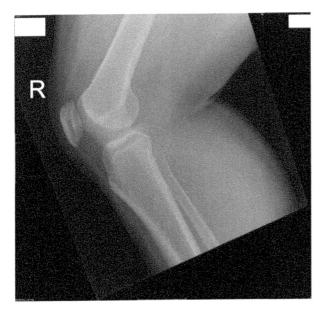

FIGURE 6.6   X-ray lateral knee.

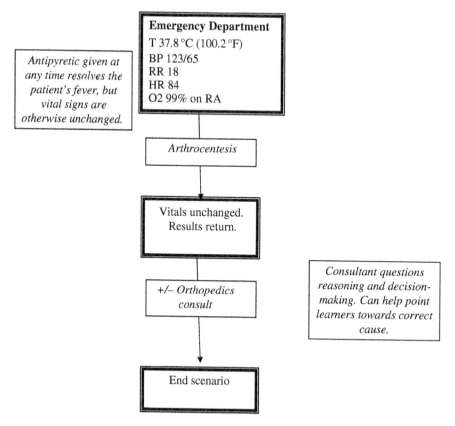

FIGURE 6.7   Flow diagram for reactive arthritis.

TABLE 6.1 Complete blood count.

Test	Value	Reference range
White blood cells ($\times 10^3/\mu l$)	14.35	4.3–10.5
Hemoglobin (g/dl)	13.8	12.0–15.5
Hematocrit (%)	41.1	36–46
Platelets ($\times 10^3/\mu l$)	3645	150–5

TABLE 6.2 Basic metabolic panel.

Test	Value	Reference range
Sodium (mEq/l)	140	136–145
Potassium (mEq/l)	4.0	3.5–5
Chloride (mEq/l)	106	98–106
CO_2 (mEq/l)	24	23–30
Blood urea nitrogen (mg/dl)	21	8–20
Creatinine (mg/dl)	1.2	0.5–1.3
Glucose (mg/dl)	107	70–99

TABLE 6.3 Urinalysis.

Test	Value	Reference range
Color	Yellow	Yellow
Appearance	Clear	Clear
Specific gravity	1.020	1.001–1.035
pH	6.0	5.0–8.0
Glucose	Negative	Negative
Bilirubin	Negative	Negative
Ketones	Negative	Negative
Blood	Negative	Negative
Protein	Negative	Negative
Nitrite	Negative	Negative
Leukocyte esterase	Small	Negative
Microscopic (/hpf):		
Red blood cells	0	0–2
White blood cells	15	0–5
Bacteria	None	None

TABLE 6.4 Complete blood count.

Test	Value	Reference range
White blood cells ($\times 10^3$/µl)	12.1	4.3–10.5
Hemoglobin (g/dl)	14.3	12.0–15.5
Hematocrit (%)	43	36–46
Platelets ($\times 10^3$/µl)	364	150–450

TABLE 6.5 Basic metabolic panel.

Test	Value	Reference range
Sodium (mEq/l)	140	136–145
Potassium (mEq/l)	4.3	3.5–5
Chloride (mEq/l)	105	98–106
CO_2 (mEq/l)	26	23–30
Blood urea nitrogen (mg/dl)	18	8–20
Creatinine (mg/dl)	0.7	0.5–1.3
Glucose (mg/dl)	98	70–99

TABLE 6.6 Inflammatory markers.

Test	Value	Reference range
Erythrocyte sedimentation rate (mm/hour)	62	0–20
C-reactive protein (mg/dl)	2.3	≤ 0.8

TABLE 6.7 Arthrocentesis panel.

Test	Value	Reference range
Color	Yellow	Clear
Clarity	Cloudy	Transparent
White blood cells (/mm³)	15 492	0–200
Polymorphonuclear cells (%)	70	< 25
Gram stain	Negative	Negative
Crystals	Negative	Negative
Culture	Pending	–

TABLE 6.8 Gonorrhea/chlamydia nucleic acid amplification test.

Test	Value	Reference range
Neisseria gonorrhoeae	Negative	Negative
Chlamydia trachomatis	Positive	Negative

CHAPTER 7

Systemic Infectious Emergencies

Donald T. Ellis, II[1,2]

[1] *Duke Children's Hospital and Health Center, Durham, NC, USA*
[2] *Department of Pediatrics, Division of Emergency Medicine, Duke University Medical Center, Durham, NC, USA*

SEPTIC SHOCK

Educational Goals

Learning Objectives

1. Recognize critical illness and potential for decompensation in a patient with septic shock (MK, PC, ICS).
2. Identify respiratory failure and demonstrate airway competence through bag-valve-mask (*BVM*) ventilation, endotracheal intubation, and confirmation of airway placement (MK, PC).
3. Demonstrate appropriate treatment with intravenous (IV) crystalloid fluid and vasoactive medication (MK, PC).
4. Order broad-spectrum antibiotics early (MK, PC).
5. Know indications for admission to an intensive care unit (*ICU*) (SBP).
6. Obtain blood and urine cultures prior to the administration of broad-spectrum antibiotics (MK).

Emergency Medicine Simulation Workbook: A Tool for Bringing the Curriculum to Life,
Second Edition. Edited by Traci L. Thoureen and Sara B. Scott.
© 2022 John Wiley & Sons Ltd. Published 2022 by John Wiley & Sons Ltd.
Companion website: www.wiley.com/go/thoureen/simulation/workbook2e

Critical Actions Checklist

☐ Order appropriate IV access (two large-bore IV cannulas) and consider central venous access for resuscitation and vasoactive medication administration (PC).
☐ Order intraosseous (*IO*) access when IV attempts are unsuccessful (MK, PC).
☐ Provide BVM ventilation for respiratory failure (PC).
☐ Perform endotracheal intubation to secure the airway and confirm placement (MK, PC).
☐ Order appropriate laboratory testing (MK).
☐ Ensure early administration of broad-spectrum antibiotics (MK, PC).
☐ Consult for admission to ICU after initial stabilization (ICS, P, SBP).

The checklist above may be altered to incorporate learners from various disciplines. For example, when hosting personnel from the emergency medical services (*EMS*), critical actions may include adherence to local EMS sepsis protocols.

Simulation Set-up

Environment: Emergency department (*ED*) treatment room. For EMS providers, the environment may begin at the patient's home.

Mannequin: Adult simulator mannequin (should be clothed). Simulated vomitus and/or stool may be present for additional realism.

Props: To be displayed on plasma/computer screen or printed and distributed as handouts in the scenario room when ordered by the learners or results released by the laboratory:

- Images (see online component for septic shock, Scenario 7.1 at `https://www.wiley.com/go/thoureen/simulation/workbook2e`):
  - Chest x-ray read as "Scattered opacities are present diffusely (right greater than left); increased size of cardiac shadow may be due to anterior-posterior technique and/or poor inspiratory effort" (Figure 7.1).
  - Abdominal x-ray which is normal (Figure 7.2).
  - Post-intubation chest x-ray demonstrating appropriate endotracheal tube placement with bilateral infiltrates (Figure 7.3).
  - Electrocardiogram (ECG) with sinus tachycardia and short PR interval (Figure 7.4).
- Laboratory tests (see online component as above):
  - Blood gas, arterial (Table 7.1).
  - Complete blood count (Table 7.2).
  - Chemistry panel (Table 7.3).

- Hepatic panel (Table 7.4).
- Lactate (Table 7.5).
- Coagulation panel, including D-dimer level (Table 7.6).
- Type and screen (Table 7.7).
- Urinalysis (Table 7.8).

Available supplies:

- Basic airway supplies and code cart.
- Medications:
  - Liter bags of 0.9% saline and lactated Ringer's solution (*LR*)

> Any imaging or laboratory results not provided above (such as a computed tomography (CT) of the head) should be verbally reported as normal if the learners order these.

- Pre-labeled syringes:
  - Rapid sequence intubation (*RSI*) medications.
  - Specific induction and paralytic medications typical of your institution.
- Pre-labeled IV bags:
  - Sedative(s) of choice at your institution (e.g., fentanyl, midazolam).
  - Broad-spectrum antibiotics.
  - Vasopressor of choice at your institution (e.g., norepinephrine, epinephrine).
- Fiberoptic scope, video-assisted laryngoscope, cricothyrotomy tray, and/or supraglottic airway device(s) (optional).

Distractor: none

Actors

- Family member (optional) is able to provide basic history.
- EMS may be represented by an actor or another learner. If represented by an actor, they should provide the scenario background as noted below.
- Patient voice may be male or female, whichever is preferred. Speech should be garbled and unintelligible. Patient is not able to engage in conversation or follow commands during assessment.
- ED nurse is able to place peripheral IV/IO lines and administer medications and IV fluids. The nursing staff has cultivated tremendous medical knowledge during their career and can cue learners if necessary.
- Medical intensivist is available via telephone consultation.

Case Narrative

Scenario Background

The patient is a 52-year old man (may substitute a woman) who presents to the ED for fever. He has been ill for several days, most notably with fever, cough, vomiting, and diarrhea. He was noted to have worsened several hours prior to arrival and seemed somewhat confused. His family became concerned and called EMS.

Chief complaint:	Fever.
Patient's medical history:	hypertension, type 2 diabetes mellitus.
Medications:	lisinopril, metformin (not compliant).
Allergies:	none.
Family history:	Father: myocardial infarction (deceased). Mother: cerebrovascular accident (deceased).
Social history:	Non-smoker, drinks up to two alcoholic beverages daily. No other drug history known. Lives with companion.

> Allergies may be changed to a history of anaphylaxis to penicillin, depending on the expertise of the learners and the educational objectives of the instructors.

Initial Scenario Conditions

Middle-aged man arriving via EMS. He is in apparent extremis and is incoherent.

> Case may begin with EMS arriving "on scene" as described above.

Vital signs:	Temperature 102.7°F (39.2°C), HR 128, RR 24, BP 98/63, SpO$_2$ 93% on non-rebreather mask.
General:	Recumbent, non-cooperative, middle-aged man in apparent distress.
Head:	Atraumatic.
Eyes:	Pupils are 3 mm bilaterally and equally reactive to light.
Mouth/throat:	Dry oral mucosa.
Neck:	Supple, no goiter.
Heart:	Tachycardic, regular rhythm; no murmurs, rubs, or gallops. Dorsalis pedis pulses are diminished (1+) bilaterally with capillary refill of approximately four seconds.
Lungs:	Tachypneic, labored respirations with bilateral crackles.
Abdomen:	Non-distended. Bowel sounds are absent. No bruit present. There is generalized tenderness over the abdomen without palpable organomegaly or mass. No rebound tenderness is present.

Genitourinary: Normal-appearing adult male (or female) external genitalia.
Extremities: Decreased tone, no pitting edema.
Skin: Pale, diaphoretic, and without rash.
Neurologic: Withdraws and moans in response to painful stimuli. Eyes are closed. Speech is incomprehensible.

Physical exam findings not available to your mannequin can be reported verbally if requested by the learners. For example, if your mannequin cannot simulate diaphoresis, you may simply report the change verbally when learners are examining the skin or request the skin exam.

See Flow Diagram (Figure 7.5) for additional scenario changes described below.

Case Narrative, Continued

All learners should perform an initial assessment and prioritize obtaining IV/IO access as well as begin to provide IV fluid. The team leader should recognize impending airway failure and institute assisted ventilations before securing the airway with an endotracheal tube (and confirming its position). Depending on the expertise of the learner and capability of specific simulator used, you may include a difficult airway component. Participants may attempt bilevel positive airway pressure, but the patient will vomit and potentially aspirate if this treatment path is pursued. Failure to secure the airway will result in significant clinical deterioration and will culminate in pulseless electrical activity within seven minutes if not corrected.

Following successful endotracheal intubation, the patient will improve temporarily; however, after several minutes, he will become unresponsive to fluid resuscitation and require vasoactive medications to maintain homeostatic blood pressure. Failure to institute therapies such as norepinephrine or epinephrine will result in marked decline and ultimately in simulator arrest.

Learners should also order broad-spectrum antibiotics (after obtaining blood and urine cultures) and contact an intensivist to arrange for transfer to an ICU. Depending on the expertise of the learner you may add pertinent allergy history (e.g., a history of anaphylaxis to penicillin) to make the choice of antibiotics more challenging.

Advanced learners should both order appropriate diagnostics (laboratory testing and imaging) and observe for clinical worsening. Of note, if the learner attempts to obtain CT imaging before the patient is stabilized (e.g., if the mean arterial blood pressure is less than 65 mmHg and not trending upward, the patient will deteriorate.

The case is successfully completed when the patient is stabilized, treated with broad-spectrum antibiotics, and accepted for transfer to the ICU.

Instructor Notes

Pathophysiology

- Sepsis represents a clinical syndrome of altered inflammation in the setting of infection and features both pro- and anti-inflammatory mechanisms [1].

Clinical Features

- Organ dysfunction and inflammatory dysregulation may be manifested by a multitude of abnormalities including one or more of the following [1]:
  - Temperature abnormalities (fever or hypothermia).
  - Tachycardia.
  - Hypotension.
  - Respiratory failure.
  - Thrombocytopenia.
  - Hyperbilirubinemia.
  - Altered mental status.
  - Renal insufficiency/failure (elevated creatinine).

Diagnosis

- There is no "gold standard" test for sepsis, although laboratory testing (e.g., complete blood count, blood gas, lactate, creatinine, d-dimer) may be helpful [1].
- The Sepsis-3 Task Force convened on the topic in 2016.
- Sepsis is defined as "life-threatening organ dysfunction caused by a dysregulated host response to infection" [1].
- Septic shock is defined as "a subset of sepsis in which underlying circulatory, cellular, and metabolic abnormalities are associated with a greater risk of mortality than sepsis alone" [1, 2].
  - Adults with septic shock must have hypotension requiring vasopressor therapy to maintain mean arterial blood pressure $\geq$ 65 mmHg and have a serum lactate level > 2 mmol/l after adequate fluid resuscitation" [2].
- The Quick Sequential [Sepsis-related] Organ Failure Assessment (*qSOFA*) score calculated as follows:
  - Glasgow Coma Scale (*GCS*) score < 15 (1 point).
  - Systolic blood pressure $\leq$ 100 mmHg (1 point).
  - Respiratory rate $\geq$ 22/minute (1 point).
  - A qSOFA score $\geq$ 2 has been demonstrated to reliably predict increased potential for morbidity and mortality in adults with sepsis [1, 3].

Management

- Fluid management:
  - Crystalloids (30 ml/kg ideal body weight) within the first three hours [4].
  - No benefit of colloid solution (e.g., albumin) over crystalloids [4].
- Airway/breathing:
  - Patients in respiratory failure should receive 100% oxygen via BVM.
  - Endotracheal intubation for patients in respiratory failure and/or presenting with inadequate airway protection.
- Medications:
  - Vasoactive medications, particularly epinephrine and norepinephrine to treat fluid-refractory hypotension.
  - Broad-spectrum antibiotics, may also include antifungal agents (e.g., with activity against *Candida* species) and/or antiviral agents (e.g., agents with activity against influenza, herpes simplex virus).
- Isolation
  - Strict adherence to isolation policies may reduce the risk of transmission of infections to patients, staff, and visitors.

Debriefing Plan

Plan for approximately 20–30 minutes for discussion.

Potential Questions for Discussion

- What are the competing definitions/terms applied to sepsis?
- If IO access is needed, what are the preferred sites?
- Should all septic patients have central IV access?
- If a patient has an allergy (for example, penicillin), what are acceptable alternative antibiotics?

REFERENCES FOR SEPTIC SHOCK

1. Singer, M., Deutschman, C.S., Seymour, C.W. et al. (2016). The third international consensus definitions for sepsis and septic shock (Sepsis-3). *JAMA*. 315 (8): 801–810.
2. Shankar-Hari, M., Phillips, G.S., Levy, M.L. et al. (2016). Developing a new definition and assessing new clinical criteria for septic shock: for the third international consensus definitions for sepsis and septic shock (Sepsis-3). *JAMA*. 315 (8): 775–787.
3. Seymour, C.W., Liu, V.X., Iwashyna, T.J. et al. (2016). Assessment of clinical criteria for sepsis: for the third international consensus definitions for sepsis and septic shock (Sepsis-3). *JAMA*. 315 (8): 762–774.

4. Rhodes, A., Evans, L.E., Alhazzani, W. et al. (2017). Surviving sepsis campaign: international guidelines for management of sepsis and septic shock: 2016. *Intensive Care Med.* 43 (3).

SELECTED READINGS FOR SEPTIC SHOCK

Jarczak, D., Kluge, S., and Nierhaus, A. (2021). Sepsis-pathophysiology and therapeutic concepts. *Front. Med. (Lausanne)* 8: 628302.

Wasyluk, W. and Zwolak, A. (2021). Metabolic alterations in sepsis. *J. Clin. Med.* 10 (11): 2412.

BACTERIAL MENINGITIS

Educational Goals

Learning Objectives

1. Recognize the potential for bacterial meningitis in a child without meningismus (MK, PC, ICS).
2. Understand the importance of administering broad-spectrum antibiotics early in the patient encounter (MK, PC).
3. Obtain cultures from blood and urine in addition to cerebrospinal fluid (*CSF*) when considering the diagnosis of bacterial meningitis (MK).
4. Identify the most common bacterial pathogens responsible for meningitis in children over the age of one month (MK).
5. Demonstrate knowledge of the indications for admission to a pediatric ICU (*PICU*) (SBP).

Critical Actions Checklist

- ☐ Obtain appropriate IV/IO access (PC).
- ☐ Obtain weight via length-based resuscitation tape or scale (PC).
- ☐ Order appropriate laboratory testing (MK).
- ☐ Order appropriate broad-spectrum antibiotics (MK, PC).
- ☐ Perform lumbar puncture (optional) (PC).
- ☐ Consult pediatric critical care for admission to a PICU after initial stabilization (ICS, P, SBP).

Simulation Set-up

Environment: ED treatment room.

Mannequin: Pediatric simulator mannequin (should be approximately eight years of age and wearing casual clothing).

Props: To be displayed on plasma/computer screen or printed and distributed as handouts in the scenario room when ordered by the learners or results released by the laboratory:

- Images (see online component for bacterial meningitis, Scenario 9.2 https://www.wiley.com/go/thoureen/simulation/workbook2e):
  - Chest x-ray (Figure 7.6) which demonstrates bilateral streaking
  - Post-intubation chest x-ray (Figure 7.7) demonstrating appropriate endotracheal tube placement and worsening bilateral opacities. Use if the exercise incorporates respiratory failure.

- Head CT without contrast (Figure 7.8). If ordered by participant(s), report preliminary reading is as follows: "No acute intracranial process, including but not limited to mass, edema, hemorrhage, herniation, or shunting."
- Laboratory tests (see online component as above):
  - Point-of-care ("fingerstick") glucose (Table 7.9).
  - Complete blood count (Table 7.10).
  - Differential white blood cell count (Table 7.11).
  - Chemistry panel (Table 7.12).
  - Blood gas (Table 7.13).
  - Lactate (Table 7.14).
  - Urinalysis (Table 7.15).
  - Rapid streptococcal test (Table 7.16).
  - Rapid influenza test (Table 7.17).

Available supplies:

- Pediatric airway supplies and code cart (including a length-based resuscitation tape).
- Pediatric lumbar puncture task trainer/simulator (optional).
- Medications:
  - Liter bags of 0.9% saline and LR.
  - Pre-labeled syringes:
    - RSI medications. The specific induction and paralytic medications typically used at your institution.
  - Pre-labeled IV bags:
    - Medications of choice for continuing sedation, typically used at your institution (e.g., fentanyl, midazolam).
    - Broad-spectrum antibiotics.

Distractor: None.

Actors

- Parent is able to provide detailed history.
- Patient voice may be female or male. Speech should be intelligible; crying intermittently. Patient is sleepy and confused but answers rudimentary questions appropriately. They follow simple commands despite discomfort during assessment.
- ED nurse is able to place peripheral IV lines (may also place IO lines if desired) and administer medications and IV fluids. The nurse possesses extensive medical knowledge and may cue learners if necessary.
- Pediatric intensivist is available via phone consultation.

Case Narrative

Scenario Background

The patient is an eight-year old (female pronouns will be used, but the simulation may substitute a male patient) who presents to the ED for evaluation of fever. She has been ill for the past 72 hours, with a cough and sore throat. The illness was also associated with anorexia. Within the past 12 hours, she has developed a headache (global in location; unable to describe quality of the pain; rated by her parent as moderate-to-severe), vomiting, and profound fatigue. She was evaluated by her primary care provider and referred to the ED.

Chief complaint:	fever.
Patient's medical history:	None.
Medications:	acetaminophen (160 mg, most recently administered six hours prior to the current evaluation).
Allergies:	None.
Family history:	Both parents are living and healthy.
Social history:	Attends school. No specific sick contacts are identified when asked.

Initial Scenario Conditions

School-aged girl (or boy) arriving via private automobile. She was carried by her parent from triage to the examination room. She appears uncomfortable and is tearful throughout the encounter.

Vital signs:	Temp 104.4°F (40.2°C), HR 148, RR 30, BP 118/83, SpO$_2$ 99% on room air.
Weight:	26 kg via length-based resuscitation tape.
General:	School-aged girl with eyes closed. She appears uncomfortable and cries frequently, even while attempting to cooperate. She prefers the examination room to remain darkened.
Head:	Atraumatic. Face is symmetric.
Eyes:	Pupils 4 mm bilaterally and equally reactive to light. No dysconjugate gaze, +photophobia.
Ears:	Tympanic membranes slightly erythematous without purulent effusion or perforation. Normal pneumatic otoscopy. Hearing intact to voice.
Nose:	Moderate clear rhinorrhea.
Mouth/throat:	Oropharyngeal mucosa erythematous without exudate or petechiae. Palatine tonsils mildly enlarged but symmetric. Uvula and tongue midline.
Neck:	Supple, no meningismus.
Heart:	Tachycardic, regular rhythm; no murmurs, rubs, or gallops. Dorsalis pedis pulses 2+ bilaterally. Capillary refill < 2 seconds.

Lungs: Tachypneic, non-labored respirations. Good air exchange without crackles, rhonchi, or wheezing.

Abdomen: Non-distended. Bowel sounds are normal. Mild non-focal tenderness over the abdomen without palpable organomegaly or mass. No rebound.

Extremities: No gross deformities, pitting edema, or focal tenderness.

Skin: Pale, diaphoretic, and without rash.

Neurologic: Sleepy yet awakens easily. Confused but somewhat cooperative. Speech is truncated but readily interpreted by the examiner. Sensation to light touch is grossly intact. Motor strength is grossly intact, although examination is limited by the patient's cooperation. She refuses to ambulate.

Physical exam findings not available to your mannequin can be reported verbally if requested by the learners. For example, the ear exam can be reported verbally if requested by the learner.

See flow diagram (Figure 7.9) for additional scenario changes described.

Case Narrative, Continued

All learners should perform an initial assessment and prioritize obtaining IV/IO access as well as begin to provide IV fluid. The team leader should recognize the patient as being ill-appearing and act quickly to address this infectious disease emergency.

All learners should order broad-spectrum antibiotics (after obtaining blood and urine cultures) *early* in the course of the encounter. They should also perform a lumbar puncture once the patient is stable, but antibiotics must not be delayed for diagnostic purposes. If the patient has not been stabilized and has not received broad-spectrum antibiotics before obtaining a CT or transferring from the ED, she will rapidly deteriorate.

For advanced learners, despite appropriate management, the patient will decompensate and develop respiratory failure requiring endotracheal intubation. After intubation, she becomes hypotensive despite IV fluids and requires vasoactive medications to maintain adequate blood pressure. Failure to order vasopressors will result in marked decline and ultimately in cardiac arrest.

The case is successfully completed when the patient is stabilized, treated with broad-spectrum antibiotics, and accepted for transfer to a PICU.

If a lumbar puncture simulator is unavailable, learners may simply indicate that they would perform the procedure and describe the steps involved.

Instructor Notes

Pathophysiology

- Bacterial meningitis is an infection involving the meninges.
- In the absence of effective antibiotic therapy, it is almost uniformly fatal [1–3].

Clinical Features

- The classic presentation of fever, neck stiffness (meningismus), and altered mental status is absent in around half of adults with bacterial meningitis.
- This triad is even less common in children [4].
- According to a 2015 study, the most common symptoms in children ages 5–17 years were [4]:
  - Fever (86%).
  - Headache (71%).
  - Nausea or vomiting (61%).
  - Altered mental status (46%).
  - Hyperalgesia (25%).
  - Photophobia (21%).
  - Fatigue (21%).
- Younger patients, particularly those under one year of age, often present with nonspecific signs.

Diagnosis

- CSF analysis is essential.
  - CSF should be sent for culture, Gram stain, cell count (with differential white blood cell count), protein and glucose levels.
    - Qualitative polymerase chain reaction (*PCR*) panels performed on CSF may increase the likelihood of identifying common bacterial, fungal and viral pathogens.
    - PCR panels do not provide information on susceptibilities to antibiotics [1, 5].
  - Contraindications to performing lumbar puncture. include [6]:
    - Elevated intracranial pressure (e.g., hydrocephalus, intracranial mass).
    - Bleeding disorder (e.g., severe thrombocytopenia, uncorrected hemophilia, active anticoagulation).
    - Cellulitis, abscess, or other soft tissue infection over the puncture site.

- Although cerebral herniation may still occur, even in the presence of normal head imaging, recent consensus guidelines list indications for obtaining CT imaging prior to performing lumbar puncture as [7]:
  - Focal neurologic deficits (other than abnormalities of the cranial nerves).
  - New-onset seizures.
  - GCS of 9 or less.
  - Significant immunocompromise.

Management

- Fluid management:
  - Crystalloid fluid should be given, especially if there is concomitant dehydration or shock.
  - Monitor urine output and serum electrolytes, particularly for the onset of syndrome of inappropriate antidiuretic hormone.
- Airway/breathing:
  - Monitor for respiratory failure and for inability to protect the airway.
  - Provide supplemental oxygen or perform endotracheal intubation for hypoxia or respiratory failure, respectively.
- Medications:
  - Broad-spectrum antibiotics should be given early, although it is acceptable to obtain cultures first, if doing so will not significantly delay their administration.
  - For children over one month of age, vancomycin plus ceftriaxone is one of the most common combinations.
  - May substitute other (ideally bactericidal) choices if the patient has an allergy or if the selection is unavailable. Options may vary depending on institution and include but are not limited to one or more of the following: aztreonam, meropenem, chloramphenicol, trimethoprim-sulfamethoxazole, and a fluoroquinolone. Consultation with pediatric infectious disease is highly recommended in cases of severe allergy to penicillin, cephalosporins, and/or vancomycin [3].
  - Patients with concurrent septic shock may require vasopressors.
- Isolation and chemoprophylaxis:
  - Universal precautions should be employed for any patient.
  - Droplet precautions should be added for those with suspected *Neisseria* or *Haemophilus influenza* type B (HiB) meningitis "until 24 hours after initiation of effective antimicrobial therapy" [8].
  - Household members and other close contacts of patients with meningococcal meningitis should receive chemoprophylaxis. Exposure to pneumococcal disease does not typically warrant the same except in specific cases of immunocompromise [3].

Debriefing Plan

Plan for approximately 30 minutes for discussion.

Potential Questions for Discussion

- How long is it acceptable to withhold antibiotics if obtaining IV access proves difficult?
- How long does it take for broad-spectrum antibiotics to sterilize the CSF, rendering the culture ineffective?
- What are the most common pathogens responsible for bacterial meningitis in children?
- Who should receive chemoprophylaxis after exposure to a patient with bacterial meningitis?

REFERENCES FOR BACTERIAL MENINGITIS

1. Kaplan, S.L. (2020). Bacterial meningitis in children older than one month: Clinical features and diagnosis. *UpToDate*. https://www.uptodate.com/contents/bacterial-meningitis-in-children-older-than-one-month-clinical-features-and-diagnosis?topicRef=1289&source=see_link (accessed 2 September 2021).
2. Hasbun, R. (2020). Pathogenesis and pathophysiology of bacterial meningitis. *UpToDate*. https://www.uptodate.com/contents/pathogenesis-and-pathophysiology-of-bacterial-meningitis?topicRef=5968&source=see_link (accessed 2 September 2021).
3. Kaplan, S.L. (2020). Bacterial meningitis in children older than one month: Treatment and prognosis. *UpToDate*. https://www.uptodate.com/contents/bacterial-meningitis-in-children-older-than-one-month-treatment-and-prognosis?topicRef=1289&source=see_link (accessed 2 September 2021).
4. Johansson Kostenniemi, U., Norman, D., Borgström, M. et al. (2015). The clinical presentation of acute bacterial meningitis varies with age, sex and duration of illness. *Acta Paediatr.* 104 (11): 1117.
5. Liesman, R.M., Strasburg, A.P., Heitman, A.K. et al. (2018). Evaluation of a commercial multiplex molecular panel for diagnosis of infectious meningitis and encephalitis. *J. Clin. Microbiol.* 56 (4): e01927-17.
6. Engelborghs, S., Niemantsverdriet, E., Struyfs, H. et al. (2017). Consensus guidelines for lumbar puncture in patients with neurological diseases. *Alzheimers Dement. (Amst).* 8: 111–126.
7. van de Beek, D., Cabellos, C., Dzupova, O. et al. (2016). ESCMID guideline: diagnosis and treatment of acute bacterial meningitis. *Clin. Microbiol. Infect.* 22 (Suppl 3): S37–S62.

8. American Academy of Pediatrics (2015). Haemophilus influenzae infections. In: *Red Book: 2015 Report of the Committee on Infectious Diseases*, 30e (eds. D.W. Kimberlin, M.T. Brady, M.A. Jackson and S.S. Long), 368–547. Elk Grove Village, IL: American Academy of Pediatrics.

SELECTED READINGS FOR BACTERIAL MENINGITIS

Alamarat, Z. and Hasbun, R. (2020). Management of acute bacterial meningitis in children. *Infect. Drug Resist.* 13: 4077–4089.

Biondi, E.A., Lee, B., Ralston, S.L. et al. (2019). Prevalence of bacteremia and bacterial meningitis in febrile neonates and infants in the second month of life: a systematic review and meta-analysis. *JAMA Netw. Open.* 2 (3): e190874.

Zainel, A., Mitchell, H., and Sadarangani, M. (2021). Bacterial meningitis in children: neurological complications, associated risk factors, and prevention. *Microorganisms* 9 (3): 535.

EBOLA

Educational Goals

Learning Objectives

1. Recognize hemorrhagic fever as a potential public health emergency (MK, PC, ICS).
2. Select appropriate level of isolation for potential Ebola virus disease (*EVD*) (MK, SBP).
3. Select appropriate personal protective equipment (*PPE*) and demonstrate correct donning and doffing technique (MK, PC, SBP).
4. Recognize a potential emerging infectious disease threat (MK, SBP).
5. Identify appropriate resources and reporting agencies for emerging infectious disease threats (SBP).
6. Institute supportive care while maintaining strict isolation (MK, PC).

Critical Actions Checklist

- ☐ Institute immediate, appropriate isolation (MK).
- ☐ Don appropriate PPE (PC).
- ☐ Order appropriate IV access (PC).
- ☐ Begin supportive care with IV fluid resuscitation (PC).
- ☐ Notify Hospital Infection Control and the public health officials of the potential patient with EVD (ICS, P, SBP).

Simulation Set-Up

Environment: ED treatment room

Mannequin: Adult male simulator mannequin, moulaged with simulated vomitus and/or hematochezia.

Props: To be displayed on plasma/computer screen or printed and distributed as handouts in the scenario room when ordered by the learners or results released by the laboratory:

- Images (see online component for ebola, Scenario 7.3 at https://www.wiley.com/go/thoureen/simulation/workbook2e):
  - Chest x-ray (normal) (Figure 7.10).
- Laboratory tests (see online component as above):
  - Point-of-care (fingerstick) glucose (Table 7.18).
  - Blood gas, arterial (Table 7.19).
  - Complete blood count (Table 7.20).

- Differential white blood cell count (Table 7.21).
- Chemistry panel, including magnesium (Table 7.22).
- Hepatic panel (Table 7.23).
- Lactate (Table 7.24).
- Coagulation panel, including D-dimer and fibrinogen (Table 7.25).
- Type and screen (Table 7.26).
- Urinalysis (Table 7.27).

Available supplies:

- Basic airway and resuscitation supplies.
- PPE as available at your institution.
- Medications:
  - Liter bags of 0.9% saline and/or LR solution.
  - Vasopressors (norepinephrine, epinephrine, vasopressin, etc.) in prelabeled bags or syringes.

Distractor: none

Actors

- Patient voice is male. Speech is appropriate.
- ED nurse is able to place peripheral IV lines (may also place IO lines if desired) and administer medications and IV fluids. The nurse possesses significant medical knowledge and may cue learners if necessary.
- An infectious disease expert is available via telephone.

Case Narrative

Scenario Background

A 19-year old male university student presents to the ED for evaluation of fever. He developed fever and abdominal pain after returning from visiting family five days ago. (NOTE: if learners ask a travel history, they will be informed that the patient has visited the Democratic Republic of the Congo, DRC). Fever is subjective and has been treated periodically with ibuprofen. The abdominal pain is diffuse, most notably in the epigastrium, and worsening over the past one to two days. In the past 24 hours, he has developed non-bloody, non-bilious vomiting, and profuse, bloody diarrhea. Other complaints include malaise, fatigue, and headache. Earlier today, he was evaluated at the university's student health clinic where he was referred to the ED of your institution.

Chief complaint:	Fever.
Patient's medical history:	None.
Meds:	ibuprofen (400 mg approximately four hours prior to the visit to the ED).
Allergies:	acetaminophen (rash).
Family history:	His parents and two siblings are living and reportedly healthy.
Social history:	He attends a local university and is from the DRC (where he was visiting just prior to becoming ill). He denies drug use and is sexually active with one female partner.

Initial Scenario Conditions

Adult man, ambulatory on arrival.

Vital signs:	Temp 38.7 °C (101.2 °F), HR 132, RR 22, BP 93/61, SpO$_2$ 97% on room air.
General:	Well-developed but ill-appearing young adult man.
Head:	Atraumatic.
Eyes:	Pupils 3 mm bilaterally reactive to light, +conjunctival injection.
Mouth/throat:	Dry mucous membranes. Oropharynx without erythema, exudate, or petechiae.
Neck:	Supple, no meningismus.
Heart:	Tachycardic, regular rhythm; no murmurs, rubs, or gallops. Dorsalis pedis pulses 2+ bilaterally with capillary refill of two to three seconds.
Lungs:	Tachypneic, mildly increased work of breathing. Good air exchange without crackles, rhonchi, or wheezing.
Abdomen:	Atraumatic, non-distended. Bowel sounds are hyperactive. Tenderness to palpation diffusely, particular.rly over the epigastrium. No palpable organomegaly or mass. No rebound tenderness
Genitourinary:	Normal adult male external genitalia with descended, non-edematous, non-tender testicles without any palpable hernia.
Extremities:	No gross deformities, pitting edema, or focal tenderness.
Skin:	Warm, dry, without rash.
Neurologic:	Awake, alert, appropriate, without focal deficits.

Physical exam findings not available to your mannequin can be reported verbally if requested by the learners. For example, if your mannequin does not have the capability to demonstrate abdominal exam findings, they can be reported verbally.

See flow diagram (Figure 7.11) for additional scenario changes described.

Case Narrative, Continued

As described above, the patient is ill-appearing on presentation. However, he is not sufficiently toxic to preclude obtaining a complete history. If not asked by the interviewer, he adds that he has recently returned from the DRC. If asked to elaborate, the patient will add that he attended several gatherings of family and friends, one of which was a funeral for a distant relative whose cause of death remains unknown. There are no other sick contacts.

With knowledge of the patient's travel, the learners must immediately order the highest level of isolation, notify their institution's infection control program and the local health department, and don appropriate PPE.

All learners should perform an initial assessment, obtain IV/IO access, and initiate IV fluids. Additionally, learners should order appropriate diagnostic testing and observe for clinical decline (based on subsequent history, learners may request additional laboratory tests). If IV fluids are administered, the patient will improve temporarily. If IV fluids are not given, the patient's heart rate will increase, and he will ultimately develop frank hypotension, followed by cardiac arrest.

The case ends successfully when the patient is stabilized, and appropriate control measures are in place.

> Depending on the level of learner and specific objectives, demonstration of appropriate doffing of PPE could also be a learning objective and critical action.

Instructor Notes

Pathophysiology

- Based on its ability to cause widespread morbidity and mortality, Ebola and its related filoviruses represent an incredibly challenging public health crisis [1, 2].
- Transmitted through contact with mucous membranes or broken skin [2].
- Incubation period of approximately 8–12 days.

Clinical Features

- Nonspecific manifestations (particularly fever) [3].
- Within approximately one week of developing initial symptoms, vomiting and diarrhea emerge as predominant features [3, 4].
- Common signs and symptoms are as follows [2, 3]:
  - Fever.
  - Anorexia.
  - Weakness.

- Malaise.
- Dyspnea.
- Nausea and vomiting.
- Diarrhea.
- Abdominal pain.
- Myalgias.
- Conjunctival injection.
- Headache.
- Seizure.
- Unusual bleeding or hemorrhage (less common that previously reported).
- Hypoxemia.
- Seen in approximately half of patients with EVD treated in Europe and the United States [1].
  - Mortality often occurs one to two weeks after clinical illness begins.
  - Survivors often begin to recover within the first week, although full recovery may be lengthy [3].

Diagnosis

- High index of suspicion with suggestive clinical history in combination with travel history. For current advisories, review recommendations from the Centers for Disease Control and Prevention (see Selected Reading for Ebola).
- Testing for EVD is performed in cooperation with public health officials [5].

Management

- Fluid management:
  - Massive gastrointestinal losses often require up to 10 l of crystalloid per day [2, 4].
  - Monitor urine output and serum electrolytes, particularly sodium, potassium, calcium, magnesium [1].
- Airway/breathing:
  - Noncardiogenic pulmonary edema may require endotracheal intubation and mechanical ventilation [1, 6].
- Medications:
  - There is currently no vaccine or antiviral medication approved by the Food and Drug Administration (*FDA*).
  - Consider contacting the FDA for single-patient authorization of investigational drug(s) for EVD.
  - Mainstay of treatment is supportive care.

- Patients with concurrent septic shock may require vasopressors and broad-spectrum antibiotics [3, 4, 6].
- Isolation:
  - Extreme caution must be used to prevent contact with the patient, their bodily fluids, and any objects contaminated by bodily fluids [7].
  - Detailed information from the Centers for Disease Control and Prevention is available online [7].

Debriefing Plan

Plan for approximately 30 minutes for discussion.

Potential Questions for Discussion

- Where did the virus originate?
- How many people have been treated for EVD in the United States?
- How do I notify this facility's infection control program and the local health department if there is a suspected case of EVD?
- If I care for a patient with EVD, what is my risk of developing the disease?
- What is the current mortality rate for cases of EVD?
- Is there a current outbreak of EVD anywhere in the world?

REFERENCES FOR EBOLA

1. Uyeki, T.M., Mehta, A.K., Davey, R.T. Jr. et al. (2016). Clinical management of Ebola virus disease in the United States and Europe. *N. Engl. J. Med.* 374 (7): 636.
2. Baseler, L., Chertow, D.S., Johnson, K.M. et al. (2017). The pathogenesis of Ebola virus disease. *Annu. Rev. Pathol.* 12: 387.
3. Ebola virus disease (EVD) information for clinicians in U.S. healthcare settings. https://www.cdc.gov/vhf/ebola/clinicians/evd/clinicians.html (accessed 22 September 2020).
4. American Academy of Pediatrics (2015). Hemorrhagic fevers caused by filoviruses: Ebola and Marburg. In: *Red Book: 2015 Report of the Committee on Infectious Diseases*, 30e (eds. D.W. Kimberlin, M.T. Brady, M.A. Jackson and S.S. Long), 364–369. Elk Grove Village, IL: American Academy of Pediatrics.
5. Centers for Disease Control and Prevention (2016). Identify, isolate, inform: Emergency department evaluation and management for patients under investigation (PUIs) for Ebola virus disease (EVD). https://www.cdc.gov/vhf/ebola/clinicians/emergency-services/emergency-departments.html (accessed 3 September 2021).

6. Wolf, T., Kann, G., Becker, S. et al. (2015). Severe Ebola virus disease with vascular leakage and multiorgan failure: treatment of a patient in intensive care. *Lancet* 385: 1428–1435.

7. Centers for Disease Control and Prevention (2018). Infection prevention and control recommendations for hospitalized patients under investigation (PUIs) for Ebola virus disease (EVD) in US Hospitals. `https://www.cdc.gov/vhf/ebola/clinicians/evd/infection-control.html` (accessed 3 September 2021).

SELECTED READINGS FOR EBOLA

Centers for Disease Control and Prevention (2015). Ebola report: by the numbers. `https://www.cdc.gov/about/ebola/ebola-by-the-numbers.html` (accessed 3 September 2021).

Infectious Disease Society of America (2021). Ebola resources. `https://www.idsociety.org/public-health/ebola/ebola-resources` (accessed 3 September 2021).

APPENDIX

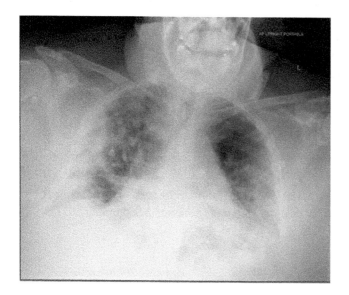

FIGURE 7.1 Chest x-ray with scattered opacities.

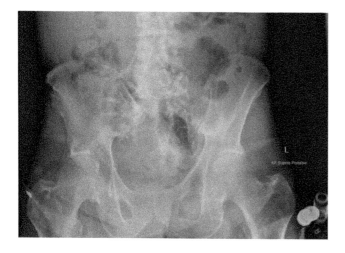

FIGURE 7.2 Abdominal x-ray (normal).

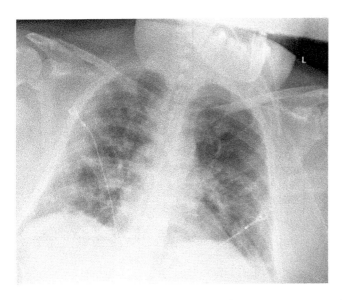

FIGURE 7.3 Post-intubation chest x-ray demonstrating appropriate endotracheal tube placement with bilateral infiltrates.

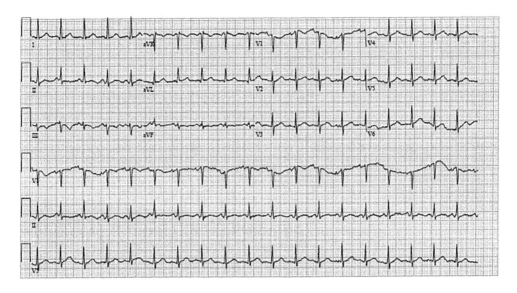

FIGURE 7.4 Electrocardiogram with sinus tachycardia and short PR interval.

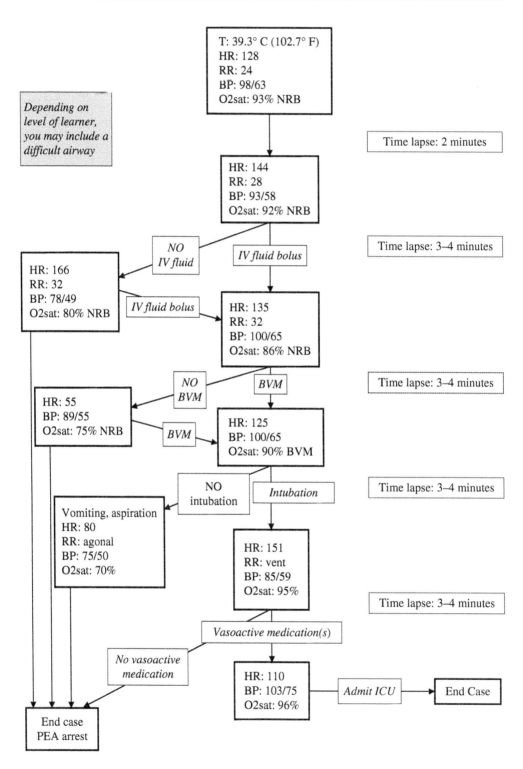

FIGURE 7.5   Flow diagram for sepsis.

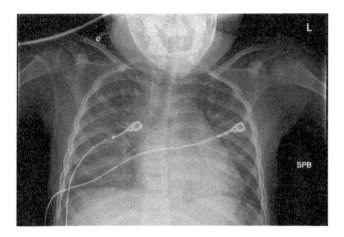

FIGURE 7.6   Chest x-ray preintubation, demonstrating bilateral streaking.

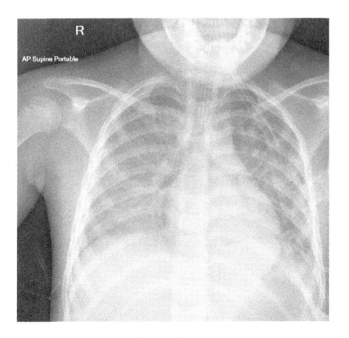

FIGURE 7.7   Post-intubation chest x-ray.

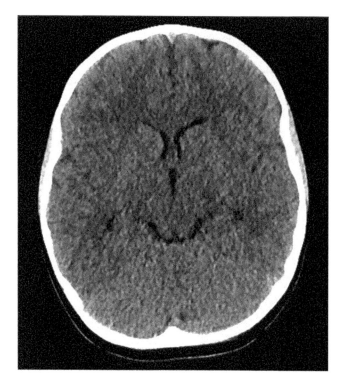

FIGURE 7.8   Computed tomography of the head without contrast.

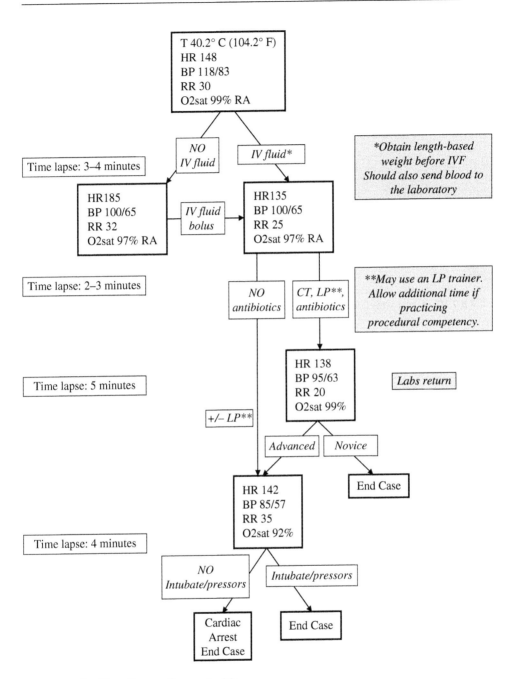

FIGURE 7.9   Flow diagram for meningitis.

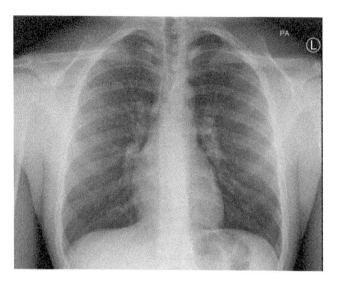

FIGURE 7.10   Chest x-ray (normal).

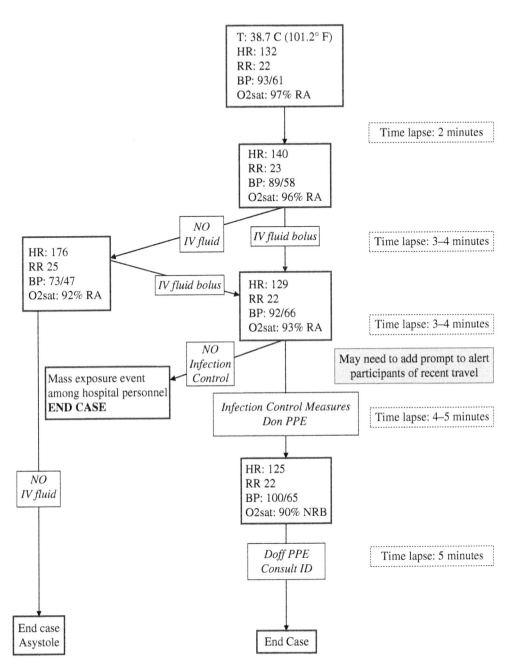

FIGURE 7.11 Flow diagram for Ebola.

TABLE 7.1 Arterial blood gas.

Test	Value	Reference range
pH	7.22	7.35–7.45
$PaCO_2$ (mmHg)	22	35–45
PaO_2 (mmHg)	70	75–100
Base excess (mmol/l)	−6	−3–3
Bicarbonate (mmol/l)	12	20–28
Hemoglobin O_2 (%)	94	94–99

TABLE 7.2 Complete blood count.

Test	Value	Reference range
White blood cells (× 10^9/l)	15.1	3–10
Hemoglobin (g/dl)	11.9	14–17
Hematocrit (%)	35.8	39–49
Platelets (× 10^9/l)	479	150–450
Mean corpuscular hemoglobin (fl)	76	80–100

TABLE 7.3 Chemistry panel.

Test	Value	Reference range
Sodium (mmol/l)	134	135–145
Potassium (mmol/l)	3.3	3.5–5.5
Chloride (mmol/l)	109	98–110
Carbon dioxide (mmol/l)	14	21–30
Blood urea nitrogen (mg/dl)	40	7–20
Creatinine (mg/dl)	1.8	0.6–1.2
Glucose (mg/dl)	242	70–140
Calcium (mg/dl)	9.7	8.7–10
Magnesium (mg/dl)	2.1	1.8–2.5
Phosphorus (mg/dl)	4.2	2.3–4.5

TABLE 7.4 Hepatic panel.

Test	Value	Reference range
Aspartate aminotransferase (iu/l)	35	15–40
Alanine aminotransferase (iu/l)	54	15–60
Bilirubin (mg/dl)	1.3	0.5–1.5
Alkaline phosphatase (iu/l)	88	25–100
Albumin	3.8	3.5–4.8
Total protein	6.5	6.2–8

TABLE 7.5 Lactate.

Test	Value	Reference range
Lactate (mmol/l)	4.8	0.5–2

TABLE 7.6 Coagulation panel.

Test	Value	Reference range
Prothrombin time (seconds)	16.2	9–13
International normalized ratio	1.4	0.9–1.1
Partial thromboplastin time (seconds)	36	27–37
Fibrinogen (mg/dl)	110	200–450
d-Dimer (ng)	875	< 500

TABLE 7.7 Blood type and screen.

Test	Value	Reference range
ABO Rh type	O positive	O, A, B, AB (positive, negative)
Antibody	Negative	Negative

TABLE 7.8   Urinalysis.

Test	Value	Reference range
Color	Amber	Colorless–dark yellow
Clarity	Cloudy	Clear
Specific gravity	1.035	1.005–1.030
Protein	2+	Negative
Glucose	1+	Negative
Ketones	2+	Negative
Blood	Trace	Negative
pH	5.4	5–8
Nitrite	Negative	Negative
Bilirubin	Negative	Negative
Urobilinogen (mg/dl)	0.4	0.2–1
Leukocyte esterase	Negative	Negative

TABLE 7.9   Point-of-care (fingerstick) glucose.

Test	Value	Reference range
Glucose (mg/dl)	72	70–140

TABLE 7.10   Complete blood count.

Test	Value	Reference range
White blood cells (× 10^9/l)	24	4–13
Hemoglobin (g/dl)	15	11–16
Hematocrit (%)	43.1	35–46
Platelets (× 109/l)	398	150–450
Mean corpuscular hemoglobin (fl)	92	80–100

TABLE 7.11 Differential white blood cell count.

Test	Value	Normal range
Segmented neutrophil (%)	78	25–50
Band (%)	14	0–5
Lymphocyte (%)	7	45–70
Monocyte (%)	1	1–10
Eosinophil (%)	0	0–10

TABLE 7.12 Chemistry panel.

Test	Value	Reference range
Sodium (mmol/l)	140	135–145
Potassium (mmol/l)	4.2	3.5–5.5
Chloride (mmol/l)	103	98–110
Carbon dioxide (mmol/l)	12	21–30
Blood urea nitrogen (mg/dl)	32	7–20
Creatinine (mg/dl)	1.1	0.4–0.8
Glucose (mg/dl)	83	70–140
Calcium (mg/dl)	9.9	8.7–10

TABLE 7.13 Table blood gas, arterial.

Test	Value	Reference range
pH	7.21	7.35–7.45
$PaCO_2$ (mmHg)	38	35–45
PaO_2 (mmHg)	88	75–100
Base excess (mmol/l)	7	−3–3
Bicarbonate (mmol/l)	10	20–28
Hemoglobin O_2	98	94–99

TABLE 7.14 Lactate.

Test	Value	Reference range
Lactate (mmol/l)	5.9	0.5–2

TABLE 7.15 Urinalysis.

Test	Value	Reference range
Color	Dark yellow	Colorless–dark yellow
Clarity	Turbid	Clear
Specific gravity	1.040	1.005–1.030
Protein	2+	Negative
Glucose	Negative	Negative
Ketones	2+	Negative
Blood	Negative	Negative
pH	6	5–8
Nitrite	Negative	Negative
Bilirubin	Negative	Negative
Urobilogen (mg/dl)	0.3	0.2–1
Leukocyte esterase	Negative	Negative

TABLE 7.16 Rapid streptococcal test.

Test	Value	Reference range
Streptococcal antigen	Negative	Negative

TABLE 7.17 Rapid influenza test.

Test	Value	Reference range
Influenza	Negative	Negative

TABLE 7.18 Point-of-care (fingerstick) glucose.

Test	Value	Reference range
Glucose (mg/dl)	65	70–140

TABLE 7.19 Arterial blood gas.

Test	Value	Reference range
pH	7.14	7.35–7.45
$PaCO_2$ (mmHg)	30	35–45
PaO_2 (mmol/l)	90	75–100
Base excess (mmol/l)	5	−3–3
Bicarbonate (mmol/l)	15	20–28
Hemoglobin O_2 (%)	96	94–99

TABLE 7.20 Complete blood count.

Test	Value	Reference range
White blood cells (× 10⁹/l)	2.1	3–10
Hemoglobin (g/dl)	11.8	14–17
Hematocrit (%)	35	39–49
Platelets (× 10⁹/l)	147	150–450
Mean corpuscular hemoglobin (fl)	85	80–100

TABLE 7.21 Differential white blood cell count.

Test	Value	Reference range
Segmented neutrophil (%)	60	25–50
Band (%)	5	0–5
Lymphocyte (%)	15	45–70
Monocyte (%)	15	1–10
Eosinophil (%)	5	0–10

TABLE 7.22 Chemistry panel (including magnesium).

Test	Value	Reference range
Sodium (mmol/l)	133	135–145
Potassium (mmol/l)	4.4	3.5–5.5
Chloride (mmol/l)	110	98–110
Carbon dioxide (mmol/l)	12	21–30
Blood urea nitrogen (mg/dl)	34	7–20
Creatinine (mg/dl)	1.4	0.6–1.2
Glucose (mg/dl)	68	70–140
Calcium (mg/dl)	8.2	8.7–10
Magnesium (mg/dl)	1.5	1.7–2.2

TABLE 7.23 Hepatic panel.

Test	Value	Reference range
Aspartate aminotransferase (iu/l)	642	15–40
Alanine aminotransferase (iu/l)	445	15–60
Bilirubin (mg/dl)	1.7	0.5–1.5
Alkaline phosphatase (iu/l)	102	25–100
Albumin (g/dl)	3.2	3.5–4.8
Protein, total (g/dl)	5.9	6.2–8

TABLE 7.24 Lactate.

Test	Value	Reference range
Lactate (mmol/l)	6.9	0.5–2

TABLE 7.25 Coagulation panel.

Test	Value	Reference range
Prothrombin time (seconds)	16	9–13
International normalized ratio	1.3	0.9–1.1
Partial thromboplastin time (seconds)	49	27–37
Fibrinogen (mg/dl)	112	200–450
d-Dimer (ng)	884	< 500

TABLE 7.26 Blood type and screen.

Test	Value	Reference range
ABO Rh type	A negative	O, A, B, AB (positive, negative)
Antibody	Negative	Negative

TABLE 7.27 Urinalysis.

Test	Value	Reference range
Color	Dark yellow	Colorless–dark yellow
Clarity	Cloudy	Clear
Specific gravity	1.038	1.005–1.030
Protein	1+	Negative
Glucose	Negative	Negative
Ketones	2+	Negative
Blood	2+	Negative
pH	7.3	5–8
Nitrite	Negative	Negative
Bilirubin	Negative	Negative
Urobilinogen (mg/dl)	0.4	0.2–1
Leukocyte esterase	Negative	Negative

CHAPTER 8

Nontraumatic Musculoskeletal Emergencies

Andrew Ortega and Nur-Ain Nadir

Department of Emergency Medicine, Kaiser Permanente Modesto Medical Center, Modesto, CA, USA

RHABDOMYOLYSIS

Educational Goals

Learning Objectives

1. Identify risk factors for rhabdomyolysis (MK, PC).
2. Evaluate for rhabdomyolysis by ordering a creatine kinase (*CK*) (MK, PC).
3. Identify the clinical features of compartment syndrome (MK, PC).
4. Demonstrate appropriate consultation with nephrology for acute renal failure secondary to severe rhabdomyolysis (MK, PC, ICS).
5. Demonstrate appropriate consultation with a surgical specialist for fasciotomy (MK, PC, ICS).

Critical Actions Checklist

☐ Obtain appropriate intravenous (IV) access (2 large-bore cannulas) (PC).
☐ Obtain pertinent history from emergency medical services (EMS) and family (ICS, P).

Emergency Medicine Simulation Workbook: A Tool for Bringing the Curriculum to Life, Second Edition. Edited by Traci L. Thoureen and Sara B. Scott.
© 2022 John Wiley & Sons Ltd. Published 2022 by John Wiley & Sons Ltd.
Companion website: www.wiley.com/go/thoureen/simulation/workbook2e

☐ Appropriately treat pain (PC, MK).
☐ Order a CK level (PC, MK).
☐ Initiate IV fluids with at least one liter of 0.9% saline (PC, MK).
☐ Perform compartment pressure measurement (MK, PC).
☐ Consult vascular/orthopedic surgery (ICS, P, SBP).

Simulation Set-Up

Environment: May begin on scene at apartment (for prehospital learners) and transitions to the emergency department (ED). Alternatively, may start in an ED treatment room.

Mannequin: Male simulator mannequin in clothing. The patient has track marks moulaged on bilateral arms and feet, this can be done with make-up.

Props: To be displayed on plasma screen/computer screen or printed out on handouts in scenario room when asked for/return from lab:

- Images (see online component for *Rhabdomyolysis*, Scenario 8.1, at https://www.wiley.com/go/thoureen/simulation/workbook2e):
  - Right tibia fibula x-ray (normal) (Figure 8.1).
  - Right knee x-ray (normal) (Figure 8.2).
  - Chest x-ray (normal) (Figure 8.3).
  - Computed tomography (CT) of the head (representative slice, normal) (Figure 8.4).
- Laboratory tests (see online component as above):
  - Complete blood count (Table 8.1).
  - Complete metabolic panel (Table 8.2).
  - Lactate (Table 8.3).
  - Creatine kinase (Table 8.4).
  - Arterial blood gas (Table 8.5).
  - Urinalysis (Table 8.6).
  - Urine microscopy (Table 8.7).
  - Urine drug test (Table 8.8).

Available supplies:

- Basic airway and code cart.
- Medications:
  - Liter bags of 0.9% and/or lactated Ringer's solution (*LR*).
  - Pre-labeled syringes:

- Analgesic medication.
- Tetanus toxoid.
- Procedure tray with handheld intracompartmental pressure monitoring device, betadine, chlorhexidine, scalpel, and gauze (optional). An orange can be used as an inexpensive trainer for the procedure.

Distractor: None.

Actors

- Patient voice is male. Patient should sound lethargic. He complains of pain in his right leg. He is able to follow commands and answer questions.
- EMS may be an actor or another learner.
- Patient's parent is able to provide history of the initial presentation of the patient and pertinent medical history, but is unaware of the patient's drug use.
- ED nurse can administer medications/fluids. The nurse does have medical knowledge and may cue learners if needed.
- Nephrology, vascular surgery, and orthopedic surgery available via telephone consultation.

Case Narrative

Scenario Background

A 22-year-old man is brought in by EMS after his parents went to his apartment and found him passed out in a chair. The parent had last spoken to him last night, and reports he was studying for an exam this week. The parent called this morning and when he did not answer, they went to his apartment. Patient was unresponsive and his parent called 911. The patient is now responsive. EMS reports that they administered naloxone en route. The patient is complaining of right leg pain.

Chief complaint:	Decreased responsiveness.
Patient's medical history:	None.
Medications:	None.
Allergies:	None.
Family history:	Hypertension in father.
Social history:	Alcohol on the weekends. No tobacco. Tried heroin at a party a month ago and use has been increasing to three to four times a week.

Initial Scenario Conditions

Young man brought in by EMS sleepy, but responsive. Patient is moaning in pain.

> Case may start with EMS receiving this case on scene and performing their objectives to initiate treatment and transport. Patient exam will show 2 mm pupils.
>
>   Alternatively, case background may be presented prior to case as an EMS medical consult or by EMS on arrival.

Vital signs:	Temp 97.7°F (36.5°C), HR 100, RR 18, BP 116/88, SpO_2 100% on room air.
General:	Lying on bed moaning.
HEENT:	Head is atraumatic. Pupils 4 mm and reactive.
Neck:	Supple, full range of motion.
Cardiovascular:	Tachycardic and regular, no palpable pulse in right lower extremity.
Lungs:	Tachypneic, lungs clear.
Abdomen:	Abdomen, soft and nondistended. Diminished bowel sounds.
Extremities:	No gross deformities, right lower extremity extremely tender to palpation. If the learner asks, the calf feels firm to palpation.
Skin:	No rashes. Track marks in antecubital regions and bilateral feet noted.
Neurologic:	Sleepy, slow to respond, but appropriate, Glasgow Coma Scale score is 15.

> Physical exam findings not available on your mannequin can be reported verbally if asked for by learners; for example, if your mannequin is unable to simulate differential pulses, you can report this finding verbally when the learner performs the pertinent portion of the exam.

See flow diagram (Figure 8.5) for further scenario changes described below.

Case Narrative, Continued

Learners of all levels (EMS, students and postgraduate learners) should perform a primary survey, obtain appropriate IV access, and appropriately administer IV fluids and pain medication. Prehospital learners should identify the need for naloxone in the field. Failure to obtain pertinent history or to provide naloxone by EMS, will result in decompensation with respiratory decline and/or pulseless electrical activity arrest. All other learners should obtain pertinent history of naloxone given prior to arrival and order appropriate labs and imaging.

  Following appropriate initial management, there is an initial period of stabilization. During this time, any ordered imaging/labs return. The case may end here with consultation of nephrology for student learners.

For advanced learners, after diagnostics return, the patient begins to complain of severe pain. Despite adequate pain medication the patient continues to have worsening pain. Learners should identify pain out of proportion and consider use of intracompartmental pressure monitoring. If they do not recognize that the pain represents compartment syndrome, the nurse can prompt them, saying, "Doctor, why is this patient in so much pain?" If they still do not recognize the problem, the nurse can say, "His foot feels cool and I can't feel a pulse." After compartment syndrome is recognized, learners should consult vascular/orthopedic surgery. Optionally, learners may also obtain intracompartmental pressure measurement using an orange as a trainer.

The case ends when the patient is stabilized and dispositioned to the operating room for fasciotomy.

Instructor Notes

Etiologies

- Traumatic or muscle compression:
  - Crush syndrome.
  - Prolonged acute immobilization.
  - Restraints or abuse.
  - High-voltage electrical injury.
- Nontraumatic and exertional:
  - Deconditioned individual with subsequent prolonged exertion.
  - Exertion in extremely hot, humid conditions.
  - Impaired normal heat loss.
  - Increased metabolic demand:
    - Seizures.
    - Psychotic agitation.
    - Amphetamine overdose.
- Nontraumatic and nonexertional:
  - Drugs:
    - Alcohol.
    - Opioids.
    - Statins.
    - Volatile anesthetics.
  - Toxins:
    - Metabolic poisons (cyanide).
    - Snake venom.
    - Insect venom.
    - Mushrooms poisoning.

- Infections.
- Electrolyte disorders.
- Endocrine disorders.

Pathophysiology

- Condition of muscle necrosis causing:
  - Increased intracellular ionized calcium.
  - ATP depletion.
  - Myocyte injury and death:
    - Release of cytotoxic chemicals.
    - Capillary leak → third spacing of fluids.
    - Acidosis and electrolyte abnormalities.
  - Renal tubule injury results from myoglobin, acidosis and hypovolemia.

Clinical Features

- Characteristic triad of muscle pain, weakness, and dark urine.
- If rhabdomyolysis is severe, patient may also complain of:
  - Malaise
  - Fever
  - Dysrhythmias
  - Nausea and vomiting
  - Abdominal pain
  - Oliguria/anuria.
- If compartment syndrome present:
  - Tense wood-like feeling of affected extremity/compartment.
  - The five Ps:
    - Pain out of proportion of exam.
    - Pulselessness.
    - Paresthesia.
    - Paralysis.
    - Pallor.
- Laboratory abnormalities may include:
  - Elevated serum creatine kinase.
  - Elevated serum and/or urine myoglobin.
  - Electrolyte abnormalities:
    - Hyperkalemia.
    - Hyperphosphatemia.

- Hypocalcemia.
- Metabolic acidosis: elevated anion gap may be present.
- Hyperuricemia
- Elevated creatinine
- Elevated alanine aminotransferase and aspartate aminotransferase.
- Findings suggestive of disseminated intravascular coagulation:
  - Decreased platelets.
  - Elevated prothrombin time, partial prothromboplastin time, and international normalized ratio.
  - Schistocytes.
- Hematuria on urine dipstick with only 0–5 red blood cells/high power field on urine microscopy:
  - May indicate myoglobinuria.

Diagnosis

Elevated creatine kinase > 5 times upper limit of normal.

Management

- Fluid management: isotonic solution:
  - Initiate 1–2 l/hour.
  - Maintenance to establish urine output of 200–300 ml/hour.
- Medications:
  - Analgesics.
  - Sodium bicarbonate:
    - Use in patients with a creatine kinase > 5000
    - 130 mEq/l (150 ml of 8.4% sodium bicarbonate in 1 l of water) at an infusion rate of 200 ml/hour until urine pH is > 6.5.
    - Arterial pH should be monitored every two hours.
    - Discontinue bicarbonate if pH > 7.5.
    - Do not administer if hypocalcemia present or serum bicarbonate > 30.
  - Diuretics:
    - Mannitol and loop diuretics have not been proven to have any significant benefit [1].
- Consultation:
  - Nephrology for fluid management and acute kidney injury.
  - Surgical specialty for compartment syndrome (if p:resent).
  - Compartment pressure measurement (typically measured with a manometer):

- 15–20 mmHg requires serial intracompartmental pressure measurements.
- 20–30 mmHg should be admitted and the surgical team should be consulted.
- >30 mmHg suggests compartment syndrome and need for fasciotomy.

Debriefing Plan

Plan for approximately 30 minutes for discussion.

Potential Questions for Discussion

- How do you diagnose a patient with rhabdomyolysis?
- What is the appropriate fluid management in a patient with severe rhabdomyolysis?
- What are the signs and symptoms of compartment syndrome?
- What is the diagnostic criteria for compartment syndrome?

REFERENCE FOR RHABDOMYOLYSIS

1. Chavez, L.O., Leon, M., Einav, S., and Varon, J. (2016). Beyond muscle destruction: a systematic review of rhabdomyolysis for clinical practice. *Crit. Care* 20 (1): 135.

SELECTED READINGS FOR RHABDOMYOLYSIS

Cone, J. and Inaba, K. (2017). Lower extremity compartment syndrome. *Trauma Surg. Acute Care Open* 2 (1): e000094.

Huerta-Alardín, A.L., Varon, J., and Marik, P.E. (2005). Bench-to-bedside review: rhabdomyolysis – an overview for clinicians. *Crit. Care* 9 (2): 158–169.

McMillan, T.E., Gardner, W.T., Schmidt, A.H., and Johnstone, A.J. (2019). Diagnosing acute compartment syndrome-where have we got to? *Int. Orthop.* 43 (11): 2429–2435.

SLIPPED CAPITAL FEMORAL EPIPHYSIS

Educational Goals

Learning Objectives

1. Identify the risk factors for slipped capital femoral epiphysis (*SCFE*) (MK, PC).
2. Evaluate for SCFE (MK, PC).
3. Demonstrate appropriate dosing of analgesia in a pediatric patient (MK, PC).
4. Discuss management with orthopedic surgery (PC, ICS, P).
5. Discuss the diagnosis and management plan to parent (P, PC, and ICS).
6. Demonstrate effective communication with an agitated parent. (P, ICS).

Critical Actions Checklist

☐ Obtain pertinent history from parent (ICS, P).
☐ Administer adequate analgesic medication (PC, MK).
☐ Identify SCFE on hip x-ray (MK, PC).
☐ Consult orthopedic surgery (ICS, P, SBP).

Simulation Set-Up

Environment: ED exam room.

Mannequin: Male pediatric simulator mannequin (elementary-aged size), in a hospital gown. Obesity can be moulaged with a pediatric obesity suit such as the SimUSuit®.

Props: To be displayed on plasma screen/computer screen or printed out on handouts in scenario room when asked for/return from lab:

- Images (see online component for SCFE, Scenario 10.2 at https://www.wiley.com/go/thoureen/simulation/workbook2e):
  - Right hip x-ray showing SCFE (Figure 8.6).
  - Right knee x-ray (normal) (Figure 8.7).
- Laboratory tests (see online component as above):
  - Complete blood count (Table 8.9).
  - Basic metabolic panel (Table 8.10).
  - Urinalysis (Table 8.11).
  - Erythrocyte sedimentation rate (Table 8.12).
  - C-reactive protein (Table 8.13).

Available supplies:

- Basic airway and code cart
- Medications:
  - Liter bags of 0.9% saline and/or LR.
  - Labeled syringes:
    - Analgesic medication (e.g. ketorolac, fentanyl, morphine).
    - *Distractor:* If the patient does not receive appropriate analgesia the parent will become more insistent and upset and insist on pain control for patient.

Actors

- Patient voice is male. He should be alert and complaining of pain.
- Parent is agitated about the amount of pain his/her son is in and becomes verbally aggressive if his pain is not addressed.
- ED nurse can administer medications/fluids. The nurse does have medical knowledge and may cue learners if needed.
- Orthopedic surgery available via telephone consultation.

Case Narrative

Scenario Background

A 10-year-old boy is brought in by a parent. He is complaining of right knee pain for the past 5 days. Parent states that the patient was recently diagnosed with "strep throat" two weeks ago. He had taken all his antibiotics as prescribed and had improved. Over the past five days, he began to have progressive right knee pain after visiting a trampoline park with friends. He has not had fever or rash.

Chief complaint:	Right knee pain.
Patient's medical history:	On calorie restricted diet by pediatric dietician. (Mom will answer for patient about medical history "his only problem has been his weight; he is overweight and the dietician has asked us to watch his diet closely").
Medications:	None.
Allergies:	None.
Family history:	Obesity and diabetes in father and mother.
Social history:	fourth-grade student, no recreational drug use, no smoking or alcohol.

Initial Scenario Conditions

Young obese boy brought in with moderate pain, but acting appropriately.

Vital signs:	Temp 100.2°F (37.9°C), HR 115, RR 22, BP 106/74, SpO$_2$ 99% on room air.
Weight:	47 kg.
General:	Awake, alert.
HEENT:	Head is atraumatic, Pupils 3 mm and reactive. Normal pharynx.
Neck:	Supple, full range of motion.
Cardiovascular:	Regular rate rhythm, normal symmetric distal pulses.
Lungs:	Normal effort, lungs clear.
Abdomen:	Abdomen soft, nondistended, no hernias.
Extremities:	Right knee normal range of motion, no tenderness on palpation, no effusion, no erythema. Pain with movement of right hip with moderate tenderness to palpation.
Skin:	No rashes.
Neurologic:	Alert and appropriate. Sensation intact distally.

Physical exam findings not available on your mannequin can be reported verbally if asked for by learners; for example, if you do not have an obesity suit for your mannequin, you can report this finding to the learners when they ask about the general appearance of the patient.

See flow diagram (Figure 8.8) for further scenario changes described.

Case Narrative, Continued

Learners of all levels (EMS, students and postgraduate learners) should initially perform a primary survey, obtain appropriate IV access, and administer pain medication. Appropriate studies should be ordered.

Following appropriate initial assessment and pain management, there is an initial period of stabilization. During this time, any ordered imaging/lab results return. The case may end here with correct recognition of SCFE and consultation of orthopedic surgery for junior learners and students.

For advanced learners, after approximately three minutes, pain can worsen, causing the parent to become agitated. The parent can make statements like "My child is in pain, this is absolutely unacceptable, I want to talk to a supervisor." The acknowledgment of parental concern, in conjunction with reassurance and adequate pain management, will resolve the parent's agitation.

The case ends when the patient is stabilized and orthopedic surgery is consulted for admission.

Instructor Notes

Pathophysiology

- Displacement of a portion of the proximal femur distal to the physis (growth plate).
- Occurs when shearing forces applied to the femoral head exceed the strength of the capital femoral physis.
- Most often idiopathic.
- May be associated with certain endocrine disorders:
  - Hypothyroidism.
  - Hyperthyroidism.
  - Growth hormone deficiency.

Epidemiology

- Most common hip pathology in adolescents and pre-adolescents.
- Risk factors:
  - Obesity.
  - Male sex.
  - Recent growth spurt.
  - Radiation therapy.

Clinical Features

- Pain in the hip, groin, thigh or knee.
- May have altered gait.

Diagnosis

Imaging:
- Plain radiographs – x-ray hip:
  - Bilateral AP and lateral (frog leg) view (abnormalities most easily seen on lateral view).
  - Posterior displacement of femoral epiphysis (ice cream slipping off of a cone).
  - Widening and irregularity of the physis, with thinning of the proximal epiphysis (early change)
- CT:
  - Useful for chronic slips.
- Magnetic resonance imaging (*MRI*):
  - Useful if normal x-ray but clinical suspicion is high.
  - May show widening of physis with edema (diagnostic of disease)

Management

- Pain management:
  - Oral/IV analgesia.
  - Fascia iliaca nerve block.
- Consult orthopedic surgery:
  - Operative stabilization
  - Non-weight-bearing while awaiting definitive management.

Debriefing Plan

Plan for approximately 30 minutes for discussion.

Potential Questions for Discussion

- What are risk factors for SCFE?
- What is the differential diagnosis for pediatric hip/knee pain?
- What are imaging findings associated with SCFE?

SELECTED READINGS FOR SLIPPED CAPITAL FEMORAL EPIPHYSIS

Green, D.W., Reynolds, R.A.K., Khan, S.N., and Tolo, V. (2005). The delay in diagnosis of slipped capital femoral epiphysis: a review of 102 patients. *HSS J.* 1: 103–106.

Millis, M.B. (2017). SCFE: clinical aspects, diagnosis, and classification. *J. Child Orthop.* 11 (2): 93–98.

Mooney, J.F. et al. (2005). Management of unstable/acute slipped capital femoral epiphysis: : results of a survey of the POSNA membership. *J. Pediatr. Orthop.* 25: 2, 162–166.

CAUDA EQUINA SYNDROME

Educational Goals

Learning Objectives

1. Recognize risk factors for cauda equina syndrome (MK, PC).
2. Perform pertinent physical exam for evaluation of lower back pain (MK, PC).
3. Recognize the clinical features of urinary retention and use a bladder scan or foley catheter for diagnosis appropriately (MK, PC).
4. Discuss with a spine surgeon for emergent decompression (MK, PC, and ICS).

Critical Actions Checklist

☐ Obtain pertinent history from patient (PC, MK, ICS).
☐ Administer appropriate pain control (PC, MK).
☐ Perform/request a full neurological exam, including reflexes in the lower extremities (PC, MK).
☐ Perform/order bladder scan/ultrasound to evaluate for urinary retention (PC, MK).
☐ Order emergent MRI of the lumbar spine (MK, PC).
☐ Consult a spine surgeon (depending on the protocol at your institution) (ICS, P).

> Physical exam findings not available on your mannequin can be reported verbally if asked for by learners; for example, for reflexes, you can report this finding verbally when the learner performs or asks about the pertinent portion of the exam.

Simulation Set-Up

Environment: ED treatment room.

Mannequin: Male adult simulator mannequin, in hospital gown.

Props: To be displayed on plasma screen/computer screen or printed out on handouts in scenario room when asked for/return from lab:

- Images (see online component for cauda equina, Scenario 8.3 at https://www.wiley.com/go/thoureen/simulation/workbook2e):
  - Lumbar x-ray (normal) (Figure 8.9).
  - MRI lumbar spine report stating cauda equina compression (Figure 8.10).
- Laboratory tests (see online component as above):
  - Complete blood count (Table 8.14).

- Basic metabolic panel (Table 8.15).
- Urinalysis (Table 8.16).
- Erythrocyte sedimentation rate (Table 8.17).
- C-reactive protein (Table 8.18).

Available supplies:

- Basic airway and code cart.
- Medications:
  - Liter bags of 0.9% saline and/or LR.
  - Pre-labeled syringes:
    - Analgesic medication (e.g. fentanyl, morphine).
- Foley catheter bag filled with 1500 ml yellow fluid

Distractor: None

Actors

- Patient voice is male. The patient should be distressed secondary to pain. He is agitated when answering questions.
- EMS may be an actor or another learner
- ED nurse can administer medications/fluids. The nurse does have medical knowledge and may cue learners if needed.
- Spinal surgeon available via telephone consultation.

Case Narrative

Scenario Background

A 54-year-old man is brought in by EMS. The patient states that he has been having some trouble urinating. He saw his doctor yesterday, and was told it was likely due to benign prostatic hypertrophy. He has also been feeling like his legs have been weak over the past two weeks and he has been having difficulty walking; this has gotten significantly worse since last night. He reports that his chronic back pain has significantly worsened over the past 24 hours.

Chief complaint:	Trouble urinating, back pain.
Patient's medical history:	Chronic back pain and benign prostatic hypertrophy.
Medications:	Tamsulosin.
Allergies:	None.
Family history:	Coronary artery disease in mother.
Social history:	None.

Initial Scenario Conditions

Middle-aged man brought in moaning due to pain.

Vital signs: Temp 98.9°F (37.2°C), HR 106, RR 16, BP 148/88, SpO$_2$ 99% on room air.
General: Alert.
HEENT: Head is atraumatic, pupils 4 mm, reactive.
Neck: Supple, full range of motion.
Cardiovascular: Tachycardic and regular, palpable pulses in lower extremities.
Lungs: Clear.
Abdomen: Abdomen soft, with suprapubic distention and moderate guarding/tenderness.
Extremities: No gross deformities.
Skin: No rashes.
Back: Midline tenderness to palpation of lumbar-sacral spine. No deformities or step-offs palpated. No erythema, warmth noted.
Neurologic: Oriented. 3/5 strength of the bilateral lower extremities, 0/4 bilateral patella and ankle reflexes. Diminished rectal tone and sensation. No anal wink.

> Learners should specifically ask for each individual component of the exam, specifically regarding the neurologic exam. Physical exam findings not available on your mannequin can be reported verbally if asked for by learners; for example, If you mannequin cannot simulate reflexes or motor, you can verbally report the exam when it is requested.

See flow diagram (Figure 8.11) for further scenario changes described.

Case Narrative, Continued

Learners of all levels (EMS, students and postgraduate learners) should initially perform a primary survey, obtain appropriate IV access, and appropriately administer pain medication. Failure to appropriately manage the patient's pain will lead to agitation of the patient and the patient will refuse to participate in further history or exam.

Appropriate labs and imaging should be ordered. Following analgesic administration, there is some improvement of vital signs.

If urinary retention is not identified, the patient becomes agitated and complains of trouble urinating. The patient will begin to have worsening urinary retention with suprapubic pain requiring urinary catheter placement. The MRI technician may prompt learners regarding increasing abdominal pain preventing completion of MRI, if urinary catheter is not requested. After urinary catheter placement, the MRI report will return.

If the learner does not consult with spine surgery, the patient will start to cue consultation by asking probing questions of the learners: "Will this ever get better? Will I be able to urinate without a catheter? Is there someone who can fix this?"

The case ends when the patient is stabilized and spine surgery has been consulted.

Instructor Notes

Pathophysiology

- The cauda equina consists of 18 nerve roots.
- Cauda equina syndrome is caused by loss of function of two or more of the 18 nerve roots.
- Typical causes include:
  - Disc disease (most common cause).
  - Malignancy.
  - Spinal trauma.
  - Spinal stenosis.
  - Infection.

Clinical Features

- Back pain:
Radicular pain may reflect dorsal nerve involvement.
  - Urinary incontinence/ retention:
> 500 ml is > 90% sensitive for the diagnosis.
  - Neurologic deficits:
    - Usually bilateral symptoms/signs.
    - Depends on spinal level of nerve root compression.
    - Loss of strength:
      - May affect hip, knee, ankle, toe flexion or extension.
      - Bladder and rectal sphincter paralysis:
      - Reflects involvement of S3–S5 nerve roots.
      - Correlates to urinary retention and bowel incontinence.
    - Loss of reflexes:
      - Achilles tendon, patellar tendon, bulbocavernosus or anal wink.
    - Sensory loss:
      - Classically in the perineal distribution ("saddle anesthesia").

Diagnosis

Imaging:
- Lumbar spine x-ray

- • Typically n.ormal
- • MRI:
- • Typically non-contrast.
  - • If infectious etiology is suspected IV contrast may be required.
  - • Demonstrates compression of the cauda equina.
- • CT myelogram:
  - • Indicated for patients with contraindications for MRI.
  - • Invasive procedure requiring injection of contrast into the subarachnoid space.

Management

- • Pain management.
- • Urinary catheter placement:
  - • If urinary retention present.
- • High-dose steroids:
  - • May be indicated for metastatic or malignant lesions.
- • Consultation of spine surgeon for operative management.

Debriefing Plan

Plan for approximately 30 minutes for discussion.

Potential Questions for Discussion

- • What are the causes of cauda equina syndrome? What is the most common cause?
- • What are possible exam abnormalities for a patient with cauda equina syndrome?
- • What is imaging modality of choice for evaluation of cauda equina syndrome?
- • What is the management of cauda equina syndrome?

SELECTED READINGS FOR CAUDA EQUINA SYNDROME

Chamberlain, M.C. (2012). Neoplastic meningitis and metastatic epidural spinal cord compression. *Hematol. Oncol. Clin. North Am.* 26 (4): 917–931.

Heyes, G., Jones, M., Verzin, E. et al. (2018). Influence of timing of surgery on cauda equina syndrome: outcomes at a national spinal centre. *J. Orthop.* 5 (1): 210–215.

Jailoh, I. and Minhas, P. (2007). Delays in the treatment of cauda equina syndrome due to its variable clinical features in patients presenting to the emergency department. *Emerg. Med. J.* 24: 33–34.

Seecharan, D. and Arnold, P. (2014). Spinal cord injuries and syndromes. In: *Textbook of the Cervical Spine* (eds. F. Shen, D. Samartzis and R. Fessler), 192–196. Philadelphia, PA: Saunders.

APPENDIX

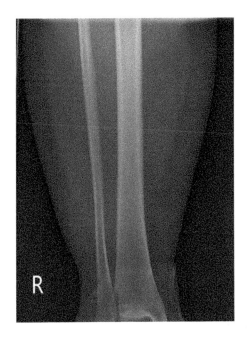

FIGURE 8.1   Right tibia/fibula x-ray (normal).

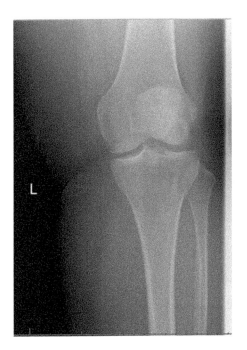

FIGURE 8.2   Right knee x-ray (normal).

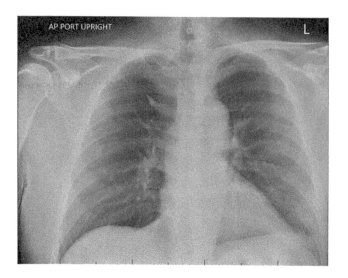

FIGURE 8.3   Chest x-ray (normal).

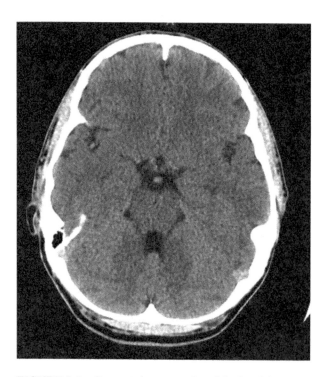

FIGURE 8.4   Computed tomography of the head (representative slice, normal).

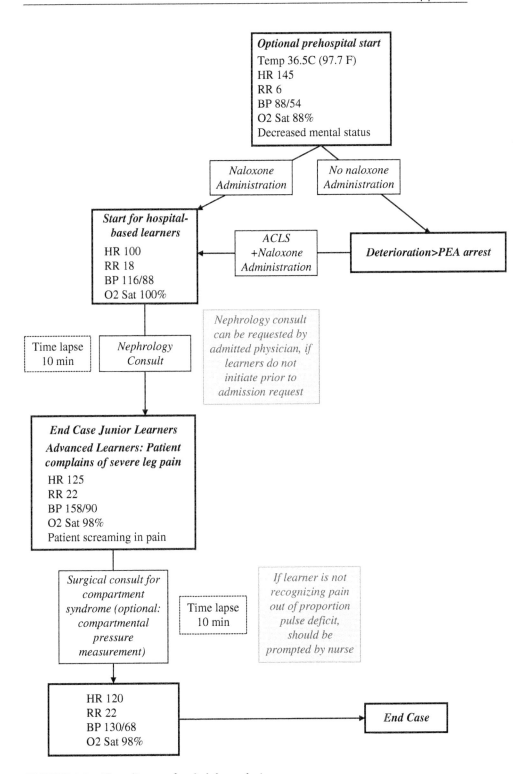

FIGURE 8.5 Flow diagram for rhabdomyolysis.

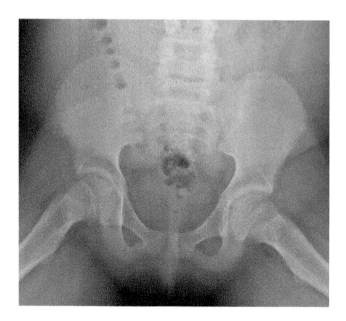

FIGURE 8.6   Right hip x-ray showing slipped capital femoral epiphysis.

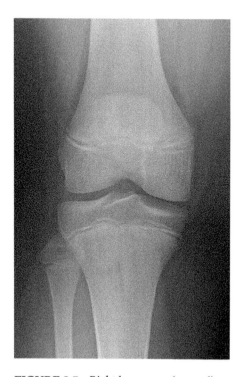

FIGURE 8.7   Right knee x-ray (normal).

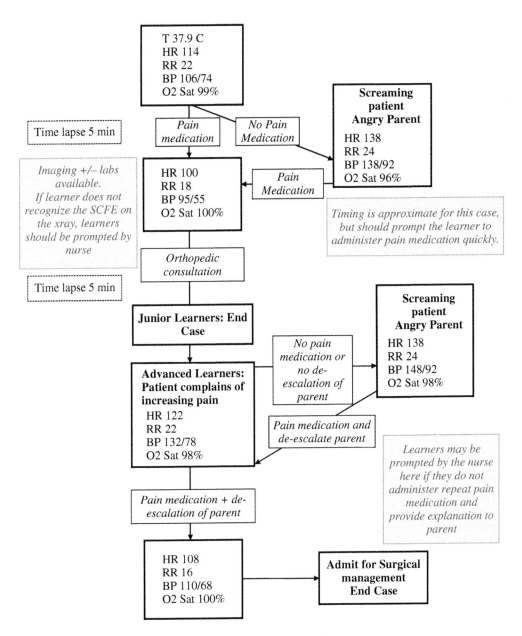

FIGURE 8.8 Flow diagram for slipped capital femoral epiphysis.

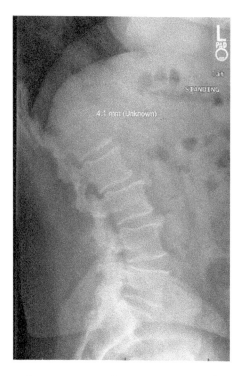

FIGURE 8.9   Lumbar x-ray (normal).

Lumbar MRI Report

Impression:
1. Multilevel degenerative changes including disc osteophyte complexes and facet and ligamentum flavum hypertrophy. The findings contribute to mild spinal canal stenosis at L1-L2. Mild multilevel neural foraminal narrowing.

2. Severe right paracentral disc extrusion at the L3-L5 causing compression of the cauda equina. Findings consistent with cauda equina syndrome. Recommend spinal surgery consultation.

FIGURE 8.10   Magnetic resonance imaging report, which states cauda equina compression.

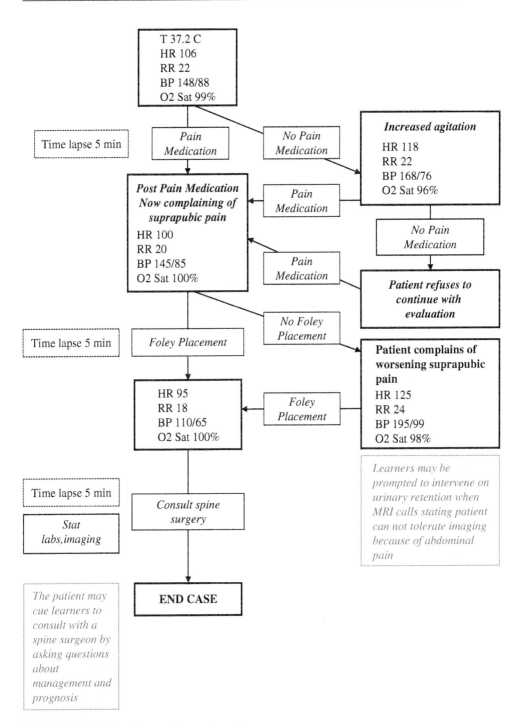

FIGURE 8.11   Flow diagram for cauda equina.

TABLE 8.1 Complete blood count.

Test	Values	Reference range
White blood cell count (× 10 000/μl)	18.00	4.8–10.8
Hemoglobin (g/dl)	9.4	12.6–17.4
Hematocrit (%)	18.7	37.0–51.0
Platelets (× 10³/μl)	245	130–400

TABLE 8.2 Complete metabolic panel.

Test	Value	Reference range
Sodium (mmol/l)	135	136–136
Potassium (mmol/l)	5.5	3.5–5.0
Chloride (mmol/l)	106	95–110
Bicarbonate	15	22–26
Blood urea nitrogen (mg/dl)	60	8–21
Creatinine (mg/dl)	3.5	0.6–1.2
Glucose (mg/dl)	216	70–100
Calcium (mg/dl)	9.2	8.5–10.5
Total protein (g/dl)	6.4	6.0–8.5
Albumin (g/dl)	3.5	3.5–4.8
Total bilirubin (mg/dl)	1.0	0–1.2
Aspartate aminotransferase (iu/l)	482	0–40
Alanine aminotransferase (iu/l)	554	0.32

TABLE 8.3 Lactate level.

Test	Value	Reference range
Lactate (mEq/l)	4.4	< 2.0

TABLE 8.4 Creatine kinase.

Test	Value	Reference range
Creatine kinase (iu/l)	75 000	22–198

TABLE 8.5   Arterial blood gases.

Test	Value	Reference range
pH	7.29	7.35–7.45
pCO_2 (mmHg)	59	35–45
pO_2 (mmHg)	68	80–100
Bicarbonate (mEq/l)	27	22–28

TABLE 8.6   Urinalysis.

Test	Value	Reference range
Glucose	Negative	Negative
Protein	Negative	Negative
Ketones	Negative	Negative
Bilirubin	Negative	Negative
Nitrates	Negative	Negative
Leukocyte esterase	Negative	Negative
Blood	+++	Negative

TABLE 8.7   Urine microscopy.

Test	Value	Reference range
White blood cell count (/hpf)	0–2	0–5
Red blood cell count (/hpf)	0–2	0–5
Bacteria (/hpf)	0	0
Epithelial cells (/hpf)	0	0

TABLE 8.8   Urine drug screen.

Test	Value	Reference range
Cannabinoids	Negative	Negative
Opiates	Positive	Negative
Benzodiazepines	Negative	Negative
Cocaine	Negative	Negative
Amphetamines	Negative	Negative
Barbituates	Negative	Negative
Phencyclidine	Negative	Negative

TABLE 8.9 Complete blood count.

Test	Values	Reference range
White blood cell count (× 10³/μl)	11.00	4.8–10.8
Hemoglobin g/dl)	12.6	12.6–17.4
Hematocrit (%)	28.3	37.0–51.0
Platelets (× 10³/μl)	335	130–400

TABLE 8.10 Basic metabolic panel.

Test	Value	Reference range
Sodium (mEq/l)	135	136–136
Potassium (mEq/l)	4.2	3.5–5.0
Chloride (mEq/l)	106	95–110
Bicarbonate	20	22–26
Blood urea nitrogen (mg/dl)	15	8–21
Creatinine (mg/dl)	0.8	0.6–1.2
Glucose (mg/dl)	116	70–100
Calcium (mg/dl)	9.2	8.5–10.5

TABLE 8.11 Urinalysis.

Test	Value	Reference range
White blood cell count (/hpf)	0–2	0–5
Rred blood cell count (/hpf)	0–2	0–5
Glucose	Negative	Negative
Protein	Negative	Negative
Ketones	Negative	Negative
Bilirubin	Negative	Negative
Nitrates	Negative	Negative
Leukocyte esterase	Negative	Negative

TABLE 8.12 Erythrocyte sedimentation rate.

Test	Value	Reference range
Erythrocyte sedimentation rate	5	< 20

TABLE 8.13 C-reactive protein.

Test	Value	Reference range
C-reactive protein	< 1.0	< 0.3

TABLE 8.14 Complete blood count.

Test	Value	Reference range
White blood cells (× 10³/μl)	7.00	4.8–10.8
Hemoglobin (g/dl)	14.2	12.6–17.4
Hematocrit (%)	29.7	37.0–51.0
Platelets (× 10³/μl)	324	130–400

TABLE 8.15 Basic metabolic panel.

Test	Value	Reference range
Sodium (mEq/l)	135	136–136
Potassium (mEq/l)	4.2	3.5–5.0
Chloride (mEq/l)	106	95–110
Bicarbonate (mEq/l)	18	22–26
Blood urea nitrogen (mEq/l)	22	8–21
Creatinine (mg/dl)	1.1	0.6–1.2
Glucose (mg/dl)	108	70–100
Calcium (mg/dl)	9.2	8.5–10.5

TABLE 8.16 Urinalysis.

Test	Value	Reference range
White blood cells (/hpf)	0–2	0–5
Red blood cells (/hpf)	0–2	0–5
Glucose	Negative	Negative
Protein	Negative	Negative
Ketones	Negative	Negative
Bilirubin	Negative	Negative
Nitrates	Negative	Negative
Leukocyte esterase	Negative	Negative

TABLE 8.17 Erythrocyte sedimentation rate.

	Value	Reference range
Erythrocyte sedimentation rate(mm/hour)	7	< 20

TABLE 8.18 C-reactive protein.

Test	Value	Reference range
C-reactive protein	< 1.0	< 0.3

CHAPTER 9

Obstetric/Gynecologic Emergencies

Catherine M. Wares and Mark J. Bullard

Department of Emergency Medicine, Carolinas Medical Center, Atrium Health, Charlotte, NC, USA

BREECH DELIVERY

Educational Goals

Learning Objectives

1. Demonstrate ability to perform an obstetric cervical check (MK, PC).
2. Recognize frank breech presentation (MK, PC).
3. Perform appropriate maneuvers to deliver an infant in breech presentation (MK, PC, SBP, ICS).
4. Appropriately consult obstetric and pediatric services (ICS, P, SBP).

Critical Actions Checklist

- ☐ Perform appropriate history and physical exam, including genitourinary exam (PC).
- ☐ Recognize signs of a frank breech presentation (MK, PC).
- ☐ Perform indicated maneuvers for a successful breech delivery (MK, PC).

Emergency Medicine Simulation Workbook: A Tool for Bringing the Curriculum to Life,
Second Edition. Edited by Traci L. Thoureen and Sara B. Scott.
© 2022 John Wiley & Sons Ltd. Published 2022 by John Wiley & Sons Ltd.
Companion website: www.wiley.com/go/thoureen/simulation/workbook2e

☐ Consult obstetric and pediatric consultant for additional support (ICS, P, SBP).
☐ Discuss medical care with patient (ICS, P, MK).

Critical actions can be changed to address the educational needs of the learner. An emergency medical services (EMS) provider may have objectives related to EMS protocols for imminent delivery and subsequent emergency department (ED) transfer.

Simulation Set-Up

Environment: ED resuscitation bay. Alternatively for EMS providers, this may also start "on scene" and transition to a hospital setting.

Mannequin:

- Option 1: Birthing simulator mannequin, at term, in active labor with frank breech presentation.
- Option 2: Adult simulator mannequin moulaged with gravid abdomen and a birthing simulator task trainer set-up with a frank breech presentation.
- Option 3: Adult simulator mannequin moulaged with gravid abdomen. A separate newborn mannequin is optional.

Props: To be displayed on monitor or printed out on handouts in scenario room when asked:

- Images (see online component for breech delivery, Scenario 9.1 at https://www.wiley.com/go/thoureen/simulation/workbook2e):
  - Neonatal heart monitor strip (heart rate 86) (Figure 9.1).
  - Neonatal heart monitor strip (heart rate 48) (Figure 9.2).
- Laboratory tests (see online component as above):
  - Maternal complete blood count (Table 9.1).
  - Maternal basic metabolic panel (Table 9.2).
  - Maternal blood type (Table 9.3).
  - Neonatal heel stick glucose (Table 9.4).

Any imaging or lab work not provided can be verbally reported as normal if the learners order the study.

Available supplies:

- Basic adult and neonatal airway supplies (nasal cannula, non-rebreather, bag-valve mask).
- Medications:
  - Liter bags of 0.9% saline and lactated Ringer's solution (*LR*).

Distractor: None.

Actors

- EMS may be an actor.
- Patient voice is female.
- ED nurse can administer medications/fluids and may cue learners if needed. Additionally, the nurse may act as a second set of hands for the scenario.

Case Narrative

Scenario Background

A 22-year-old woman (gravida 2 para 1), 37 weeks pregnant, presents with signs of labor. She has an upcoming appointment to see an obstetrician, but admits to having had no prenatal care. She had no problems with her first delivery. She came to the ED when she felt her "water break."

Patient's medical history:	Negative.
Medications:	Prenatal vitamins.
Allergies:	No known drug allergies.
Family history:	Mother living with hypertension. Father living with diabetes.
Social history:	No tobacco, drugs, or alcohol. Patient lives at home with her spouse.

Initial Scenario Conditions

A 22-year old woman is brought in by EMS, gravid, in moderate distress.

> Case may start with EMS receiving this case on scene as presented, and adhering to EMS protocols for treatment/evaluation of stability, and transport.

Vital signs:	Temp 98.6°F (37°C), HR 114, RR 26, BP 100/60, RA SpO$_2$ 99%.
Head:	Normocephalic/atraumatic.
Eyes:	Pupils 4 mm and reactive.
Neck:	Supple, no lymphadenopathy, no thyromegaly.
Heart:	Tachycardic and regular, distal pulses palpable.
Lungs:	Clear breath sounds bilaterally.

Abdomen:	Soft, gravid (37-week uterus), mild tenderness.
Genitourinary:	No vaginal bleeding; frank breech.
Extremities:	No gross deformities, bilateral trace edema.
Skin:	Normal skin exam.
Neurologic:	Awake, non-focal, oriented × 4.

> Physical exam findings not available on your mannequin can be reported verbally if asked for by learners; for example, if your mannequin does not have birth simulation capabilities, you can moulage your adult mannequin with a gravid abdomen and use a separate birthing simulator. Alternatively, you may report the genitourinary findings verbally.

See flow diagram (Figure 9.3) for further scenario changes described.

Case Narrative, Continued

Depending on the learner level, the scenario will either take place at a facility with available obstetric services or a community ED without obstetric services. The learner will be called to the room for a patient in active labor The term infant will demonstrate frank breech presentation and delivery will be imminent. Depending on the desired scenario complexity the neonate may also require resuscitation.

Learners of all levels (EMS, novice and advanced learners) should initially perform a primary history and physical exam and obtain appropriate IV access. Depending on learner level, the scenario will require delivery of a term breech neonate.

If a birthing simulator mannequin or task trainer is unavailable, when asked for the cervical exam, the nurse can report that the learner can palpate soft tissue consistent with the fetal buttocks.

If learners request a bedside ultrasound, the nurse can verbally report that the head does not appear to be down.

The novice learner is only required to recognize frank breech presentation with the expectation of immediate consultation to obstetric services at the same location for emergent caesarean section.

For advanced learners, the scenario will take place at a facility without obstetric services and thus will require breech vaginal delivery. The learner will be expected to manage the delivery appropriately (verbalize and/or perform various maneuvers as delivery proceeds). Additionally, the scenario can be complicated with the need for neonatal resuscitation.

The case ends when the patients are stable and transfer has been arranged to a hospital with neonatology/obstetric services

Instructor Notes

Pathophysiology

- General:
  - 3–4% of singleton term deliveries are breech.
  - 10% of preterm fetuses will present breech.
  - Perinatal mortality and morbidity are estimated 3× that of vertex delivery [1].
  - Planned caesarean section is the best method of delivering a known singleton term breech:
    - Decreased fetal morbidity and mortality.
    - No increased risk of maternal morbidity.
  - Most breech presentations are planned for caesarean section, but patients may present to the ED unexpectedly:
    - Nearly 10% of women who plan for caesarean section deliver vaginally.
    - Labor and delivery may occur at a site where caesarean section is unavailable.
    - Patients without prenatal care (unknown presentation).
- Types:
  - Frank or extended breech:
    - Most common (60–70%).
    - Lower extremities fully flexed at hip and fully extended at the knee.
    - Presenting part (buttocks/sacrum) may fit snugly into lower segment.
    - Cord prolapse uncommon.
  - Complete or flexed breech:
    - Least common (10%).
    - Both hips and knees are flexed.
    - Presenting part more variable and prolapsed cord slightly more common.
  - Incomplete breech or footling breech:
    - 20–25% of term breech presentation.
      Most common preterm presentation
    - One or both hips not completely flexed.
    - Presenting part is one, or both, feet or knee/s.
    - Presenting part may slip through an incompletely dilated cervix increasing the chance of entrapment of the infant's shoulders or head.

Management

- Preparation:
  - Obtain IV access, place on oxygen and cardiac monitor. Monitor fetal heart rate (if available).

- Check for umbilical cord prolapse and manually elevate presenting part if identified.
- Assess if cervix is fully dilated.
- Provide adequate analgesia.
- Delivery:
  - Consider episiotomy.
  - Never pull from below.
  - Do nothing until the infant's umbilicus is visible.
    - At this point, umbilical cord usually becomes compressed.
    - Aim for delivery within two to three minutes.
  - Keep the infant's back anterior.
  - Delivery of arms.
  - Delivery of head (Mauriceau–Smellie–Veit technique):
    - Suprapubic pressure promotes flexion of head.
    - Fetus placed on supinated left arm.
    - Middle and index fingers of left hand placed over fetus' maxilla to promote head flexion.
    - Fingers of pronated right hand placed on fetus' suboccipital region promoting head flexion.
    - Gentle downward and backward traction of fetus until delivery achieved.

Debriefing Plan

Plan for approximately 30 minutes for discussion.

Potential Questions for Discussion

- Why do EM providers need to have an understanding of breech delivery?
- What are the various types of breech presentation?
- What complications could you expect from the different types of breech presentations?
- How does the type of breech presentation affect management?
- What is the Mauriceau–Smellie–Veit technique?

REFERENCE FOR BREECH DELIVERY

1. Mukhopadhyay, S. and Arulkumaran, S. (2002). Breech delivery. *Best Pract. Res. Clin. Obstet. Gynaecol.* 16 (1): 31–42.

SELECTED READINGS FOR BREECH DELIVERY

Borhart, J. and Voss, K. (2019). Precipitous labor and emergency department delivery. *Emerg. Med. Clin. North Am.* 37 (2): 265–276.

Robertson, J., Braude, D., Stonehocker, J., and Moreno, J. (2015). Prehospital breech delivery with fetal head entrapment: a case report and review. *Prehosp. Emerg. Care* 19 (3): 451–456.

Tunde-Byass, M. and Hannah, M. (2003). Breech vaginal delivery at or near term. *Semin. Perinatol.* 27 (1): 34–45.

SHOULDER DYSTOCIA

Educational Goals

Learning Objectives

1. Recognize clinical signs of imminent delivery (MK, PC).
2. Recognize clinical signs of shoulder dystocia (MK, PC).
3. Demonstrate specific maneuvers to relieve shoulder dystocia (MK, PC).
4. Discuss the case with obstetric and neonatal/pediatric consultants (ICS, P, SBP).
5. Demonstrate professionalism and appropriate communication with the nurse, consultants, and the patient (ICS, P).

Critical Actions Checklist

- ☐ Perform focused history and exam (PC).
- ☐ Perform a cervical check (*PC*).
- ☐ Identify shoulder dystocia (MK, PC).
- ☐ Perform maneuvers for successful delivery of shoulder dystocia (MK, PC).
- ☐ Consult obstetrics and neonatal/pediatric teams for admission (ICS, P, SBP).

Critical actions can be changed to address the educational needs of the learner. For example, learner can identify and address nuchal cord or perform uncomplicated precipitous delivery.

Simulation Set-Up

Environment: ED treatment room in a hospital with no in-house obstetrician.

Mannequin: Maternal birthing mannequin or adult mannequin moulaged to portray a full-term gravid abdomen.

If a pregnant mannequin is unavailable, a gravid uterus can be simulated by placing a pillow under clothes or a commercial pregnancy simulator (The Empathy Belly®) can be used.

Props: To be displayed on plasma screen/computer screen or printed out on handouts in scenario room when asked for/return from lab:

- Images (see online component for shoulder dystocia, Scenario 9.2 at https://www.wiley.com/go/thoureen/simulation/workbook2e):

  - Crowning fetal head (Figure 9.4).
  - Head delivered (Figure 9.5).
- Laboratory tests (see online component as above):
  - Basic metabolic panel (Table 9.5).
  - Complete blood count (Table 9.6).
  - ABO blood type (Table 9.7).
  - Neonatal heelstick glucose (Table 9.8).
- Videos (see online component as above):
  - Video clip with turtle sign (Video 9.1).

Available supplies:

- Personal protective equipment (gown, shoe covers, sterile gloves).
- Medications:
  - Liter bags of 0.9% saline and LR.
  - Labeled syringes of analgesia medication (e.g. morphine).
- Cord clamps or hemostats, surgical scissors (optional).

Distractor: None.

Actors

- Patient voice is a female screaming, "I need to push!"
- ED nurse will administer medications and assist with shoulder dystocia maneuvers.
- Obstetrician and neonatal/pediatric specialists are available by telephone consultation.

Case Narrative

Scenario Background

A 22-year-old woman (gravida 2 para 1) at 39 weeks and 5 days of gestation presents in labor. She reports that her waters broke at home and her contractions are now two minutes apart. She has had routine prenatal care without complications.

Background can be presented by EMS provider, nurse, or can be provided by a triage sheet.

Patient's medical history:	Prior full-term pregnancy with no complications
Medications:	Prenatal vitamins
Allergies:	No known drug allergies.
Family history:	Non-contributory.
Social history:	No tobacco, alcohol, or drug use.

Initial Scenario Conditions

The learner will be called to the room for a patient in active labor. The patient presents as a pregnant woman who appears full term, yelling "I need to push!"

> The case may start with EMS on scene as presented above while performing their objectives to identify and deliver an infant with shoulder dystocia with subsequent ED transport of the patients.

Vital signs:	Temp 98.6°F (37°C), HR 116 RR 28, BP 120/60, RA SpO$_2$ 99%.
Head:	Head normocephalic and atraumatic.
Heart:	Tachycardic with regular rate.
Lungs:	Clear bilaterally.
Abdomen:	Gravid.
Genitourinary:	Fully dilated, crowning fetal head.
Neurologic:	Alert and oriented × 4.

> Physical exam findings not available on your mannequin can be visually displayed (Figure 9.2, Video 9.1) or verbally reported by your nurse.

See flow diagram (Figure 9.6) for further scenario changes described.

Case Narrative, Continued

If the learner does not quickly perform a cervical check and realize that delivery is imminent, the patient will repeatedly scream "I NEED TO PUSH!" Within minutes, the learner should be prepared for delivery.

Once the infant's head has delivered, the infant will become stuck and the shoulders will not deliver. If the learner does not recognize shoulder dystocia, the nurse can note "It looks like the head is turtling." or "Do you think the shoulders are stuck?"

The learner should perform maneuvers to aid successful delivery of the infant, which may include the McRoberts maneuver and/or suprapubic pressure.

For advanced learners, entry maneuvers can be applied.

The case ends when maneuvers to relieve shoulder dystocia are successful, the infant is delivered, and the learner has communicated with an accepting physician at another facility.

Instructor Notes

Pathophysiology

- Shoulder dystocia occurs when the head is delivered but the anterior shoulder becomes lodged behind the maternal pubic symphysis and there is an inability to deliver the anterior shoulder with gentle downward traction on the fetal head.
- Occurs in around 2% of cephalic vaginal deliveries.

Clinical Features

- The "turtle sign," is when the head delivers then quickly retracts.
- Predictive factors include:
  - Advanced fetal weight.
  - Gestational diabetes.
  - Previous history of shoulder dystocia.
- Complications of shoulder dystocia:
  - Maternal:
    - Postpartum hemorrhage from atony.
    - Fourth-degree lacerations.
  - Fetal:
    - Brachial plexus injury (5–15% of cases) but usually resolves within one year.
    - Clavicle (15%) and humeral fractures (<1%), which normally heal without intervention.
    - Hypoxic encephalopathy.
    - Death.

Diagnosis

- Primarily clinical.

Management

- The head–body delivery time matters to avoid fetal acidosis and hypoxic ischemic encephalopathy; goal is for delivery within five minutes.
- The Advanced Life Support in Obstetrics course uses the HELLPERR mnemonic to assist providers in addressing shoulder dystocia in a systematic way [1].

- Note – pulling harder is not a maneuver and can result in significant fetal trauma; continue *gentle* traction during the entire process:
  - **H:** Call for help.
  - **E:** Evaluate for episiotomy – typically not useful and has fallen out of favor.
  - **L:** Legs for McRoberts maneuver:
    - Recommended as the first maneuver.
    - Extreme lithotomy position; flexing maternal hips so thighs are on the abdomen.
    - Increases the inlet diameter and decreases lumbosacral lordosis.
  - **P:** Pressure (suprapubic) aka Rubin I maneuver:
    - Pressure applied suprapubically is directed to the fetal anterior shoulder.
    - When used in conjunction with the McRoberts maneuver, relieves majority of dystocias.
  - **E:** Entry maneuvers:
    - Shift infant to rotate the anterior shoulder under the maternal pubic symphysis.
    - Rubin II:
      - Put fingers behind most accessible fetal shoulder and cause shoulder adduction; push shoulder toward face/chest to decrease shoulder width.
    - Wood's screw and reverse screw maneuvers:
      - Use fingers to apply force either to posterior or anterior surface of posterior shoulder to rotate the infant from under the maternal pubic symphysis.
  - **R:** Remove the posterior arm:
    - Deliver the posterior arm first then hand should be visualized first.
    - Flex the elbow (to prevent humeral fracture) of the posterior arm until forearm can be gripped and swept across the chest and pulled out.
  - **R:** Roll the patient (Gaskin maneuver):
    - Placing the patient in an "all fours" position can open the canal.
    - One of the most successful of all maneuvers.
- If all HELPERR maneuvers are unsuccessful, consider:
  - Deliberate clavicle fracture by applying pressure anteriorly and superiorly away from infant's lung.
  - Zavenelli maneuver: push head back in and hold pressure until caesarean section can be performed.

Debriefing Plan

Plan for approximately 30 minutes for discussion.

Potential Questions for Discussion

- What are signs of imminent delivery?
- What physical exam findings can determine the gestational age of pregnancy?

- How should a cervical check be performed?
- What is shoulder dystocia and the clinical signs of shoulder dystocia?
- How does shoulder dystocia increase fetal morbidity?
- What are the maneuvers used to relieve dystocia?

REFERENCE FOR SHOULDER DYSTOCIA

1. Baxley, E. and Gobbo, R. (2004). Shoulder dystocia. *Am. Fam. Physician* 69: 1707–1714.

SELECTED READINGS FOR SHOULDER DYSTOCIA

Borhart, J. and Voss, K. (2019). Precipitous labor and emergency department delivery. *Emerg. Med. Clin. North Am.* 37 (2): 265–266.

Del Portal, D.A., Horn, A.E., Vilke, G.M. et al. (2014). Emergency department management of shoulder dystocia. *J. Emerg. Med.* 46 (3): 378–382.

Hart, D., Nelson, J., Moore, J. et al. (2017). Shoulder dystocia delivery by emergency medicine residents: a high-fidelity versus a novel low-fidelity simulation model – a pilot study. *AEM Educ. Train.* 23 (10): 357–362.

POSTPARTUM HEMORRHAGE AFTER PRECIPITOUS DELIVERY WITH OR WITHOUT NEONATAL RESUSCITATION

Educational Goals

Learning Objectives

1. Identify and manage hemorrhagic shock (MK, PC, SBP).
2. List the possible causes of postpartum hemorrhage (PPH) (MK).
3. Demonstrate appropriate management of PPH (MK, PC).
4. Assess a newborn (optional for advanced learners) (MK, PC).
5. Resuscitate a term neonate (optional for advanced learners) (MK, PC).
6. Discuss care with patient (ICS).
7. Demonstrate appropriate consultation with obstetrician (ICS, P, SBP).

Critical Actions Checklist

- ☐ Manage PPH with appropriate medications (MK, PC).
- ☐ Administer blood products (PC).
- ☐ Administer RhoGAM (PC).
- ☐ Resuscitate newborn (MK, PC).
- ☐ Obtain bedside glucose of neonate and manage appropriately (MK, PC).
- ☐ Consult appropriate services and transfer patients (ICS, P, SBP).

> Critical actions can be changed to address the learner's educational needs. For more advanced learners, the case may include assessment and resuscitation of newborn. EMS providers may have objectives related to therapies during transport to ED including blood product management, tranexamic acid administration, field delivery with airway management, neonatal resuscitation, etc.

Simulation Set-Up

Environment: Resuscitation room in ED in a hospital with no in-house obstetrician. This scenario may start on scene and transition to the hospital setting for EMS providers.

Mannequin: Adult female simulator mannequin, post-delivery with moulaged vaginal bleeding. Simulated blood may be used on dressings under mannequin. In addition, may have optional neonatal mannequin for advanced learning objectives.

Props: To be displayed on monitor or printed out on handouts in scenario room:

- Images (see online component for PPH with or without term neonatal resuscitation, Scenario 9.3 at `https://www.wiley.com/go/thoureen/simulation/workbook2e`):
  - Neonatal heart monitor strip (heart rate 46) (Figure 9.2).
  - Complete placenta (Figure 9.7).
  - Ultrasound showing no retained products of conception (Figure 9.8).
- Laboratory tests (see online component as above):
  - Maternal complete blood count (Table 9.9).
  - Maternal basic metabolic panel (Table 9.10).
  - Maternal blood type (Table 9.11).
  - Maternal coagulation panel (Table 9.12).
  - Maternal fibrinogen (Table 9.13).
  - Neonatal heelstick glucose (Table 9.14).

Available supplies:

- Basic adult and neonatal airway supplies (nasal cannula, nonrebreather, face mask, bag–valve mask).
- Medications:
  - Liter bags of 0.9% saline and LR.
  - Packed Red blood cells.
  - Fresh frozen plasma.
  - Cryoprecipitate.
  - Pre-labeled syringes:
    - Uterotonic agents:
      - Oxytocin.
      - Methergine.
      - Hemabate.
      - Misoprostol.
    - Tranexamic acid.
    - Analgesic medication (e.g. morphine).

Distractor: none

Actors

- EMS may be an actor.
- Patient voice is female.

- ED nurse can administer medications/fluids/blood products and may cue learners if needed.
- Depending on the complexity of the scenario, learners may need additional personnel for instructed tasks (e.g., fundal massage while learner is caring for neonate).

Case Narrative

Scenario Background

A 26-year-old woman presents to the ED after a precipitous home delivery. She will report that she was approximately 37 weeks pregnant without prenatal care other than an initial visit verifying her pregnancy. The patient complains of continued vaginal bleeding and lightheadedness. Placenta was delivered prior to arrival, but was brought in with the patient (Figure 9.7).

Patient's medial history:	Negative
Medications:	Prenatal vitamins
Allergies:	No knowd drug allergies.
Family history:	Mother living with hypertension. Father living with diabetes.
Social history:	No tobacco, drugs or alcohol. Patient lives at home with her mother and father.

Initial Scenario Conditions

A 26-year old woman is brought in by EMS, in moderate distress.

> Case may start with EMS receiving this case on scene as presented and adhering to EMS protocols for treatment/evaluation of stability, and transport.

Vital signs:	Temp 98.6°F (37°C), HR 114, RR 26, BP 100/60, RA SpO$_2$ 99%.
Head:	Normocephalic/atraumatic.
Eyes:	Pupils 4 mm, reactive.
Neck:	Supple, no lymphadenopathy, no thyromegaly.
Heart:	Tachycardic and regular, distal pulses palpable.
Lungs:	Clear breath sounds bilaterally.
Abdomen:	Soft, mild suprapubic tenderness, boggy uterus.
Genitourinary:	Vaginal bleeding.
Extremities:	Bilateral trace edema, no unilateral leg swelling.
Skin:	Normal skin exam.
Neurologic:	Awake, non-focal, oriented to person, place, time, and situation.

> Physical exam findings not available on your mannequin, such as boggy uterus, can be reported verbally if asked for by learners.

See flow diagram (Figure 9.9) for further scenario changes described.

Case Narrative, Continued

Learners of all levels should initially take a history, perform a physical exam, and obtain IV access. The mother will continue to hemorrhage post-delivery and will become unstable.

For novice learners, the neonate was taken to the local pediatric ED, and the sole focus of their case will be the mother, who will need emergent evaluation and intervention for PPH.

Learners should consider all possible etiologies of PPH, however the etiology will be uterine atony. An image of a complete placenta, ultrasound images of an empty uterus and laboratory values will be available to the learner, if asked. The patient will become stable upon receiving two uterotonic agents.

For advanced learners, in addition to caring for maternal PPH, the learner will also need to resuscitate a term infant. The neonate will be cyanotic, minimally responsive to stimulation, and will require aggressive stimulus, warming and bag-valve mask ventilation (per Neonatal Resuscitation Program) The hemodynamics of the infant will improve gradually (Figure 9.9). Learners will also be expected to order a bedside glucose of the neonate which will be normal.

The case ends when patients are stable, and transfer has been arranged to a hospital with neonatology/obstetrics.

Instructor Notes

Pathophysiology

- Definition of PPH: blood loss > 500–1000 ml or blood loss accompanied by shock.
- Up to 5% incidence in United States.
- 10% recurrence in subsequent deliveries.
- Causes: (4 Ts: tone, trauma, tissue, thrombin).
  - Tone: uterine atony – most common (80%):
    - Uterine atony prevents constriction of spiral arteries in the myometrium.
    - Risk factors:
      - Prolonged second stage of labor.
      - Overdistension of uterus.
      - Medications (nifedipine, magnesium, and halogenated anesthetic agents).
      - Chorioamnionitis.
      - Leiomyoma.
      - 20% of PPH occur with no risk factors.

- Trauma: lacerations, hematoma, uterine rupture.
- Tissue: retained placenta.
- Thrombin: congenital or acquired coagulopathy:
  - Disseminated intravascular coagulopathy.
  - Associated with placental abruption and amniotic fluid embolism.

Diagnosis

- Primarily clinical:
  - Visually estimated blood loss is often inaccurate.
  - Tachycardia and hypotension are late findings and represent substantial blood loss.
- Ultrasound:
  - Examine for retained products.
- Intrauterine examination:
  - If considering retained placenta (e.g. placenta accreta).
- Inspection of placenta for completeness after delivery.

Management

- Will differ depending on etiology of hemorrhage.
- Uterine atony:
  - Prevention
    - Use oxytocin routinely at time of anterior shoulder delivery or immediately after delivery of placenta.
    - Uterine massage.
  - Treatment:
    - Uterine massage.
    - Uterotonic agents
      - First line: oxytocin. If unsuccessful, add additional agent.
      - Second line: methergine, carboprost tromethamine (Hemabate®), misoprostol.
      - No compelling data to use one second-line agent over another.
      - Carboprost contraindicated in asthmatics.
  - Placement of Foley catheter into the bladder:
    - A full bladder may contribute to uterine atony.
  - Uterine tamponade:
    - Uterine packing.
    - Bakri tube.
    - Gastric balloon from Blakemore tube.

- Emergent hysterectomy:
  - Trauma:
    - Laceration repair.
    - Ice/conservative management of hematoma.
  - Tissue:
    - Manual extraction of retained placenta.
    - Placenta accreta (placenta does not detach manually).
    - Requires surgical correction;
  - Thrombin:
    - Massive transfusion protocol (1 : 1 : 1 blood product ratio).
    - Add cryoprecipitate if fibrinogen low.
- General adjuncts for all postpartum hemorrhage:
  - Tranexamic acid-reduction of mortality from obstetric hemorrhage.
  - Risk of thrombosis is not higher in this population.
- Other considerations:
  - Inverted uterus manual replacement.

Neonatal Resuscitation [1]

- Initial assessment:
  - Infant tone, breathing/crying.
  - If poor tone, not breathing/crying → warm, dry, stimulate, position airway clear secretions.
  - If still has apnea/gasping or heart rate <100 beats/minute after 30 seconds:
    - Positive pressure ventilation with room air, place on oxygen saturation monitor, consider electrocardiogram monitor
    - Oxygen saturation probe should be preductal on right upper extremity.
    - Initial oxygen saturation of 60–65% is expected, increasing to 85–95% over the first 10 minutes as the infant transitions from fetal circulation.
    - Attempt to use minimal supplemental oxygen unless clearly needed.
  - If after another 30 seconds, heart rate <100 beats/minute:
    - Ventilation corrective steps.
    - Consider intubation or placement of laryngeal mask airway.
  - If heart rate <60 beats/minute despite steps above:
    - Intubate (if not already performed).
    - Chest compressions at a rate of 120/minute.
  - If heart rate still <60 beats/minute despite all steps above:

- Epinephrine.
- Consider hypovolemia/pneumothorax.

Debriefing Plan

Plan for approximately 30 minutes for discussion.

Potential Questions for Discussion

- What are common causes of PPH?
- What uterotonic agents are available?
- What uterotonic agent is first line therapy?
- In addition to uterotonics, what adjunct agents are available?
- What imaging and laboratory values are important for diagnosis and therapy?
- When should chest compressions and positive pressure ventilation be started in neonatal resuscitation?

REFERENCE FOR POSTPARTUM HEMORRHAGE

1. Aziz, K., Lee, H.C., Escobedo, M.B. et al. (2020). American Heart Association guidelines for cardiopulmonary resuscitation and emergency cardiovascular care. *Pediatrics* 2020: e2020038505E.

SELECTED READINGS FOR POSTPARTUM HEMORRHAGE

Committee on Practice Bulletins-Obstetrics. Practice bulletin no. 183: Postpartum hemorrhage. *Obstet. Gynecol.* 2017; 130 (4): e168–e186.

Escobedo, M., Shah, B., Song, C. et al. (2019). Recent recommendations and emerging science in neonatal resuscitation. *Pediatr. Clin. North Am.* 66 (2): 309–320.

Evensen, A., Anderson, J., and Fontaine, P. (2017). Postpartum hemorrhage: prevention and treatment. *Am. Fam. Physician* 95 (7): 442–449.

Manley, B., Owen, L., Hooper, S. et al. (2017). Toward evidence-based resuscitation of the newborn infant. *Lancet* 389 (10079): 1639–1648.

Su, C.W. (2012). Postpartum hemorrhage. *Prim. Care* 39 (1): 167–187.

APPENDIX

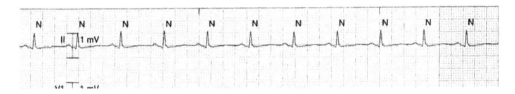

FIGURE 9.1   Neonatal heart monitor strip (heart rate 86).

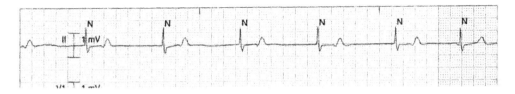

FIGURE 9.2   Neonatal heart monitor strip (heart rate 48).

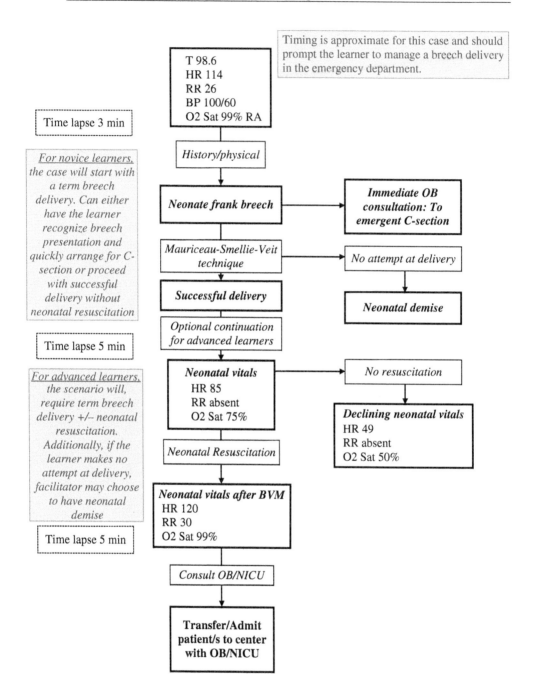

FIGURE 9.3   Breech flow diagram.

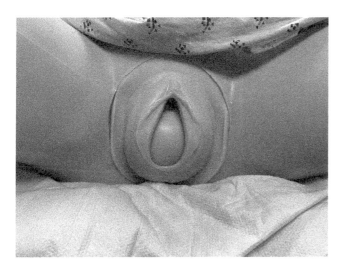

FIGURE 9.4 Crowning fetal head.

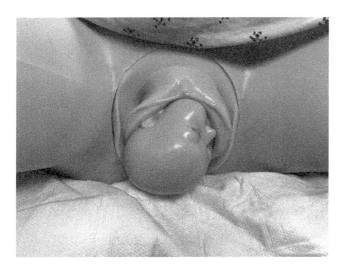

FIGURE 9.5 Head delivered.

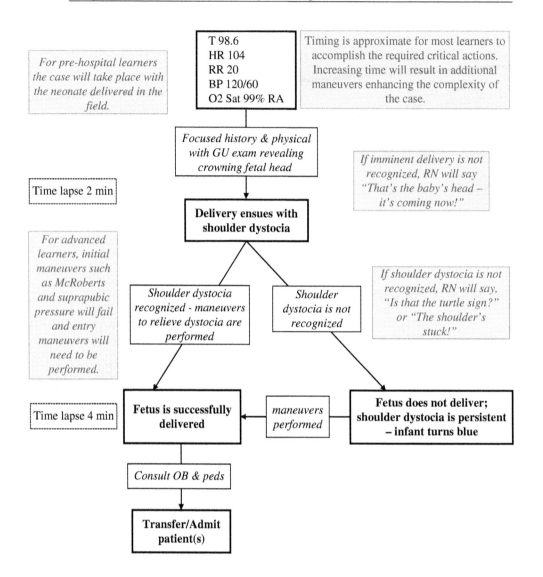

FIGURE 9.6 Shoulder dystocia flow diagram.

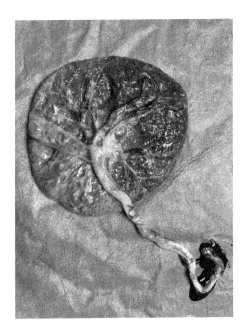

FIGURE 9.7 Complete placenta.

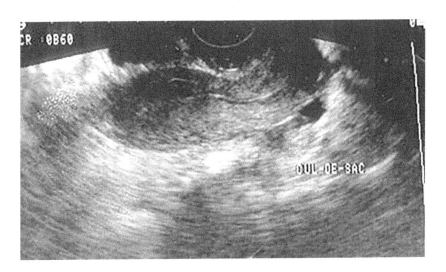

FIGURE 9.8 Ultrasound of uterus with no retained products.

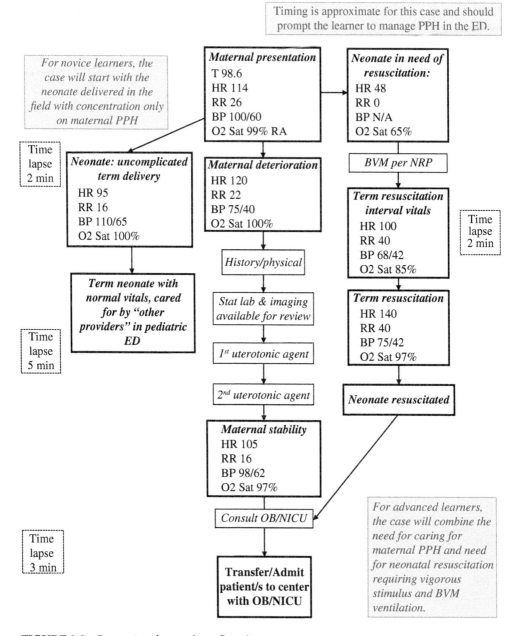

FIGURE 9.9   Postpartum hemorrhage flow diagram.

TABLE 9.1   Maternal complete blood count.

Test	Value	Reference range
White blood cells (k/μl)	7.4	3.5–11.0
Hemoglobin (g/dl)	8.0	10.5–15.0
Hematocrit (%)	26	32–45
Mean corpuscular volume (fl)	92	81–100
Platelets (k/μl)	211	150–400

TABLE 9.2   Maternal basic metabolic panel.

Test	Value	Reference range
Sodium (mmol/l)	138	135–145
Potassium (mmol/l)	3.8	3.6–5.1
Chloride (mmol/l)	108	98–110
CO_2 (mmol/l)	24	20–30
Blood urea nitrogen (mg/dl)	18	6–24
Creatinine (mg/dl)	0.9	0.4–1.3
Glucose (mg/dl)	118	67–109

TABLE 9.3   Maternal blood type.

Test	Value	Reference range
ABO/Rh (D)	A negative	–

TABLE 9.4   Neonatal heelstick glucose.

Test	Value	Reference range
Heelstick glucose (mg/dl)	78	70–109

TABLE 9.5   Basic metabolic panel.

Test	Value	Reference range
Sodium (mmol/l)	138	135–145
Potassium (mmol/l)	3.8	3.6–5.1
Chloride (mmol/l)	108	98–110
CO_2 (mmol/l)	24	20–30
Blood urea nitrogen (mg/dl)	18	6–24
Creatinine (mg/dl)	0.9	0.4–1.3
Glucose (mg/dl)	118	67–109

TABLE 9.6   Complete blood count.

Test	Value	Reference range
White blood cells (k/μl)	8.4	3.5–11.0
Hemoglobin (g/dl)	10.4	10.5–15.0
Hematocrit (%)	36	32–45
Mean corpuscular volume (fl)	92	81–100
Platelets (k/μl)	211	150–400

TABLE 9.7   Blood type.

Test	Value	Reference range
ABO/Rh (D)	O positive	–

TABLE 9.8   Neonatal heelstick glucose.

Test	Value	Reference range
Fingerstick glucose (mg/dl)	118	70–109

TABLE 9.9 Maternal complete blood count.

Test	Value	Reference range
White blood cells (k/µl)	7.4	3.5–11.0
Hemoglobin (g/dl)	8.0	10.5–15.0
Hematocrit (%)	26	32–45
Mean corpuscular volume (fl)	92	81–100
Platelets (k/µl)	211	150–400

TABLE 9.10 Maternal basic metabolic panel.

Test	Value	Reference range
Sodium (mmol/l)	138	135–145
Potassium (mmol/l)	3.8	3.6–5.1
Chloride (mmol/l)	108	98–110
CO_2 (mmol/l)	24	20–30
Blood urea nitrogen (mg/dl)	18	6–24
Creatinine (mg/dl)	0.9	0.4–1.3
Glucose (mg/dl)	118	67–109

TABLE 9.11 Maternal blood type.

Test	Value	Reference range
ABO/Rh (D)	A negative	–

TABLE 9.12 Coagulation panel.

Test	Value	Reference range
Prothrombin time (seconds)	10.5	9.4–11.5
International normalized ratio	1.0	0.9–1.2
Partial thromboplastin time (seconds)	28.0	24.2–32.0

TABLE 9.13 Maternal fibrinogen.

Test	Value	Reference range
Fibrinogen (mg/dl)	258	200–400

TABLE 9.14 Neonatal heelstick glucose.

	Value	Reference range
Heelstick glucose (mg/dl)	68	70–109

CHAPTER 10

Nervous System Emergencies

Danya Khoujah[1,2] and Wan-Tsu W. Chang[2]

[1] Emergency Medicine, MedStar Franklin Square Hospital, Baltimore, MD, USA
[2] Department of Emergency Medicine, University of Maryland School of Medicine, Baltimore, MD, USA

ACUTE ISCHEMIC STROKE

Educational Goals

Learning Objectives

1. Recognize signs and symptoms of acute ischemic stroke (*AIS*) (MK).
2. Use the National Institutes of Health Stroke Scale (*NIHSS*) in the evaluation of a patient with AIS (MK, PC).
3. Explain risks and benefits of intravenous (*IV*) thrombolytics to patient/family (MK, PC, ICS).
4. Demonstrate effective communication of relevant clinical information to consultants (ICS, P).
5. Identify and manage large vessel occlusion (*LVO*) (optional, for advanced learners) (MK, PC).

Critical Actions Checklist

- ☐ Obtain fingerstick glucose (MK).
- ☐ Obtain non-contrast computed tomography (CT) of the head (MK).

Emergency Medicine Simulation Workbook: A Tool for Bringing the Curriculum to Life, Second Edition. Edited by Traci L. Thoureen and Sara B. Scott.
© 2022 John Wiley & Sons Ltd. Published 2022 by John Wiley & Sons Ltd.
Companion website: www.wiley.com/go/thoureen/simulation/workbook2e

☐ Perform focused neurological exam including NIHSS (MK, PC).

☐ Obtain pertinent history including contraindications to tissue plasminogen activator (MK).

☐ Use appropriate antihypertensive medications for blood pressure control (MK, PC).

☐ Obtain CT angiography (*CTA*) for evaluation of LVO without delaying administration of tPA (MK, PC).

☐ Obtain informed consent for tPA (MK, PC).

☐ Novice learner: consult a neurologist or intensivist for admission (ICS, P, SBP).

☐ Advanced learner: consult a neurologist for transfer to thrombectomy-capable facility (ICS, P, SBP).

☐ Designate a leader, maintain assigned role, and use closed-loop communication (ICS, P).

Simulation Set-Up

Environment: ED treatment area at a primary stroke center without thrombectomy capability. Magnetic resonance imaging (*MRI*) is not immediately available at this clinical site.

Standardized patient: Female on a stretcher or hospital bed.

Props: Display on computer screen or as handouts:

- Images (see online component for AIS, Scenario 10.1 at [https://www.wiley.com/go/thoureen/simulation/workbook2e]):
  - Electrocardiogram (ECG) showing normal sinus rhythm (Figure 10.1).
  - Chest x-ray which is normal (Figure 10.2).
  - NCHCT showing dense left middle cerebral artery sign (Figure 10.3, Video 10.1).
  - CTA showing no LVO for novice learners (Figure 10.4, Video 10.2).
  - CTA showing left M1 occlusion for advanced learners (Figure 10.5, Video 10.3).
- Laboratory tests (see online component as above):
  - Complete blood count (Table 10.1).
  - Chemistry panel (Table 10.2).
  - Troponin (Table 10.3).
  - Coagulation panel (Table 10.4).
  - Alcohol level (Table 10.5).

Available supplies:

- Basic adult airway and code cart.
- Medications:
  - 0.9%, lactated Ringer's solution (*LR*) in liter bags.
  - Pre-labeled syringes:

- Antihypertensives: hydralazine, labetalol.
- Intubation medications commonly used at your institution.
- Pre-labeled IV bags:
- Antihypertensives: clevidipine, nicardipine.
- Premixed vial of thrombolytic medication typically used at your institution.
- NIHSS form (Figure 10.6).

Distractor: None

Actors

- Standardized patient: female dressed in regular clothes with abnormal neurological exam (refer to Figure 10.7 and physical exam described below).
- Nurse may cue learners on the availability of resources if needed. The nurse asks advanced learners to clarify the rationale behind medical decisions.
- Available by phone:
  - Neurologist.
  - Radiologist.
  - Intensivist.

Case Narrative

Scenario Background

A 65-year-old woman was heard falling in the shower and was found by her son with right-sided weakness. She reports no loss of consciousness, headache, or vomiting. The emergency medical services (EMS) attending reports that she was well 30 minutes prior when she had breakfast with her son (only provided if the learner specifically asks). Patient's son is on his way to the emergency department (ED).

Patient's medical history: Hypertension, diabetes.
Medications: Aspirin, lisinopril, metformin.
Allergies: None.
Family history: Hypertension, diabetes.
Social history: Former smoker. No alcohol or drugs. Patient lives with her son.

Initial Scenario Conditions

Older adult female brought in by EMS. Patient is awake with mild word-finding difficulty but can provide most of the history.

EMS may present the background as a medical consult or on arrival to ED.

Vital signs:	Temp 98.6°F (37°C), HR 74, RR 16, BP 205/120, SpO$_2$ 99% on room air.
Weight:	80 kg.
Head:	Atraumatic.
Eyes:	Pupils 4 mm, equal and reactive to light. Extraocular movements are intact.
Neck:	Supple, no lymphadenopathy or swelling, no midline cervical spine tenderness.
Heart:	Regular rate, distal pulses normal.
Lungs:	Clear breath sounds bilaterally.
Chest:	No signs of trauma or tenderness.
Abdomen:	Soft, nontender, normal bowel sounds.
Extremities:	No deformities, full range of motion.
Skin:	No rash or abrasions.
Neurologic:	Awake, alert, oriented × 3, mild word-finding difficulty, moves left arm and leg 5/5 strength, right face, arm, and leg 2/5 weakness, diminished right-sided sensation. Figure 10.7 details complete NIHSS of 12.

> Nurse can report exam findings not available on the standardized patient if learners specifically ask.

See flow diagram (Figure 10.8) for scenario changes described.

Case Narrative, Continued

All learners should initially perform a primary survey (ABCD) including a fingerstick glucose. Learners should initially:

- Perform a focused neurological exam.
- Obtain laboratory tests, including platelet count and coagulation panel.
- Obtain NCHCT to rule out intracranial hemorrhage.
- Calculate the NIHSS.

Learners should evaluate eligibility for IV thrombolytics by asking about contraindications and confirm last known well. Learners will discuss risks/benefits and obtain consent for IV thrombolytic; the patient should inquire about the risk of bleeding if not offered.

Blood pressure should be lowered to less than 185/110 mmHg prior to IV thrombolytic administration. Medication dosage, route, and target blood pressure should be specified. Blood pressure will only be controlled with a continuous infusion of an antihypertensive medication.

Learners will then administer IV thrombolytic; dose and rate should be specified by the learner. Neurology (if consulted) may call back after thrombolytic administration. Neurology consultation should include a discussion of imaging findings, patient's NIHSS, vital signs, interventions and response.

CTA can be obtained simultaneously with non-contrast head CT or after initiation of IV thrombolytic (may be prompted by neurology). CT perfusion and MRI are not available. Radiology will provide imaging findings based on level of learner:

- For novice learners:
  - No LVO identified. Learners should consult neurology and intensivist for disposition. Case ends here.
- For advanced learners:
  - Left M1 occlusion identified. Learners should review eligibility for thrombectomy including any pre-existing disability and request transfer to an appropriate facility. Case ends here.

Instructor Notes

Pathophysiology

- Caused by thrombotic/embolic occlusion or dissection of a cerebral artery.
- Symptoms may not reflect the entirety of at-risk brain (penumbra) if there is good collateral circulation.

Clinical Features

- Abrupt onset of neurological signs and symptoms which may include:
  - Dysarthria
  - Aphasia
  - Extremity weakness
  - Numbness
  - Facial droop
  - Limb ataxia
  - Visual field deficit
  - Extinction/inattention
  - Vertigo.

Diagnosis

- NIHSS quantifies severity.
- Neuroimaging directs management and rules out other diagnoses:
  - Non-contrast head CT may show early ischemic changes or alternate diagnosis (e.g., intracranial hemorrhage or edema).
  - CTA: can help to diagnose LVO or arterial dissection.
  - CT perfusion/magnetic resonance imaging (MRI) provides information on size of ischemia/infarct mismatch.

Management

- Laboratory tests:
  - Fingerstick glucose should be obtained on all patients with acute neurological symptoms.
  - Include platelet count, coagulation panel, and pregnancy test (if applicable).
- Blood pressure management:
  - <220/120 mmHg if not receiving thrombolytic/thrombectomy.
  - <185/110 mmHg to administer thrombolytic, then maintain <180/105 mmHg after.
  - Blood pressure post-thrombectomy depends on recanalization.
- Reperfusion therapies:
  - IV thrombolytic.
  - Risks [1]:
    - 6.4% symptomatic intracranial hemorrhage.
    - 1.6% major systemic hemorrhage.
    - 1.3–5.1% angioedema.
  - Benefits [2]:
    - 30–50% improvement to no or minimal disability at three months compared with 30% with no treatment.
  - Indications [3]:
    - Acute neurological symptoms secondary to presumed ischemia within a specific time window of last known well:
    - <3 hours
    - 3–4.5 hours: NIHSS > 25 is a relative contraindication.
    - >4.5 hours: in select patients with diffusion-positive, fluid-attenuated inversion recovery (FLAIR) negative MRI.
  - Contraindications [3]:
    - Ischemic stroke, significant head trauma, or intracranial/intraspinal surgery within three months.
    - History of intracranial hemorrhage or neoplasm.
    - Gastrointestinal malignancy or hemorrhage within 21 days.
    - Symptoms suggestive of subarachnoid hemorrhage, infective endocarditis, or aortic dissection.
    - Blood pressure > 185/110 mmHg.
    - Coagulopathy: platelets $<100 \times 10^3/\mu l$, international normalized ratio > 1.7, activated partial thromboplastin time > 40 seconds, or prothrombin time > 15 seconds.
    - Use of low-molecular-weight heparin within 24 hours, direct thrombin/factor Xa inhibitors within 48 hours, glycoprotein IIb/IIIa inhibitors.

- Although controversy exists regarding the efficacy of IV thrombolytic therapy, it remains standard of care [3]. Rationale for deviation from guidelines should be well-documented.
- Endovascular thrombectomy [3–5]:
- Within six hours of last-known well:
  - Age ≥ 18 years.
  - Pre-stroke modified Rankin scale score 0 or 1.
  - NIHSS ≥ 6.
  - Alberta Stroke Program early CT score ≥ 6.
  - Internal carotid artery or proximal MCA occlusion.
  - 6–24 hours of last-known well:
    - All the above *and* ischemia/infarct mismatch on CT perfusion/MRI.

Debriefing Plan

Allow approximately 30 minutes for discussion.

Potential Questions for Discussion

- How do you approach a patient presenting with acute neurological symptoms?
- What are the components of the NIHSS?
- What are contraindications for IV thrombolytics?
- What are the risks/benefits of IV thrombolytic that you discuss with patients when obtaining informed consent?
- When should you consider endovascular thrombectomy?

REFERENCES FOR ACUTE ISCHEMIC STROKE

1 Miller, D.J., Simpson, J.R., and Silver, B. (2011). Safety of thrombolysis in acute ischemic stroke: a review of complications, risk factors, and newer technologies. *Neurohospitalist.* 1 (3): 138–147.

2 National Institute of Neurological Disorders and Stroke rt-PA Stroke Study Group (1995). Tissue plasminogen activator for acute ischemic stroke. *N. Engl. J. Med.* 333: 1581–1587.

3 Powers, W.J., Rabinstein, A.A., Ackerson, T. et al. (2019). 2019 update to the 2018 guidelines for the early management of patients with acute ischemic stroke: a guideline for healthcare professionals from the American Heart Association/American Stroke Association. *Stroke* 50 (12): e344–e418.

4 Nogueira, R.G., Jadhav, A.P., Haussen, D.C. et al. (2018). Thrombectomy 6 to 24 hours after stroke with a mismatch between deficit and infarct. *N. Engl. J. Med.* 378 (1): 11–21.

5 Albers, G.W., Marks, M.P., Kemp, S. et al. (2018). Thrombectomy for stroke at 6 to 16 hours with selection by perfusion imaging. *N. Engl. J. Med.* 378 (8): 708–718.

INTRACEREBRAL HEMORRHAGE

Educational Goals

Learning Objectives

1. Assess airway, breathing, and circulation in a patient with altered mental status (MK, PC).
2. Manage elevated blood pressure in a patient with intracerebral hemorrhage (*ICH*) (MK, PC).
3. Perform reversal of coagulopathy (MK, PC).
4. Recognize signs of neurologic decline in ICH (MK, PC).
5. Demonstrate communication of relevant clinical information to consultants (ICS, P).
6. Manage a patient with signs of impending cerebral herniation (MK, PC).
7. Demonstrate effective team management in the care of a critically ill patient (ICS, P).

Critical Actions Checklist

- ☐ Perform primary assessment (MK, PC).
- ☐ Perform focused neurological exam, including the Glasgow Coma Scale (*GCS*) (MK, PC).
- ☐ Obtain pertinent history including antiplatelet/anticoagulant use (MK, ICS).
- ☐ Obtain fingerstick glucose (MK, PC).
- ☐ Obtain labs including platelet count, coagulation panel, type and screen (MK).
- ☐ Obtain Non-contrast head CT (MK).
- ☐ Use appropriate antihypertensive medications for blood pressure control (MK, PC).
- ☐ Appropriately reverse coagulopathy (advanced learner) (MK, PC).
- ☐ Treat empirically for impending cerebral herniation (MK, PC).
- ☐ Consult a neurosurgeon (ICS, P, SBP).
- ☐ Consult an intensivist for admission to intensive care (ICS, P, SBP).
- ☐ Designate a leader, maintain assigned roles, and use closed-loop communication (ICS, P).

Simulation Set-Up

Environment: ED treatment area

Mannequin: Male adult simulator, dressed in regular clothes, IV in place.

Props: Display on computer screen or as handouts:

- Images (see online component for ICH, Scenario 10.2 at https://www.wiley.com/go/thoureen/simulation/workbook2e)
  - ECG showing atrial fibrillation (Figure 10.9).

- Normal chest x-ray (Figure 10.10).
- Non-contrast CT of the head showing right basal ganglia ICH with intraventricular hemorrhage, hydrocephalus, and cerebral edema (Figure 10.11, Video 10.4).
- Laboratory tests (see online component as above):
  - Complete blood count (Table 10.6).
  - Chemistry Panel (Table 10.7).
  - Coagulation panel (Table 10.8) If you would like to alter the anticoagulant, refer to Table 10.11 for alternate coagulation panel values.
  - Thromboelastography (Table 10.9).
  - Type and screen (Table 10.10).

Nurse can report any imaging/labs not provided as normal. For novice learners the coagulation panel can be reported as normal.

Available supplies:

- Basic adult airway and code cart.
- Medications:
  - IV fluids in labeled 1 L bags: 0.9% saline, RL.
  - Blood products: platelets, fresh frozen plasma.
  - Pre-labeled syringes:
    - Antihypertensives: hydralazine, labetalol.
    - Vitamin K.
    - Intubation meds commonly used at your institution.
  - Pre-labeled IV bags:
    - Antihypertensives: clevidipine, nicardipine.
    - Prothrombin complex concentrate (*PCC*) of choice for your institution.
  - Desmopressin.
  - 3% hypertonic saline, mannitol.
  - Antiepileptics: levetiracetam, fosphenytoin.

Distractor: None

Actors

- Patient's voice is male. Patient should sound somnolent, but able to follow simple commands with stimulation.
- Nurse may cue learners if needed. The nurse may ask advanced learners to clarify the rationale behind medical decisions.

- Patient's wife is at bedside and able to provide the history.
- Consultants are available by phone, including pharmacy, blood bank, neurosurgeon, and intensivist.
- EMS provider can give report to the learners as a medical consult or on arrival to the ED.

Case Narrative

Scenario Background

A 57-year-old man with a history of atrial fibrillation and hypertension was found down at home. He was last seen normal 30 minutes prior to his wife calling EMS. On scene, the patient was awake and conversational with left-sided weakness and complaining of a headache. He is now somnolent but follows simple commands with stimulation. He is accompanied by his wife. EMS provider states "He was much more interactive at the house. He's probably just tired."

Patient's medical history:	Atrial fibrillation, hypertension.
Medications:	Aspirin (see box), metoprolol, amlodipine.
Allergies:	None.
Family history:	Hypertension.
Social history:	Lives with wife and two children. Works as a computer programmer at home.

> For advanced learners, patient is on apixaban instead of aspirin, last taken six hours ago. If alternative anticoagulants are used, please refer to Table 11.11 for coagulation panel values.

Initial Scenario Conditions

A middle-aged man is brought in by EMS. Patient is somnolent but protecting his airway. He opens his eyes and follows simple commands with stimulation. IV placed by EMS.

Vital signs:	Temp 98.9°F (37.2°C), HR 92, RR 20, BP 224/146, SpO$_2$ 98% on room air.
Weight:	80 kg.
Head:	Atraumatic.
Eyes:	Pupils 4 mm, equal, and reactive to light.
Neck:	Supple.
Heart:	Irregularly irregular, distal pulses normal.
Lungs:	Tachypneic, clear breath sounds bilaterally.
Chest:	No signs of trauma or tenderness.
Abdomen:	Soft and non-tender. Normal bowel sounds.
Extremities:	No deformities.

Skin: No rash or abrasions.

Neurologic: Half-opens eyes to stimulation. States name and follows simple commands. Left face, arm, and leg 0/5 strength and decreased sensation. Normal right-sided strength and sensation. Remainder of the NIH Stroke Scale is normal.

> The nurse can report exam findings not available on the mannequin if learners specifically ask.

See flow diagram (Figure 10.12) for scenario changes described.

Case Narrative, Continued

All learners should initially perform a primary survey, including fingerstick glucose. Learners should recognize that the patient had a neurological decline from initial EMS assessment. Patient's wife may cue learners by asking why the patient is not as responsive as he was previously.

Learners should order a non-contrast CT of the head; the nurse will clarify whether the patient is ready for transport to CT. Learners should explicitly discuss airway assessment before transport. If learners do not assess the airway or explicitly discuss airway assessment prior to transport, the patient will vomit, subsequently desaturate, and require antiemetic, supplemental oxygen, and intubation.

Learners must recognize hypertension requiring treatment, in the setting of ICH. Medication dosage, route of administration, and systolic blood pressures (SBP) parameters (140–180 mmHg) should be specified. SBP is not controlled with a bolus dose of antihypertensives and can only be controlled with an infusion of an antihypertensive.

Advanced learners must reverse coagulopathy using PCC or andexanet alfa. Learners should specify dosage. Pharmacy and blood bank are available for phone consultation, if requested.

> The case can be modified with the use of a different anticoagulant; corresponding case changes are in Table 10.11.

The patient will continue to have neurologic decline with corresponding changes in vital signs indicating impending cerebral herniation requiring empiric treatment and intubation. The nurse may prompt learners if needed. Neurosurgery is available for consultation for novice learners only. If learners do not initiate empiric treatment for impending cerebral herniation, the patient will herniate.

The case ends when the patient is stabilized and accepted for admission to an intensive care unit or if the allocated time has elapsed.

Instructor Notes

Pathophysiology

- Primary ICH occurs from rupture of small penetrating vessels due to chronic hypertension or cerebral amyloid angiopathy.
- Secondary ICH occurs from coagulopathy, sympathomimetic drugs, or underlying vascular anomalies.
- Neurologic deterioration from hematoma expansion and/or development of hydrocephalus commonly occur.

Clinical Features

- Abrupt onset of neurological symptoms.
- Headache, nausea, vomiting, and altered mental status may signal increased intracranial pressure.
  - > 20% of patients have decrease in GCS of 2 or more points from time time of EMS assessment to evaluation in the ED [1].
  - Cushing's triad → signs reflecting impending cerebral herniation:
  - Widened pulse pressure (increasing systolic, decreasing diastolic).
  - Bradycardia.
  - Irregular respirations.
- Seizures may occur depending on the location of ICH.

Diagnosis

- Non-contrast CT of the head.
- Cerebrovascular imaging may be indicated to evaluate etiology.

Management

- Assess airway, breathing, circulation and disability.
- Correct hypo/hyperglycemia, electrolyte abnormalities and coagulopathy, as needed.
- Blood pressures management:
  - Rapidly lowering blood pressures in ICH is safe [2, 3].
  - It is reasonable to target SBP 140–180 mmHg, though comorbidities and degree of chronic hypertension should be considered.
- Platelet transfusion:
  - Associated with worse outcomes, including an increased risk of death in patients taking antiplatelet medications [4].
  - This study did not include patients undergoing neurosurgical procedures [4].

- There is insufficient evidence for platelet function assays or thromboelastography to direct platelet transfusions.
- Coagulopathy reversal (Table 11.11).
- Treat elevated intracranial pressure and/or herniation.
  - Perform tiered management (Table 10.12).
- Seizure prophylaxis.
  - Not indicated in primary ICH.

Debriefing Plan

Allot approximately 30 minutes for discussion.

Potential Questions for Discussion

- How do you approach a patient presenting with altered mental status?
- What are the components of the GCS?
- How do you manage elevated blood pressure in ICH?
- What is the role of platelet transfusion in patients with ICH?
- How would you reverse coagulopathy from a factor Xa inhibitor? What about other anticoagulants?
- What are common causes for neurological deterioration in ICH?
- How would you manage increased intracranial pressure with signs of impending herniation in a patient with ICH?

REFERENCES FOR INTRACEREBRAL HEMORRHAGE

1 Moon, J.S., Janjua, N., Ahmed, S. et al. (2008). Prehospital neurologic deterioration in patients with intracerebral hemorrhage. *Crit. Care Med.* 36: 172–175.

2 Anderson, C.S., Heeley, E., and Huang, Y. (2013). Rapid blood-pressure lowering in patients with acute intracerebral hemorrhage. *N. Engl. J. Med.* 368 (25): 2355–2365.

3 Qureshi, A.I., Palesch, Y.Y., Barsan, W.G. et al. (2016). Intensive blood-pressure lowering in patients with acute cerebral hemorrhage. *N. Engl. J. Med.* 375 (11): 1033–1043.

4 Baharoglu, M.I., Cordonnier, C., Al-Shahi Salman, R. et al. (2016). Platelet transfusion versus standard care after acute stroke due to spontaneous cerebral haemorrhage associated with antiplatelet therapy (PATCH): a randomised, open-label, phase 3 trial. *Lancet* 387 (10038): 2605–2613.

5 Frontera, J.A., Lewin, J.J. 3rd, Rabinstein, A.A. et al. (2016). Guideline for reversal of antithrombotics in intracranial hemorrhage: a statement for healthcare professionals from the Neurocritical Care Society and Society for Critical Care Medicine. *Neurocrit. Care* 24: 6–46.

6 Pollack, C.V. Jr., Reilly, P.A., Eikelboom, J. et al. (2015). Idarucizumab for dabigatran reversal. *N. Engl. J. Med.* 373 (6): 511–520.

7 Connolly, S.J., Milling, T.J. Jr., Eikelboom, J.W. et al. (2016). Andexanet alfa for acute major bleeding associated with factor Xa inhibitors. *N. Engl. J. Med.* 375 (12): 1131–1141.

8 Cadena, R., Shoykhet, M., and Ratcliff, J.J. (2017). Emergency neurological life support: intracranial hypertension and herniation. *Neurocrit. Care* 27 (Suppl 1): 82–88.

SELECTED READINGS FOR INTRACEREBRAL HEMORRHAGE

Hemphill, J.C. 3rd and Lam, A. (2017). Emergency neurological life support: intracerebral hemorrhage. *Neurocrit. Care* 27 (Suppl 1): 89–101.

PEDIATRIC STATUS EPILEPTICUS

Educational Goals

Learning Objectives

1. Recognize status epilepticus (MK, PC).
2. Demonstrate appropriate management of status epilepticus (MK, PC).
3. Identify causes of provoked seizures (MK).
4. Recognize the indications for intubation in status epilepticus (MK, PC).
5. Demonstrate effective communication of clinical progress to parents/care-givers and address their concerns (ICS, P).
6. Demonstrate effective team management skills (ICS, P).

Critical Actions Checklist

- ☐ Obtain IV or intraosseous (*IO*) access (PC).
- ☐ Obtain fingerstick glucose (MK).
- ☐ Order appropriate dose of a benzodiazepine as first-line antiepileptic medication (MK, PC).
- ☐ Order appropriate dose of a second-line antiepileptic medication after patient has second seizure (MK, PC).
- ☐ Order a third-line antiepileptic medication for refractory seizures (MK, PC).
- ☐ Order noncontrast head CT and labs to evaluate cause for provoked seizures (MK).
- ☐ Perform endotracheal intubation for airway compromise or when starting IV anesthetics (MK, PC).
- ☐ Use appropriate meds for intubation (advanced learner) (MK, PC).
- ☐ Consult a pediatric intensivist for disposition (ICS, P, SBP).
- ☐ Designate a leader, maintain assigned role, and use closed-loop communication (ICS, P).

Simulation Set-up

Environment: ED treatment area.

Mannequin: Female pediatric simulator (elementary-aged size), dressed in regular clothes. IV in place for novice learners. Non-rebreather (*NRB*) mask in place. Some high-fidelity mannequins can simulate seizure. Alternatively, your nurse can cue learners to seizure activity, or you could use a vibrating object under the mattress to simulate seizure.

Props: Display on computer screen or as handouts:

- Images (see online component for SE, Scenario 10.3 at https://www.wiley.com/go/thoureen/simulation/workbook2e):
  - Chest x-ray (normal) (Figure 10.13).
  - Non-contrast head CT (normal) (Figure 10.14).
  - ECG showing sinus tachycardia (Figure 10.15).
- Laboratory tests (see online component as above):
  - Complete metabolic panel (Table 10.13).
  - Complete blood count(Table 10.14).
  - Lactate (Table 10.15).
  - Creatine kinase (Table 10.16).

The nurse can report any imaging/labs not provided as normal.

Available supplies:

- Pediatric code cart and basic airway supplies.
- Pediatric measuring tape (e.g., Broselow tape).
- Medications:
  - IV fluids in labeled 1 l bags: 0.9% saline, LR.
  - Pre-labeled syringes:
    - Benzodiazepines: lorazepam, midazolam, diazepam.
    - Intubation meds commonly used at institution.
  - Pre-labeled IV bags:
    - Antiepileptics/sedatives: (e.g., fosphenytoin, levetiracetam, and/or agents commonly used at your institution).

Distractor: None.

Actors

- Patient voice is female. Patient should sound confused and lethargic. She is not able to follow commands or answer questions.
- Nurse may cue learners if needed. The nurse asks advanced learners to clarify the rationale behind medical decisions.
- Parent is present at bedside and able to provide the history
- Pediatric neurologist and pediatric intensivist available by telephone.
- EMS crew member can give report (optional).

Case Narrative

Scenario Background

An 8-year-old girl with a history of seizures is brought in by EMS after having a two-minute seizure. She is still unresponsive, moaning intermittently, and answers questions incomprehensibly. She is accompanied by a parent.

Patient's medical history:	Epilepsy
Medications:	Levetiracetam
Allergies:	None
Family history:	Unremarkable
Social history:	Lives with parents and one younger sibling. Goes to elementary school.

Initial Scenario Conditions

Young girl brought in by EMS. Patient is moaning intermittently. NRB mask in place. EMS performed no other interventions because seizure activity terminated spontaneously. IV access established for novice learners only.

EMS may present background as a medical consult or on arrival to the ED.

Vital signs:	Temp 97.1°F (36.2°C), HR 110, RR 18, BP 120/70, O2 sat 100% on NRB.
Weight:	25 kg.
Head:	Atraumatic.
Eyes:	Pupils 4 mm and reactive to light.
Neck:	Supple, no lymphadenopathy or swelling.
Heart:	Tachycardic and regular, distal pulses normal.
Lungs:	Tachypneic, clear breath sounds bilaterally.
Chest:	No signs of trauma or tenderness.
Abdomen:	Soft and non-tender. Normal bowel sounds.
Extremities:	No deformities.
Skin:	No rash or abrasions.
Neurologic:	Eyes half-open. Moans and withdraws to pain.

Nurse can report exam findings not available on the mannequin (e.g., pupil reactivity) if learners specifically ask.

See flow diagram (Figure 10.16) for scenario changes described.

Case Narrative, Continued

All learners should initially perform a primary survey and obtain a fingerstick glucose. Patient will begin seizing one minute after the start of the scenario. Learners should recognize status epilepticus. Advanced learners will not be able to obtain IV access. They may consider IO access, but ideally will administer intramuscular (IM) midazolam. After cessation of seizure, IV access can be obtained.

Seizure will terminate within 30 seconds of benzodiazepine administration. Seizure will resume two minutes later, and not resolve with repeat doses of benzodiazepines, prompting the learners to start parenteral antiepileptic meds. Dosage and route of administration should be specified by the learners. Learners may order second-line antiepileptics at the same time as the initial benzodiazepine, prompting instructors to skip the second seizure. Inadequately treated seizures will lead to deterioration and cardiopulmonary arrest.

Seizure will terminate again within one minute of starting the appropriate second-line antiepileptic medication. There is temporary stabilization, during which learners should obtain further history and order diagnostics.

After four minutes, seizure will resume, prompting learners to induce a coma using an agent for refractory seizures. Concurrent intubation is necessary. If learners fail to manage the airway prior to inducing coma, the patient will go into cardiopulmonary arrest.

Learners may start additional antiepileptics at this time, which is acceptable but will not terminate seizure activity. Pediatric neurologist/intensivist will be available for consultation for novice learners only.

Following appropriate treatment, any ordered imaging/labs will return. The case ends when the patient is accepted for transfer to a pediatric intensive care unit.

Instructor Notes

Pathophysiology

- Seizures are disordered electrical activity in the brain manifesting in a variety of abnormal neurological symptoms.
- Caused by decreased activity at the γ-aminobutyric acid receptors and increased activity at glutaminergic receptors, such as N-methyl-d-aspartate.
- Most are self-limited and last for ≤2 minutes [1].
- Classified as "provoked" or "unprovoked."
- Provoked causes: electrolyte abnormality, infection, ICH/mass, toxic ingestion, and eclampsia.

Clinical Features

- Status epilepticus is a seizure lasting ≥5 minutes or ≥2 seizures without a return to baseline.

- Non-convulsive status epilepticus:
- No overt seizure activity but can have altered mental status, prolonged post-ictal period, and/or automatisms.
- Hyperthermia, rhabdomyolysis, and lactic acidosis can result from prolonged seizures.

Diagnosis

- Primarily clinical.
- EEG in patients concerning for non-convulsive status epilepticus.

Management

- Consult the American Epilepsy Society's treatment algorithm for older children and adults [2].
- Management of seizures in neonates is beyond the scope of this discussion.
- Assess ABCD.
- Obtain fingerstick glucose.
- In status epilepticus, causes of provoked seizures should be evaluated.
- Focused laboratory testing:
  - Electrolytes (especially sodium, glucose, and calcium).
  - Serum levels of antiepileptic drugs, if applicable.
  - Pregnancy test in patients of child-bearing age.
  - Head CT in patients with suspected trauma, compromised immune system, bleeding disorder, or history of cancer.
  - Lumbar puncture in suspected meningitis/encephalitis.
- Medications [2]:
  - First line: benzodiazepines:
    - Lorazepam 0.1 mg/kg IM/IV (max 4 mg).
    - Diazepam 0.2 mg/kg IM/IV, 0.5 mg/kg rectal (max 8 mg).
    - Midazolam 0.2 mg/kg IM/IV (max 10 mg).
  - Second line: antiepileptics
    - Fosphenytoin 20 mg/kg.
    - Valproic acid 40 mg/kg.
    - Levetiracetam 60 mg/kg.
    - Phenobarbital (15–20 mg/kg).
    - The ESETT (Established Status Epilepticus Treatment trial) showed similar efficacy among fosphenytoin, valproic acid, and levetiracetam [3].
  - Third line: coma induction [2, 4]:
    - Midazolam: 0.2 mg/kg IV bolus, 0.05–2 mg/kg/hour infusion.

- Propofol: 1–2 mg/kg IV bolus, 20–65 µg/kg/minute infusion.
- Pentobarbital: 10–15 mg/kg IV bolus, 0.5–5 mg/kg/hour infusion.
- Endotracheal intubation:
  - Not all patients will require intubation.
  - Indications:
    - Airway compromise.
    - Use of third line agents to induce coma.
    - Propofol, midazolam and pentobarbital are preferred for sedation secondary to their antiepileptic properties.
    - Insufficient evidence for depolarizing vs. non-depolarizing paralytics
    - Patients receiving long-acting paralytics should be placed on EEG to evaluate ongoing seizures

Debriefing Plan

Allot approximately 30 minutes for discussion.

Potential Questions for Discussion

- How do you manage a seizing patient?
- What is status epilepticus?
- What are second- and third-line agents for treatment of status epilepticus?
- What diagnostics should you order for a patient with status epilepticus? How might the results change management?
- What are the indications for intubation? Any special considerations when selecting a sedative or paralytic?
- What is non-convulsive status epilepticus and why is it clinically relevant?

REFERENCES FOR STATUS EPILEPTICUS

1. Chen, J.W.Y., Naylor, D.E., and Wasterlain, C.G. (2007). Advances in the pathophysiology of status epilepticus. *Acta Neurol. Scand.* 115: 7–15.
2. Glauser, T., Shinnar, S., Gloss, D. et al. (2016). Evidence-based guideline: treatment of convulsive status epilepticus in children and adults: report of the Guideline Committee of the American Epilepsy Society. *Epilepsy. Curr.* 16 (1): 48–61.
3. Kapur, J., Elm, J., Chamberlain, J.M. et al. (2019). Randomized trial of three anticonvulsant medications for status epilepticus. *N. Engl. J. Med.* 381 (22): 2103–2113.
4. Brophy, G.M., Bell, R., Claassen, J. et al. (2012). Guidelines for the evaluation and management of status epilepticus. *Neurocrit. Care.* 17 (1): 3–23.

SELECTED READINGS FOR STATUS EPILEPTICUS

Lawton, B., Davis, T., Goldstein, H., and Tagg., A. (2018). An update in the initial management of paediatric status epilepticus. *Curr. Opin. Pediatr.* 30 (3): 359–363.

Video 10.1 Non-contrast computed tomography of the head showing dense left middle cerebral artery sign. This video does not include audio commentary.

Video 10.2 CTA head. This video does not include audio commentary. CTA head showing no large vessel occlusion (LVO).

Video 10.3 Computed tomography angiography of the head showing occlusion of the left M1 segment of the middle cerebral artery. This video does not include audio commentary.

Video 10.4 Non-contrast head CT showing right basal ganglia intracerebral hemorrhage with intraventricular hemorrhage, hydrocephalus, and cerebral edema. This video does not include audio commentary.

APPENDIX

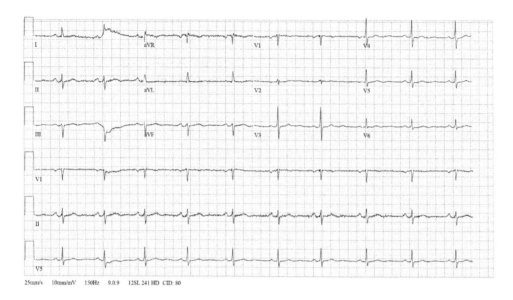

FIGURE 10.1 Electrocardiogram showing normal sinus rhythm.

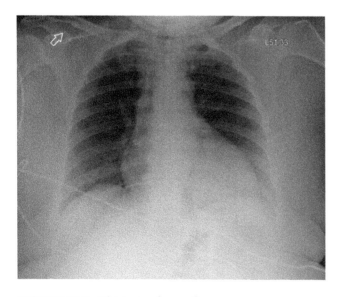

FIGURE 10.2 Chest x-ray (normal).

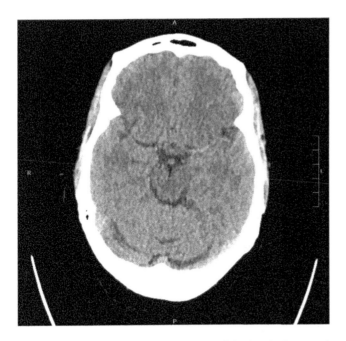

FIGURE 10.3 Computed tomography of the head, showing dense left middle cerebral artery sign.

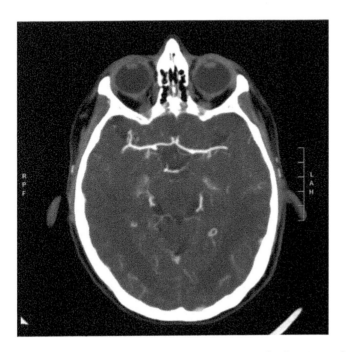

FIGURE 10.4 Computed tomography angiography showing no large vessel occlusion.

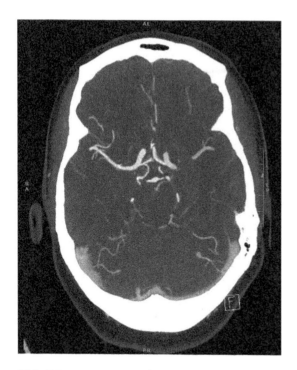

FIGURE 10.5   Computed tomography angiography showing left M1 occlusion.

N I H
STROKE
SCALE

Patient Identification. ___ ___-___ ___ ___-___ ___ ___

Pt. Date of Birth ___ ___/___ ___/___ ___

Hospital _____(___ ___-___ ___)

Date of Exam ___ ___/___ ___/___ ___

Interval: [ ] Baseline   [ ] 2 hours post treatment   [ ] 24 hours post onset of symptoms ±20 minutes [ ] 7–10 days
           [ ] 3 months   [ ] Other _____(___ ___)

Time: ___ ___:___ ___   [ ]am [ ]pm

Person Administering Scale _____

Administer stroke scale items in the order listed. Record performance in each category after each subscale exam. Do not go back and change scores. Follow directions provided for each exam technique. Scores should reflect what the patient does, not what the clinician thinks the patient can do. The clinician should record answers while administering the exam and work quickly. Except where indicated, the patient should not be coached (i.e., repeated requests to patient to make a special effort).

Instructions	Scale Definition	Score
1a. Level of Consciousness: The investigator must choose a response if a full evaluation is prevented by such obstacles as an endotracheal tube, language barrier, orotracheal trauma/bandages. A 3 is scored only if the patient makes no movement (other than reflexive posturing) in response to noxious stimulation.	0 = **Alert;** keenly responsive. 1 = **Not alert;** but arousable by minor stimulation to obey, answer, or respond. 2 = **Not alert;** requires repeated stimulation to attend, or is obtunded and requires strong or painful stimulation to make movements (not stereotyped). 3 = Responds only with reflex motor or autonomic effects or totally unresponsive, flaccid, and are flexic.	_____
1b. LOC Questions: The patient is asked the month and his/her age. The answer must be correct - there is no partial credit for being close. Aphasic and stuporous patients who do not comprehend the questions will score 2. Patients unable to speak because of endotracheal intubation, orotracheal trauma, severe dysarthria from any cause, language barrier, or any other problem not secondary to aphasia are given a 1. It is important that only the initial answer be graded and that the examiner not "help" the patient with verbal or non-verbal cues.	0 = **Answers** both questions correctly. 1 = **Answers** one question correctly. 2 = **Answers** neither question correctly.	_____
1c. LOC Commands: The patient is asked to open and close the eyes and then to grip and release the non-paretic hand. Substitute another one step command if the hands cannot be used. Credit is given if an unequivocal attempt is made but not completed due to weakness. If the patient does not respond to command, the task should be demonstrated to him or her (pantomime), and the result scored (i.e., follows none, one or two commands). Patients with trauma, amputation, or other physical impediments should be given suitable one-step commands. Only the first attempt is scored.	0 = **Performs** both tasks correctly. 1 = **Performs** one task correctly. 2 = **Performs** neither task correctly.	_____
2. Best Gaze: Only horizontal eye movements will be tested. Voluntary or reflexive (oculocephalic) eye movements will be scored, but caloric testing is not done. If the patient has a conjugate deviation of the eyes that can be overcome by voluntary or reflexive activity, the score will be 1. If a patient has an isolated peripheral nerve paresis (CN III, IV or VI), score a1. Gaze is testable in all aphasic patients. Patients with ocular trauma, bandages, pre-existing blindness, or other disorder of visual acuity or fields should be tested with reflexive movements, and a choice made by the investigator. Establishing eye contact and then moving about the patient from side to side will occasionally clarify the presence of a partial gaze palsy.	0 = **Normal.** 1 = **Partial gaze palsy;** gaze is abnormal in one or both eyes, but forced deviation or total gaze paresis is not present. 2 = **Forced deviation,** or total gaze paresis not overcome by the oculocephalic maneuver.	_____

Rev 10/1/2003

FIGURE 10.6 National Institutes of Health Stroke Scale.

Patient Identification. ___ ___-___ ___ -___ ___ ___

Pt. Date of Birth ___ __/__   /__ __

Hospital _____(__ __-__ __)

Date of Exam ___ __/__ __/__ __

Interval: [ ] Baseline   [ ] 2 hours post treatment   [ ] 24 hours post onset of symptoms ±20 minutes   [ ] 7–10 days
       [ ] 3 months   [ ] Other _____(__ __)

3. Visual: Visual fields (upper and lower quadrants) are tested by confrontation, using finger counting or visual threat, as appropriate. Patients may be encouraged, but if they look at the side of the moving fingers appropriately, this can be scored as normal. If there is unilateral blindness or enucleation, visual fields in the remaining eye are scored. Score 1 only if a clear-cut asymmetry, including quadrantanopia, is found. If patient is blind from any cause, score 3. Double simultaneous stimulation is performed at this point. If there is extinction, patient receives a 1, and the results are used to respond to item 11.	0 = **No visual loss.** 1 = **Partial hemianopia.** 2 = **Complete hemianopia.** 3 = **Bilateral hemianopia** (blind including cortical blindness).	_____
4. Facial Palsy: Ask – or use pantomime to encourage – the patient to show teeth or raise eyebrows and close eyes. Score symmetry of grimace in response to noxious stimuli in the poorly responsive or non-comprehending patient. If facial trauma/bandages, orotracheal tube, tape or other physical barriers obscure the face, these should be removed to the extent possible.	0 = **Normal** symmetrical movements. 1 = **Minor paralysis** (flattened nasolabial fold, asymmetry on smiling). 2 = **Partial paralysis** (total or near-total paralysis of lower face). 3 = **Complete paralysis** of one or both sides (absence of facial movement in the upper and lower face).	_____
5. Motor Arm: The limb is placed in the appropriate position: extend the arms (palms down) 90 degrees (if sitting) or 45 degrees (if supine). Drift is scored if the arm falls before 10 seconds. The aphasic patient is encouraged using urgency in the voice and pantomime, but not noxious stimulation. Each limb is tested in turn, beginning with the non-paretic arm. Only in the case of amputation or joint fusion at the shoulder, the examiner should record the score as untestable (UN), and clearly write the explanation for this choice.	0 = **No drift;** limb holds 90 (or 45) degrees for full 10 seconds. 1 = **Drift;** limb holds 90 (or 45) degrees, but drifts down before full 10 seconds; does not hit bed or other support. 2 = **Some effort against gravity;** limb cannot get to or maintain (if cued) 90 (or 45) degrees, drifts down to bed, but has some effort against gravity. 3 = **No effort against gravity;** limb falls. 4 = **No movement.** UN = **Amputation** or joint fusion, explain: _____ **5a. Left Arm** **5b. Right Arm**	 _____ _____
6. Motor Leg: The limb is placed in the appropriate position: hold the leg at 30 degrees (always tested supine). Drift is scored if the leg falls before 5 seconds. The aphasic patient is encouraged using urgency in the voice and pantomime, but not noxious stimulation. Each limb is tested in turn, beginning with the non-paretic leg. Only in the case of amputation or joint fusion at the hip, the examiner should record the score as untestable (UN), and clearly write the explanation for this choice.	0 = **No drift;** leg holds 30-degree position for full 5 seconds. 1 = **Drift;** leg falls by the end of the 5-second period but does not hit bed. 2 = **Some effort against gravity;** leg falls to bed by 5 seconds, but has some effort against gravity. 3 = **No effort against gravity;** leg falls to bed immediately. 4 = **No movement.** UN = **Amputation** or joint fusion, explain: _____ **6a. Left Leg** **6b. Right Leg**	 _____

Rev 10/1/2003

FIGURE 10.6   (Continued)

N I H
STROKE
SCALE

Patient Identification. ___ ___-___ ___ ___-___ ___ ___

Pt. Date of Birth ___ ___/___ ___/___ ___

Hospital _____(___ ___-___ ___)

Date of Exam ___ ___/___ ___/___ ___

Interval: [ ] Baseline   [ ] 2 hours post treatment   [ ] 24 hours post onset of symptoms ±20 minutes   [ ] 7–10 days
           [ ] 3 months   [ ] Other _____(___ ___)

7. Limb Ataxia: This item is aimed at finding evidence of a unilateral cerebellar lesion. Test with eyes open. In case of visual defect, ensure testing is done in intact visual field. The finger-nose-finger and heel-shin tests are performed on both sides, and ataxia is scored only if present out of proportion to weakness. Ataxia is absent in the patient who cannot understand or is paralyzed. Only in the case of amputation or joint fusion, the examiner should record the score as untestable (UN), and clearly write the explanation for this choice. In case of blindness, test by having the patient touch nose from extended arm position.	0 = **Absent.** 1 = **Present in one limb.** 2 = **Present in two limbs.** UN = **Amputation** or joint fusion, explain: _____	_____
8. Sensory: Sensation or grimace to pinprick when tested, or withdrawal from noxious stimulus in the obtunded or aphasic patient. Only sensory loss attributed to stroke is scored as abnormal and the examiner should test as many body areas (arms [not hands], legs, trunk, face) as needed to accurately check for hemisensory loss. A score of 2, "severe or total sensory loss," should only be given when a severe or total loss of sensation can be clearly demonstrated. Stuporous and aphasic patients will, therefore, probably score 1 or 0. The patient with brainstem stroke who has bilateral loss of sensation is scored 2. If the patient does not respond and is quadriplegic, score 2. Patients in a coma (item 1a=3) are automatically given a 2 on this item.	0 = **Normal;** no sensory loss. 1 = **Mild-to-moderate sensory loss;** patient feels pinprick is less sharp or is dull on the affected side; or there is a loss of superficial pain with pinprick, but patient is aware of being touched. 2 = **Severe to total sensory loss;** patient is not aware of being touched in the face, arm, and leg.	_____
9. Best Language: A great deal of information about comprehension will be obtained during the preceding sections of the examination. For this scale item, the patient is asked to describe what is happening in the attached picture, to name the items on the attached naming sheet and to read from the attached list of sentences. Comprehension is judged from responses here, as well as to all of the commands in the preceding general neurological exam. If visual loss interferes with the tests, ask the patient to identify objects placed in the hand, repeat, and produce speech. The intubated patient should be asked to write. The patient in a coma (item 1a=3) will automatically score 3 on this item. The examiner must choose a score for the patient with stupor or limited cooperation, but a score of 3 should be used only if the patient is mute and follows no one-step commands.	0 = **No aphasia;** normal. 1 = **Mild-to-moderate aphasia;** some obvious loss of fluency or facility of comprehension, without significant limitation on ideas expressed or form of expression. Reduction of speech and/or comprehension, however, makes conversation about provided materials difficult or impossible. For example, in conversation about provided materials, examiner can identify picture or naming card content from patient's response. 2 = **Severe aphasia;** all communication is through fragmentary expression; great need for inference, questioning, and guessing by the listener. Range of information that can be exchanged is limited; listener carries burden of communication. Examiner cannot identify materials provided from patient response. 3 = **Mute, global aphasia;** no usable speech or auditory comprehension.	_____
10. Dysarthria: If patient is thought to be normal, an adequate sample of speech must be obtained by asking patient to read or repeat words from the attached list. If the patient has severe aphasia, the clarity of articulation of spontaneous speech can be rated. Only if the patient is intubated or has other physical barriers to producing speech, the examiner should record the score as untestable (UN), and clearly write an explanation for this choice. Do not tell the patient why he or she is being tested.	0 = **Normal.** 1 = **Mild-to-moderate dysarthria;** patient slurs at least some words and, at worst, can be understood with some difficulty. 2 = **Severe dysarthria;** patient's speech is so slurred as to be unintelligible in the absence of or out of proportion to any dysphasia, or is mute/anarthric. UN = **Intubated** or other physical barrier, explain:_____	_____

Rev 10/1/2003

FIGURE 10.6   (Continued)

N I H STROKE SCALE

Patient Identification. ___ ___-___ ___ ___-___ ___ ___

Pt. Date of Birth ___ ___/___ ___/___ ___

Hospital _____ (___ ___-___ ___)

Date of Exam ___ ___/___ ___/___ ___

Interval: [ ] Baseline   [ ] 2 hours post treatment   [ ] 24 hours post onset of symptoms ±20 minutes   [ ] 7–10 days
    [ ] 3 months   [ ] Other _____(___ ___)

11. Extinction and Inattention (formerly Neglect): Sufficient information to identify neglect may be obtained during the prior testing. If the patient has a severe visual loss preventing visual double simultaneous stimulation, and the cutaneous stimuli are normal, the score is normal. If the patient has aphasia but does appear to attend to both sides, the score is normal. The presence of visual spatial neglect or anosagnosia may also be taken as evidence of abnormality. Since the abnormality is scored only if present, the item is never untestable.	0 = No abnormality. 1 = **Visual, tactile, auditory, spatial, or personal inattention** or extinction to bilateral simultaneous stimulation in one of the sensory modalities. 2 = **Profound hemi-inattention or extinction to more than one modality;** does not recognize own hand or orients to only one side of space.	_____

_____
_____

Rev 10/1/2003

FIGURE 10.6   (Continued)

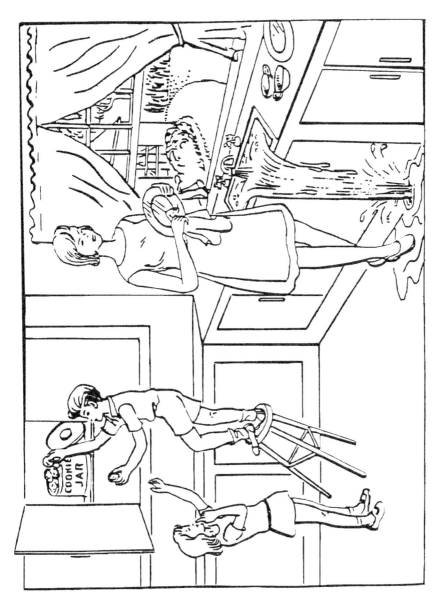

You know how.

Down to earth.

I got home from work.

Near the table in the dining
 room.

They heard him speak on the
 radio last night.

FIGURE 10.6 (Continued)

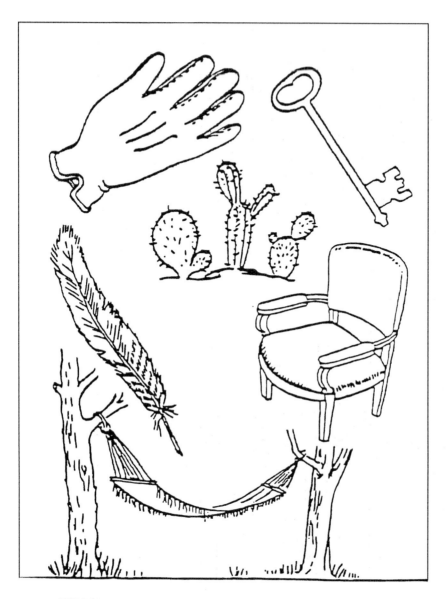

MAMA

TIP – TOP

FIFTY – FIFTY

THANKS

HUCKLEBERRY

BASEBALL PLAYER

FIGURE 10.6   (Continued)

N I H STROKE SCALE

Juanita Gonzalez

Patient Identification. ___ ___-___ ___ ___-___ ___ ___

Pt. Date of Birth ___ __/ . __/___ ___

Hospital _____(___ __-___ ___)

Date of Exam ___ __/__ __/___ ___

Interval: [ ] Baseline   [ ] 2 hours post treatment   [ ] 24 hours post onset of symptoms ±20 minutes   [ ] 7–10 days
[ ] 3 months   [ ] Other _____(___ ___)

Time: ___ ___:___ ___ [ ] am [ ] pm

Person Administering Scale_____

Administer stroke scale items in the order listed. Record performance in each category after each subscale exam. Do not go back and change scores. Follow directions provided for each exam technique. Scores should reflect what the patient does, not what the clinician thinks the patient can do. The clinician should record answers while administering the exam and work quickly. Except where indicated, the patient should not be coached (i.e., repeated requests to patient to make a special effort).

Instructions	Scale Definition	Score
1a. Level of Consciousness: The investigator must choose a response if a full evaluation is prevented by such obstacles as an endotracheal tube, language barrier, orotracheal trauma/bandages. A 3 is scored only if the patient makes no movement (other than reflexive posturing) in response to noxious stimulation.	0 = **Alert;** keenly responsive. 1 = **Not alert;** but arousable by minor stimulation to obey, answer, or respond. 2 = **Not alert;** requires repeated stimulation to attend, or is obtunded and requires strong or painful stimulation to make movements (not stereotyped). 3 = Responds only with reflex motor or autonomic effects or totally unresponsive, flaccid, and are flexic.	0
1b. LOC Questions: The patient is asked the month and his/her age. The answer must be correct - there is no partial credit for being close. Aphasic and stuporous patients who do not comprehend the questions will score 2. Patients unable to speak because of endotracheal intubation, orotracheal trauma, severe dysarthria from any cause, language barrier, or any other problem not secondary to aphasia are given a 1. It is important that only the initial answer be graded and that the examiner not "help" the patient with verbal or non-verbal cues.	0 = **Answers** both questions correctly. 1 = **Answers** one question correctly. 2 = **Answers** neither question correctly.	0
1c. LOC Commands: The patient is asked to open and close the eyes and then to grip and release the non-paretic hand. Substitute another one step command if the hands cannot be used. Credit is given if an unequivocal attempt is made but not completed due to weakness. If the patient does not respond to command, the task should be demonstrated to him or her (pantomime), and the result scored (i.e., follows none, one or two commands). Patients with trauma, amputation, or other physical impediments should be given suitable one-step commands. Only the first attempt is scored.	0 = **Performs** both tasks correctly. 1 = **Performs** one task correctly. 2 = **Performs** neither task correctly.	0
2. Best Gaze: Only horizontal eye movements will be tested. Voluntary or reflexive (oculocephalic) eye movements will be scored, but caloric testing is not done. If the patient has a conjugate deviation of the eyes that can be overcome by voluntary or reflexive activity, the score will be 1. If a patient has an isolated peripheral nerve paresis (CN III, IV or VI), score a 1. Gaze is testable in all aphasic patients. Patients with ocular trauma, bandages, pre-existing blindness, or other disorder of visual acuity or fields should be tested with reflexive movements, and a choice made by the investigator. Establishing eye contact and then moving about the patient from side to side will occasionally clarify the presence of a partial gaze palsy.	0 = **Normal.** 1 = **Partial gaze palsy;** gaze is abnormal in one or both eyes, but forced deviation or total gaze paresis is not present. 2 = **Forced deviation,** or total gaze paresis not overcome by the oculocephalic maneuver.	1

Rev 10/1/2003

FIGURE 10.7 Patient's National Institutes of Health Stroke Scale.

N I H
STROKE
SCALE

Patient Identification. ___ ___-___ ___-___ ___ ___

Pt. Date of Birth ___ ___/___ ___/___ ___

Hospital _____(___ ___-___ ___)

Date of Exam ___ ___/___ ___/___ ___

Interval: [ ] Baseline   [ ] 2 hours post treatment   [ ] 24 hours post onset of symptoms ±20 minutes   [ ] 7–10 days
  [ ] 3 months [ ] Other _____(___ ___)

3. Visual: Visual fields (upper and lower quadrants) are tested by confrontation, using finger counting or visual threat, as appropriate. Patients may be encouraged, but if they look at the side of the moving fingers appropriately, this can be scored as normal. If there is unilateral blindness or enucleation, visual fields in the remaining eye are scored. Score 1 only if a clear-cut asymmetry, including quadrantanopia, is found. If patient is blind from any cause, score 3. Double simultaneous stimulation is performed at this point. If there is extinction, patient receives a 1, and the results are used to respond to item 11.	0 = **No visual loss.** 1 = **Partial hemianopia.** 2 = **Complete hemianopia.** 3 = **Bilateral hemianopia** (blind including cortical blindness).	1 ___
4. Facial Palsy: Ask – or use pantomime to encourage – the patient to show teeth or raise eyebrows and close eyes. Score symmetry of grimace in response to noxious stimuli in the poorly responsive or non-comprehending patient. If facial trauma/bandages, orotracheal tube, tape or other physical barriers obscure the face, these should be removed to the extent possible.	0 = **Normal** symmetrical movements. 1 = **Minor paralysis** (flattened nasolabial fold, asymmetry on smiling). 2 = **Partial paralysis** (total or near-total paralysis of lower face). 3 = **Complete paralysis** of one or both sides (absence of facial movement in the upper and lower face).	2 ___
5. Motor Arm: The limb is placed in the appropriate position: extend the arms (palms down) 90 degrees (if sitting) or 45 degrees (if supine). Drift is scored if the arm falls before 10 seconds. The aphasic patient is encouraged using urgency in the voice and pantomime, but not noxious stimulation. Each limb is tested in turn, beginning with the non-paretic arm. Only in the case of amputation or joint fusion at the shoulder, the examiner should record the score as untestable (UN), and clearly write the explanation for this choice. **5a. Left Arm** **5b. Right Arm**	0 = **No drift;** limb holds 90 (or 45) degrees for full 10 seconds. 1 = **Drift;** limb holds 90 (or 45) degrees, but drifts down before full 10 seconds; does not hit bed or other support. 2 = **Some effort against gravity;** limb cannot get to or maintain (if cued) 90 (or 45) degrees, drifts down to bed, but has some effort against gravity. 3 = **No effort against gravity;** limb falls. 4 = **No movement.** UN = **Amputation** or joint fusion, explain: _____	0 ___ 3 ___
6. Motor Leg: The limb is placed in the appropriate position: hold the leg at 30 degrees (always tested supine). Drift is scored if the leg falls before 5 seconds. The aphasic patient is encouraged using urgency in the voice and pantomime, but not noxious stimulation. Each limb is tested in turn, beginning with the non-paretic leg. Only in the case of amputation or joint fusion at the hip, the examiner should record the score as untestable (UN), and clearly write the explanation for this choice. **6a. Left Leg** **6b. Right Leg**	0 = **No drift;** leg holds 30-degree position for full 5 seconds. 1 = **Drift;** leg falls by the end of the 5-second period but does not hit bed. 2 = **Some effort against gravity;** leg falls to bed by 5 seconds, but has some effort against gravity. 3 = **No effort against gravity;** leg falls to bed immediately. 4 = **No movement.** UN = **Amputation** or joint fusion, explain: _____	0 ___ 3

Rev 10/1/2003

FIGURE 10.7 (Continued)

N I H STROKE SCALE

Patient Identification. ___ __-___ ___ ___-___ ___ ___

Pt. Date of Birth ___ __/___ __/___ ___

Hospital _____(___ __-___ ___)

Date of Exam ___ __/___ __/___ ___

Interval: [ ] Baseline [ ] 2 hours post treatment   [ ] 24 hours post onset of symptoms ±20 minutes   [ ] 7–10 days
[ ] 3 months [ ] Other _____(___ ___)

7. Limb Ataxia: This item is aimed at finding evidence of a unilateral cerebellar lesion. Test with eyes open. In case of visual defect, ensure testing is done in intact visual field. The finger-nose-finger and heel-shin tests are performed on both sides, and ataxia is scored only if present out of proportion to weakness. Ataxia is absent in the patient who cannot understand or is paralyzed. Only in the case of amputation or joint fusion, the examiner should record the score as untestable (UN), and clearly write the explanation for this choice. In case of blindness, test by having the patient touch nose from extended arm position.	0 = **Absent.** 1 = **Present in one limb.** 2 = **Present in two limbs.** UN = **Amputation** or joint fusion, explain: _____	0
8. Sensory: Sensation or grimace to pinprick when tested, or withdrawal from noxious stimulus in the obtunded or aphasic patient. Only sensory loss attributed to stroke is scored as abnormal and the examiner should test as many body areas (arms [not hands], legs, trunk, face) as needed to accurately check for hemisensory loss. A score of 2, "severe or total sensory loss," should only be given when a severe or total loss of sensation can be clearly demonstrated. Stuporous and aphasic patients will, therefore, probably score 1 or 0. The patient with brainstem stroke who has bilateral loss of sensation is scored 2. If the patient does not respond and is quadriplegic, score 2. Patients in a coma (item 1a=3) are automatically given a 2 on this item.	0 = **Normal;** no sensory loss. 1 = **Mild-to-moderate sensory loss;** patient feels pinprick is less sharp or is dull on the affected side; or there is a loss of superficial pain with pinprick, but patient is aware of being touched. 2 = **Severe to total sensory loss;** patient is not aware of being touched in the face, arm, and leg.	1
9. Best Language: A great deal of information about comprehension will be obtained during the preceding sections of the examination. For this scale item, the patient is asked to describe what is happening in the attached picture, to name the items on the attached naming sheet and to read from the attached list of sentences. Comprehension is judged from responses here, as well as to all of the commands in the preceding general neurological exam. If visual loss interferes with the tests, ask the patient to identify objects placed in the hand, repeat, and produce speech. The intubated patient should be asked to write. The patient in a coma (item 1a=3) will automatically score 3 on this item. The examiner must choose a score for the patient with stupor or limited cooperation, but a score of 3 should be used only if the patient is mute and follows no one-step commands.	0 = **No aphasia;** normal. 1 = **Mild-to-moderate aphasia;** some obvious loss of fluency or facility of comprehension, without significant limitation on ideas expressed or form of expression. Reduction of speech and/or comprehension, however, makes conversation about provided materials difficult or impossible. For example, in conversation about provided materials, examiner can identify picture or naming card content from patient's response. 2 = **Severe aphasia;** all communication is through fragmentary expression; great need for inference, questioning, and guessing by the listener. Range of information that can be exchanged is limited; listener carries burden of communication. Examiner cannot identify materials provided from patient response. 3 = **Mute, global aphasia;** no usable speech or auditory comprehension.	1
10. Dysarthria: If patient is thought to be normal, an adequate sample of speech must be obtained by asking patient to read or repeat words from the attached list. If the patient has severe aphasia, the clarity of articulation of spontaneous speech can be rated. Only if the patient is intubated or has other physical barriers to producing speech, the examiner should record the score as untestable (UN), and clearly write an explanation for this choice. Do not tell the patient why he or she is being tested.	0 = **Normal.** 1 = **Mild-to-moderate dysarthria;** patient slurs at least some words and, at worst, can be understood with some difficulty. 2 = **Severe dysarthria;** patient's speech is so slurred as to be unintelligible in the absence of or out of proportion to any dysphasia, or is mute/anarthric. UN = **Intubated** or other physical barrier, explain:_____	0

Rev 10/1/2003

FIGURE 10.7   (Continued)

N I H
STROKE
SCALE

Patient Identification. ___ ___-___ ___ ___-___ ___ ___

Pt. Date of Birth ___ __/__ __/__ __

Hospital _____(__ __-__ __)

Date of Exam ___ __/__ __/__ __

Interval: [ ] Baseline   [ ] 2 hours post treatment   [ ] 24 hours post onset of symptoms ±20 minutes   [ ] 7–10 days
            [ ] 3 months   [ ] Other _____(__ __)

11. Extinction and Inattention (formerly Neglect): Sufficient information to identify neglect may be obtained during the prior testing. If the patient has a severe visual loss preventing visual double simultaneous stimulation, and the cutaneous stimuli are normal, the score is normal. If the patient has aphasia but does appear to attend to both sides, the score is normal. The presence of visual spatial neglect or anosagnosia may also be taken as evidence of abnormality. Since the abnormality is scored only if present, the item is never untestable.	0 = No abnormality. 1 = **Visual, tactile, auditory, spatial, or personal inattention** or extinction to bilateral simultaneous stimulation in one of the sensory modalities. 2 = **Profound hemi-inattention or extinction to more than one modality;** does not recognize own hand or orients to only one side of space.	0 ___

___

___

Rev 10/1/2003

FIGURE 10.7   (Continued)

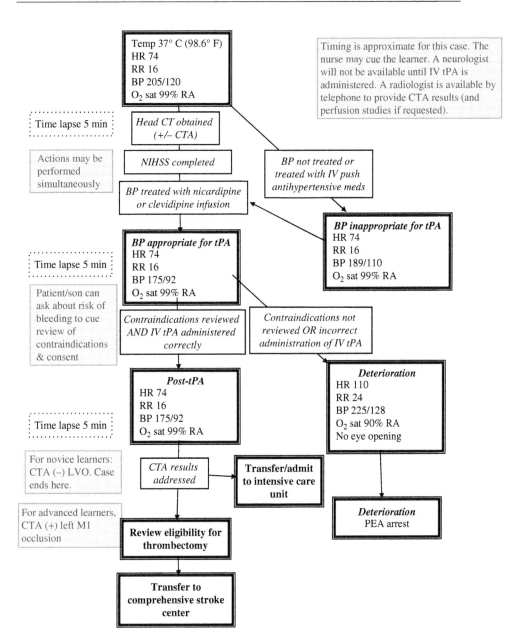

FIGURE 10.8 Flow diagram for AIS (min, minutes; RA, room air).

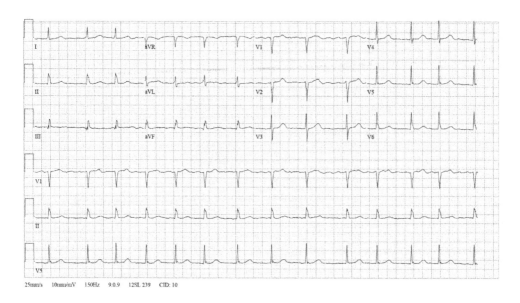

25mm/s 10mm/mV 150Hz 9.0.9 12SL 239 CID: 10

FIGURE 10.9 Electrocardiogram showing atrial fibrillation.

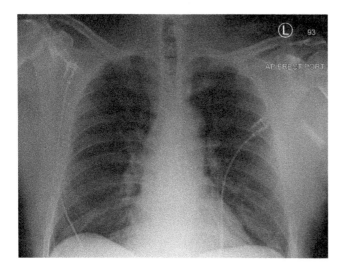

FIGURE 10.10 Chest x-ray (normal).

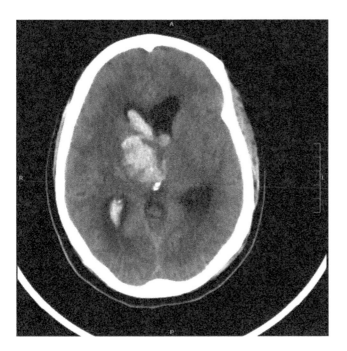

FIGURE 10.11   Computed tomography of the head showing right basal ganglia intracerebral hemorrhage with intraventricular hemorrhage, hydrocephalus, and cerebral edema.

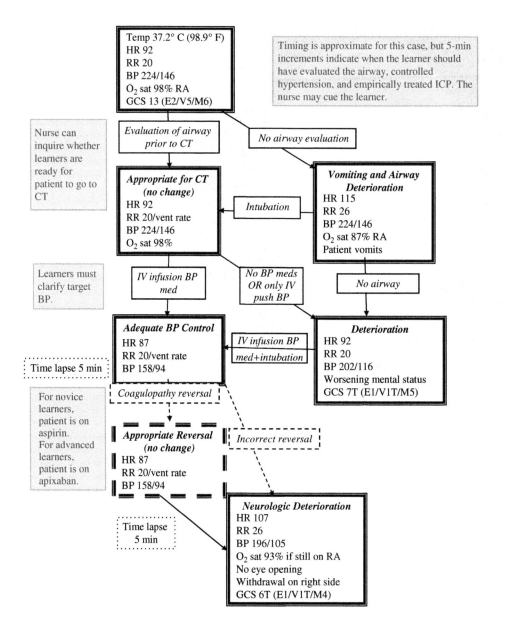

Temp 37.2° C (98.9° F)
HR 92
RR 20
BP 224/146
O₂ sat 98% RA
GCS 13 (E2/V5/M6)

Timing is approximate for this case, but 5-min increments indicate when the learner should have evaluated the airway, controlled hypertension, and empirically treated ICP. The nurse may cue the learner.

Nurse can inquire whether learners are ready for patient to go to CT

Evaluation of airway prior to CT

No airway evaluation

Appropriate for CT (no change)
HR 92
RR 20/vent rate
BP 224/146
O₂ sat 98%

Intubation

Vomiting and Airway Deterioration
HR 115
RR 26
BP 224/146
O₂ sat 87% RA
Patient vomits

Learners must clarify target BP.

IV infusion BP med

No BP meds OR only IV push BP

No airway

Adequate BP Control
HR 87
RR 20/vent rate
BP 158/94

IV infusion BP med+intubation

Deterioration
HR 92
RR 20
BP 202/116
Worsening mental status
GCS 7T (E1/V1T/M5)

Time lapse 5 min

Coagulopathy reversal

For novice learners, patient is on aspirin.
For advanced learners, patient is on apixaban.

Appropriate Reversal (no change)
HR 87
RR 20/vent rate
BP 158/94

Incorrect reversal

Time lapse 5 min

Neurologic Deterioration
HR 107
RR 26
BP 196/105
O₂ sat 93% if still on RA
No eye opening
Withdrawal on right side
GCS 6T (E1/V1T/M4)

FIGURE 10.12   Flow diagram for intracerebral hemorrhage (FFP, fresh frozen plasma; ICP, intracranial pressure; min, minutes; PCC, prothrombin complex concentrate; RA, room air).

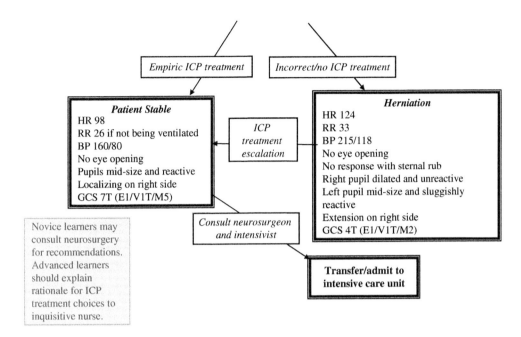

FIGURE 10.12 (Continued)

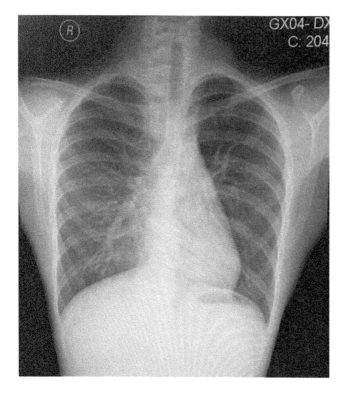

FIGURE 10.13   Chest x-ray (normal).

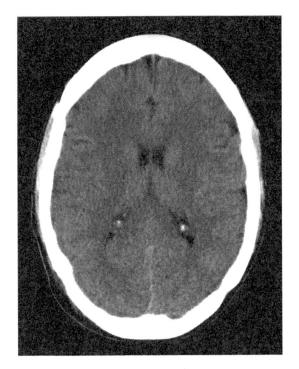

FIGURE 10.14   Computed tomography of the head (normal).

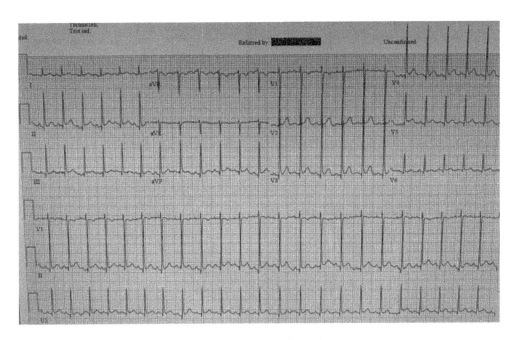

FIGURE 10.15   Electrocardiogram showing sinus tachycardia.

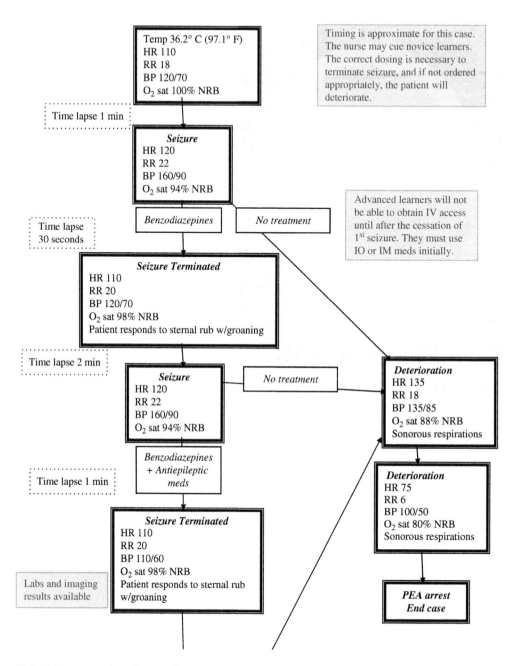

FIGURE 10.16   Flow diagram for status epilepticus in a child (FiO$_2$, fraction of inspired oxygen; min, minutes; PE, phenytoin equivalent; RA, room air).

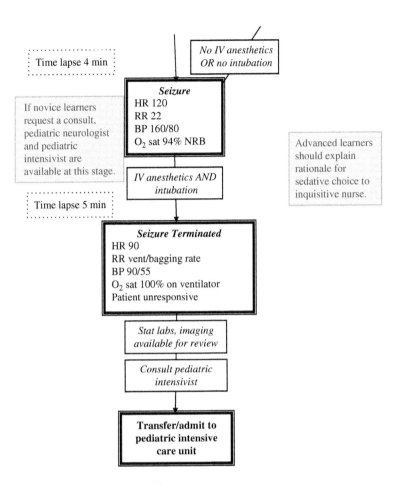

FIGURE 10.16 (Continued)

TABLE 10.1 Complete blood count.

Test	Value	Reference range
White blood cells (10³/µl)	7.2	4.5–11
Hemoglobin (g/dl)	10.8	11.9–15.7
Hematocrit (%)	34.3	35–45
Platelets (10³/µl)	213	153–367

TABLE 10.2 Chemistry panel.

Test	Value	Reference range
Sodium (mmol/l)	139	135–145
Potassium (mmol/l)	4.4	3.5–5
Chloride (mmol/l)	103	98–107
Bicarbonate (mmol/l)	25	21–30
Blood urea nitrogen (mg/dl)	22	7–17
Creatinine (mg/dl)	1.12	0.7–1.5
Glucose (mg/dl)	115	74–106
Calcium (mg/dl)	9.5	8.4–10.2
Magnesium (mg/dl)	1.7	1.6–2.3
Phosphorus (mg/dl)	3.2	2.5–4.5

TABLE 10.3 Troponin.

Test	Value	Reference range
Troponin (ng/ml)	0.03	< 0.4

TABLE 10.4 Coagulation panel.

Test	Value	Reference range
Prothrombin time (seconds)	13.7	10.8–13.3
International normalized ratio	1.0	0.9–1.1
Partial thromboplastin time (seconds)	30	31.4–48.0

TABLE 10.5 Alcohol level.

Test	Value	Reference range
Alcohol level (mg/dl)	< 10	< 10

TABLE 10.6 Complete blood count.

Test	Value	Reference range
White blood cells (103/µl)	14.0	4.5–11
Hemoglobin (g/dl)	13.0	11.9–15.7
Hematocrit (%)	39.2	35–45
Platelets (103/µl)	183	153–367

TABLE 10.7 Chemistry panel.

Test	Value	Reference range
Sodium (mmol/l)	144	135–145
Potassium (mmol/l)	3.5	3.5–5
Chloride (mmol/l)	96	98–107
Bicarbonate (mmol/l)	31	21–30
Blood urea nitrogen (mg/dl)	12	7–17
Creatinine (mg/dl)	0.82	0.7–1.5
Glucose (mg/dl)	193	74–106
Calcium (mg/dl)	9.0	8.4–10.2
Magnesium (mg/dl)	1.9	1.6–2.3
Phosphorus (mg/dl)	2.6	2.5–4.5

TABLE 10.8 Coagulation panel for advanced learners (report as normal for novice learners).

Test	Value	Reference range
Prothrombin time (s)	17.8	10.8–13.3
International normalized ratio	1.3	0.9–1.1
Partial thromboplastin time (s)	40	31.4–48.0

TABLE 10.9 Thromboelastography.

Test	Value	Reference range
Reaction time (minutes)	6	3.8–9.8
Kinetics (minutes)	3	0.7–3.4
α-angle (degrees)	60	47.8–77.7
Maximum amplitude (mm)	55	49.7–72.7
Lysis at 30 minutes (%)	4	−2.3–5.77

TABLE 10.10   Type and screen.

Test	Value
ABO-Rh	O positive
Antibody screen	Negative

TABLE 10.11   Reversal of anticoagulants in life-threatening hemorrhage [5–7].

Mechanism of action	Anticoagulant	Relevant case changes	Reversal agent	Dosage
Vitamin K antagonist	Warfarin	PT 34.25 INR 2.5	Vitamin K	10 mg IV[a]
			FFP	10–15 ml/kg IV
			PCC	25–50 units/kg IV[b,c]
LMWH	Enoxaparin	Normal coagulation profile	Protamine sulfate	Time since last dose: < 8 hours: 1 mg protamine/1 mg LMWH IV, max. 50 mg 8–12 hours: 0.5 mg protamine/1 mg LMWH IV, max. 25 mg > 12 hours: unlikely to be useful, max. 25 mg
Direct thrombin inhibitor	Dabigatran	No change	Activated PCC	50 units/kg IV
			4-factor PCC	25–50 units/kg IV
			Idarucizumab	5 g IV
			Hemodialysis	
Direct factor Xa inhibitors	Apixaban Edoxaban Rivaroxaban	No change	Activated PCC	50 units/kg IV
			4-factor PCC	25–50 units/kg IV
			Andexanet alfa	Low vs. high dose depends on dose of factor Xa inhibitor and time since last dose

FFP, fresh frozen plasma; INR, international normalized ratio; IV, intravenous; LMWH, low-molecular-weight heparin; PCC, prothrombin complex concentrate; PT, prothrombin time.

[a] Vitamin K should be co-administered with FFP or PCC.

[b] 3-factor PCC should be co-administered with FFP due to inadequate factor VII in 3-factor PCC preparation.

[c] Dosing based on factor IX component of PCC. Institutions may also specify dosing based on INR.

TABLE 10.12   Treatment of intracranial hypertension and herniation [8].

Tier	Treatments	Rationale
0	Ensure adequate ventilation and circulation	Avoid hypercarbia, hypoxia, and hypotension in brain injury
	Elevate head of bed to > 30°, maintain head in midline position	Facilitate cerebral venous drainage
	Treat fever, pain, agitation	Reduce cerebral metabolic demand
1	Administer mannitol and hypertonic saline	Improve cerebral blood flow, decrease brain water content
	If external ventricular drainage system in place, drain 5–10 ml cerebrospinal fluid	Decrease cerebrospinal fluid volume
	Use hyperventilation ONLY as a temporizing measure	Decrease cerebral blood volume through cerebral vasoconstriction
2	Administer hypertonic saline	Improve cerebral blood flow, decrease brain water content
	Administer propofol	Reduce cerebral metabolic demand
	Perform decompressive surgery if appropriate	Reduce space-occupying lesion
3	Administer pentobarbital	Reduce cerebral metabolic demand
	Induce hypothermia	Reduce cerebral metabolic demand

TABLE 10.13   Complete metabolic panel.

Test	Value	Reference range
Sodium (mmol/l)	139	135–145
Potassium (mmol/l)	4.5	3.5–5
Chloride (mmol/l)	106	101–107
Bicarbonate (mmol/l)	18	21–28
Blood urea nitrogen (mg/dl)	12	7–20
Creatinine (mg/dl)	0.33	0.26–0.61
Glucose (mg/dl)	182	70–140
Calcium (mg/dl)	9.6	9.2–10.5
Magnesium (mg/dl)	2.4	2.09–2.84
Phosphorus (mg/dl)	4.1	4.1–5.9
Alkaline phosphatase (iu/l)	210	156–369
Alanine transaminase (iu/l)	24	9–25
Aspartate aminotransferase (iu/l)	32	18–36
Albumin (g/dl)	4.0	3.5–5

TABLE 10.14 Complete blood count.

Test	Value	Reference range
White blood cells (10³/μl)	18.7	4–14.5
Hemoglobin (g/dl)	11.8	11.5–15.5
Hematocrit (%)	35.4	35–45
Platelets (10³/μl)	597	150–450
Segmented neutrophils (%)	12	32–54
Lymphocytes (%)	69.9	28–48

TABLE 10.15 Lactate.

Test	Value	Reference range
Lactate (mmol/l)	4.6	1–2.4

TABLE 10.16 Creatine kinase.

Test	Value	Reference range
Creatine kinase (iu/l)	241	26–192

CHAPTER 11

Psychobehavioral Emergencies

Afrah A. Ali[1] and Danya Khoujah[1,2]

[1] Department of Emergency Medicine, University of Maryland School of Medicine, Baltimore, MD, USA

[2] Emergency Medicine, MedStar Franklin Square Medical Center, Baltimore, MD, USA

SEXUAL ASSAULT

Educational Goals

Learning Objectives

1. Evaluate for sexual assault in a patient presenting to the emergency department (ED) after a physical assault (MK, PC, ICS).
2. Obtain pertinent history and physical examination in a patient following a sexual assault (MK, PC).
3. Discuss post-exposure prophylaxis (MK, PC, ICS).
4. Demonstrate empathy and respect while interacting with a patient (PC, P, ICS).
5. Consult with a sexual assault forensic examiner, forensic nurse examiner, or sexual assault nurse examiner (collectively referred to in this chapter as SAFE), law enforcement, and/or a social worker (P, ICS, SBP).

Emergency Medicine Simulation Workbook: A Tool for Bringing the Curriculum to Life,
Second Edition. Edited by Traci L. Thoureen and Sara B. Scott.
© 2022 John Wiley & Sons Ltd. Published 2022 by John Wiley & Sons Ltd.
Companion website: www.wiley.com/go/thoureen/simulation/workbook2e

Critical Actions Checklist

☐ Display empathy techniques using two or more of the following (PC, P, ICS).:
- Use a calm voice.
- Sit at the level of the patient.
- Pause and allow the patient to cry.
- Ask before making physical contact.

☐ Directly ask about sexual assault using non-accusatory language (PC, P, ICS).

☐ Obtain pertinent history about the assault (PC, MK, P, ICS).

☐ Assess for physical injuries (PC, MK).

☐ Counsel and offer the patient post-exposure prophylaxis for pregnancy and sexually transmitted infections (*STIs*) (PC, ICS).

☐ Communicate effectively with the care team, which may include: social work, law enforcement and/or SAFE after obtaining permission from the patient (PC, ICS, SBP).

Critical actions can be changed to address the education needs of the learner. If the learner needs to learn the methods of evidence collection and exam for a patient presenting after sexual assault, that should be included.

Simulation Set-Up

Environment: ED treatment area. A seat for the learner to use while interviewing the patient should be available.

Standardized patient: Adult female standardized patient dressed in regular clothes, sitting on the stretcher. Abrasions and bruising over multiple parts of the body as indicated in the physical examination can be made with red and brown body paint or makeup.

If educational objectives include evidence collection, female pelvic exam task trainer or standardized patient gynecological model will be needed.

Props: To be displayed on plasma screen/computer screen or printed out on handouts in scenario room when participants ask for/lab returns them:

- Laboratory tests (see online component for sexual assault, Scenario 11.1 at https://www.wiley.com/go/thoureen/simulation/workbook2e):
  - Complete blood count (Table 11.1).
  - Complete metabolic panel (Table 11.2).

- Pregnancy test (Table 11.3).
- HIV antibody test (Table 11.4).
- Rapid plasma reagin (*RPR*) test (Table 11.5).

Available supplies:

- Medications:
  - Analgesics typically used at your institution.
- Evidence collection kit (optional).

Distractor: (optional) EMS crew member states, "I think the patient was partying and is probably just drunk." If this is included the patient becomes very upset and is crying and needs to be consoled prior to obtaining history.

Actors

- Standardized female patient. She talks in a quiet voice, is tearful and answers questions in an abbreviated manner.
- ED nurse can cue learners if needed.
- Consultants can be present in person or via telephone consultation.
  - SAFE can guide the learner about deferring the evidence collection until after completion of the medical assessment.
  - Law enforcement (optional).
  - Social worker (optional).
- EMS crew member gives report to the learners (optional).

Note: A pre-brief is helpful for this case It should note that the case content can be emotionally difficult. It is essential that a safe word like "time out" is predetermined if the case becomes emotionally overwhelming for a learner, so the scenario may be paused and/or the learner may exit the scenario.

Case Narrative

Scenario Background

A 23-year-old woman presents to the ED via EMS. Patient was found in the woods by some hikers. Patient states that she had been hiking and was assaulted approximately one hour ago by an unknown male. She does not remember exactly what happened. She does not think she lost consciousness. She states, "Everything happened so fast, I don't remember it." She denies neck pain, chest/abdominal pain, or significant headache.

If the learner specifically asks, the patient was penetrated vaginally multiple times. She is unsure whether the perpetrator ejaculated during the penetration. She does not think that a condom or a foreign body was used. She has pain in her perineal area. She has not showered or changed her clothes since the incident.

Chief complaint:	Assault
Patient's medical history:	None. Tetanus, human papillomavirus (*HPV*) and hepatitis B vaccinations are up to date.
Sexual history:	Last menstrual cycle was two weeks ago. She has never been pregnant. Patient is sexually active. Her last consensual sexual activity was two weeks ago. No history of STI or HIV.
Medications:	None
Allergies:	None
Family history:	None
Social history:	No tobacco, drinks alcohol socially, no recreational drug use. She is a college student.

Initial Scenario Conditions

Patient is sitting at the edge of the stretcher.

Vital signs:	Temp 98.2°F (36.8°C), HR 110, RR 18, BP 110/70, SpO$_2$ 100% on room air.
General:	Alert and oriented; appears scared and tearful.
Head:	Abrasions and bruising on the right frontal scalp; tender when palpated.
Eyes:	Pupils equal and reactive to light. Extraocular movements intact.
Nose:	Dry, clotted blood in the right nares.
Throat:	Normal.
Neck:	Normal.
Heart:	Tachycardic, normal heart sounds.
Lungs:	Clear symmetrical breath sounds.
Abdomen:	Soft, non-tender, non-distended, normal bowel sounds; no signs of trauma.
Back:	Abrasions in the shape of nail marks noted on posterior thorax area.
Extremities:	Abrasions and bruises over both upper extremities, no swelling, no deformity, normal range of movement.
Neurologic:	Strength and sensation intact, gait steady.

Pelvic exam should only be performed on a female pelvic trainer or gynecologic model if evidence collection is one of the training goals. Physical exam findings that cannot be represented accurately can be reported verbally.

See flow diagram (Figure 11.1) for further scenario changes described.

Case Narrative, Continued

Learners should provide a calm environment to interview and examine the patient. The learners should display empathy while interacting with the patient and directly ask about the possibility of sexual assault.

Details of the assault will be volunteered to the novice learner but disclosed to the advanced learner only if specifically asked. If the learner both displays empathy and directly asks about the possibility of sexual assault, the patient will state that she was sexually assaulted by a male friend. If the learner does not display empathy, the patient will continue to cry and will not provide any further history. The nurse may prompt learners to consult the social worker if the relevant history is not obtained.

Learners should perform a complete history and physical exam. They should inquire whether the patient wants to involve law enforcement, SAFE, and/or social worker. The patient will want to file a report with law enforcement.

Learners should specifically communicate with SAFE about counseling for post-exposure prophylaxis, which SAFE will defer to the learners. The patient can cue learners by asking about the risk of contracting a disease or getting pregnant. She will choose to take prophylaxis for HIV, STIs, and pregnancy. Appropriate laboratory studies should be ordered.

The case ends when the learner has discussed the patient's disposition; is able to ensure that the patient has a safe place to go (her mother's house) and has provided the patient with the appropriate resources. This can be prompted by the nurse after 15 minutes if disposition has not been reached.

If learning objectives include performance of a sexual assault exam, the case should continue until the learner obtains the patient's informed consent and completes exam on the female pelvic trainer/gynecologic model.

Instructor Notes

Definitions and Epidemiology

- Sexual assault: sexual activity in which consent is not obtained or not freely given. It includes:
  - Rape:
    - Legal term in which there is penetration of a body orifice (mouth, vagina, or anus) involving force or the threat of force or incapacity (including drug or alcohol intoxication) [1].
    - One in five women and one in 59 men have experienced an attempted or completed rape, with much higher numbers reported for sexual assault [2].
  - Unwanted genital touching.
  - Forced viewing of or involvement in pornography.

Clinical Features

- Highly variable depending on clinical scenario.
- General body trauma occurs in more than half of rape patients presenting to the ED.
  - More frequent than genital trauma [3].
  - Defense injuries may be present and might include lacerations, bruises, abrasions on extensor surfaces of arms and medial thighs.
  - Bite marks may be present.
- Anogenital injuries:
  - Visual inspection identifies anogenital injuries in less than half of patients who have been sexually assaulted [1]. They may include:
    - Tears/abrasions of posterior fourchette.
    - Abrasions/bruising of labia minora.
    - Ecchymosis/tears of hymen.

Diagnosis

- Primarily based on history.
- Patients may not disclose certain elements of the history for fear that such details will undermine their credibility.
- Lack of injuries does not exclude sexual assault [1].

Management

- Establish support and empathy [4, 5]:
  - Use private room for interview.
  - Include social worker or SAFE, if possible, so the patient does not have to repeat the information.
  - Acknowledge the difficulty of the situation.
  - Use non-blaming, empowering language. See Box 11.1 for examples of empathetic language that can be used.
  - Ask for permission before asking intrusive questions.
  - Avoid judgmental questions, such as questioning patient's decision-making skills at the time of the assault.
  - Some patients may not want to be addressed as a "victim."
- Obtain pertinent history [1]:
  - Timing of the incident.
  - Anal, oral, or vaginal penetration with or without ejaculation.
  - Usage of foreign bodies or condoms.
  - Suspicion of drug-facilitated assault.

Box 11.1   Examples of Empathetic Language [5]

- I believe you.
- It took a lot of courage to tell me about this.
- It's not your fault.
- You didn't do anything to deserve this.
- You are not alone.
- I/We care about you and am/are here to listen or help in any way I/we can.
- I'm sorry this happened.

This shouldn't have happened to you.

- - Change in clothing or showering prior to medical presentation.
  - Past sexual, menstrual, and gynecological history.
- Physical examination
  - Obtain permission before making physical contact.
  - Strive to preserve as much evidence as possible:
    - Nothing to eat or drink.
    - If not performing the forensic examination, avoid removing clothing unless necessary for the exam.
  - Forensic examination (some details may vary based on local laws):
    - Informed consent should be obtained.
    - Evidence collection should be offered regardless of the patient's desire to involve law enforcement:
      - Ideally performed within 96 hours of the assault.
      - Evidence may be used in the future if the decision is changed.
      - Ideally performed by a SAFE [6].
      - Collect the clothes and belongings in a paper bag prior to examination.
      - Perform and document a thorough physical examination guided by the local evidence protocols and instructions in the evidence collection kit.
      - Collect swabs for DNA from areas of attempted penetration, take photographs of injury patterns, and perform a thorough vaginal and perineal examination.
  - Documentation of anogenital injuries increases the chances of successful prosecution [7].
  - Refrain from documenting assumed injury patterns and events.
- Laboratory testing:
  - Urine tests:
    - Drug screen:

- A negative routine drug screen does not exclude all potential agents used in a drug-facilitated SA. If concerned, send out labs for flunitrazepam (Rohypnol®) and gamma-hydroxybutyric acid [8].
- Pregnancy test.
- Tests for STIs:
  - Gonorrhea.
  - Chlamydia.
  - Trichomonas.
  - Syphilis.
  - Hepatitis B.
  - HIV.
- If providing HIV post-exposure prophylaxis: liver and renal function tests.
- Treatment:
  - Pregnancy and STI prophylaxis [9, 10]:
    - See Table 11.6 for medications.
    - Emergency contraception should be provided within 72 hours for non-pregnant women.
    - Hepatitis B vaccine (if the patient is unvaccinated or uncertain of vaccine status).
    - HIV:
    - Consider antiretroviral prophylaxis.
    - HPV vaccine.
    - Consider for unvaccinated women ≤ 26 years [11].
    - May extend to women through to age 45 years [12].
  - Tetanus booster if indicated [9].

Disposition and Follow-Up

- Consult with social work, SAFE and law enforcement.
- Follow-up with primary care:
  - Completion of vaccination series.
  - Serial HIV antibody tests.
- Discharge with reliable transportation and ensure patient has a safe place to go.

Debriefing Plan

Plan approximately 30 minutes for discussion.

Potential Questions for Discussion

- What is relevant history in a patient presenting for sexual assault?
- What is post-exposure prophylaxis? When is it indicated?

- What are the resources available at your institution for patients presenting following a sexual assault?
- What is the role of the SAFE?

It is important to acknowledge during the debriefing that some of the learners present may find the scenario emotional or difficult, especially if they identify with the patient. Consider offering local counseling resources for physicians.

REFERENCES FOR SEXUAL ASSAULT

1. Linden, J.A. (2011). Clinical practice: care of the adult patient after sexual assault. *N. Engl. J. Med.* 365 (9): 834–841.
2. Basile, K.C., Smith. S.G., Breiding, M.J., et al. (2014). *Sexual Violence Surveillance: Uniform definitions and recommended data elements*, version 2.0. Atlanta, GA: National Center for Injury Prevention and Control, Centers for Disease Control and Prevention.
3. Palmer, C.M., McNulty, A.M., D'Este, C., and Donovan, B. (2004). Genital injuries in women reporting sexual assault. *Sex. Health.* 1: 55–59.
4. Barron, R., Kapilevich, E., Duffy, S., and McGregor, A.J. (2016). Sexual assault: what every emergency provider needs to know. *Acad. Emerg. Med.* 23 (10): 1182.
5. Rape, Abuse and Incest National Network. Tips for talking with survivors of sexual assault. https://www.rainn.org/articles/tips-talking-survivors-sexual-assault (accessed 7 September 2021).
6. Department of Justice, Office on Violence Against Women (2018). *National Training Standards for Sexual Assault Medical Forensic Examiners*, 2e. Washington, DC: Office on Violence Against Women.
7. Gray-Eurom, K., Seaberg, D.C., and Wears, R.L. (2002). The prosecution of sexual assault cases: correlation with forensic evidence. *Ann. Emerg. Med.* 39: 39–46.
8. Bechtel, L.K. and Holstege, C.P. (2007). Criminal poisoning: drug-facilitated sexual assault. *Emerg. Med. Clin. North Am.* 25 (2): 499–525.
9. Centers for Disease Control and Prevention (2015). Sexually transmitted diseases treatment guidelines, 2015. *MMWR Recomm. Rep.* 64 (3): 1–137.
10. Cheng, L., Che, Y., and Gulmezoglu, A.M. (2012). Interventions for emergency contraception. *Cochrane Database Syst. Rev.* 8: CD001324.
11. Centers for Disease Control and Prevention (2019). Human papillomavirus (HPV): Vaccine schedule and dosing. https://www.cdc.gov/hpv/hcp/schedules-recommendations.html (accessed 7 September 2021).
12. US Food and Drug Administration (2020). Gardasil 9. https://www.fda.gov/vaccines-blood-biologics/vaccines/gardasil-9. (accessed 7 september 2021).

SELECTED READINGS FOR SEXUAL ASSAULT

Siegel, M., Gonzalez, E.C., Wijesekera, O. et al. (2017). On-the-go-training: downloadable modules to train medical students to care for adult female sexual assault survivors. *MedEdPORTAL* 13: 10656. https://doi.org/10.15766/mep_2374-8265.10656.

NON-ACCIDENTAL TRAUMA WITH AGGRESSIVE FAMILY MEMBER

Educational Goals

Learning Objectives

1. Demonstrate leadership skills in a chaotic environment (P, ICS).
2. Recognize threat to patient and staff safety and recruit additional resources (P, ICS, SBP).
3. Use verbal de-escalation techniques (P, ICS).
4. Evaluate for suspected non-accidental trauma (MK, PC, SBP).
5. Demonstrate appropriate consultation for traumatic injuries (P, ICS, SBP).

Critical Actions Checklist

- ☐ Use three or more of the following verbal de-escalation techniques:
  - Respect personal space.
  - Avoid provocation.
  - Establish verbal contact.
  - Acknowledge feelings.
  - Active listening.
  - Agree (or agree to disagree).
  - Offer choices and optimism.
  - Set clear limits (ICS, SBP, P).
- ☐ Recognize safety risk toward patient and staff and call for help (ICS, SBP, P).
- ☐ Assign roles to individuals (ICS, P).
- ☐ Consult social work or child protective services to report suspected non-accidental trauma (ICS, SBP, P).
- ☐ Obtain appropriate radiographs including a complete skeletal survey (MK, PC).
- ☐ Admit patient to appropriate service for physical injuries and further workup (MK, PC, ICS, SBP, P).

> Learning objectives/critical actions can be changed to address the educational needs of the learner. As written, this case addresses violence in the workplace and does not focus on the medical management of non-accidental trauma.

Simulation Set-Up

Environment: Pediatric ED treatment area,

Mannequin: Pediatric infant simulator mannequin, male set-up. Infant dressed in a one-sie lying in bed, crying. Moulage the right lower extremity to appear swollen and bruised.

This can be accomplished by adding an extra layer of material under the skin of the upper thigh and painting the skin with red body paint or makeup. Moulage of immersion burns to buttocks, which can be accomplished with red or brown body paint or makeup.

Props: To be displayed on plasma screen/computer screen or printed out on handouts in scenario room when participants ask for/lab returns them:

- Imaging results (see online component for aggressive family member, Scenario 11.2 at https://www.wiley.com/go/thoureen/simulation/workbook2e):
  - Chest x-ray radiology read (Figure 11.2)
  - Right femur x-ray radiology read (Figure 11.3)
  - Computed tomography of the head radiology read (Figure 11.4)
- Labs (see online component as above):
  - Complete blood count (Table 11.7).
  - Complete metabolic panel (Table 11.8).

Any imaging or lab work not provided can be verbally reported as normal if the learners order the study.

Available supplies:

- Pediatric code cart and pediatric airway supplies
- Medications
  - 100 ml bags of 0.9%.
  - Analgesics commonly used at your institution.

Distractors: For advanced learners, the mother's boyfriend can be introduced in the scenario. The father and the boyfriend will get into a verbal argument that will escalate to physical assault if not addressed.

Actors

- Patient is crying.
- Patient's father is visibly worried, argumentative and impatient. He constantly keeps asking, "What is wrong with him, why is he crying?" He eventually becomes angry and violent.

- Patient's mother is tearful and soft-spoken.
- ED nurse can administer medications/fluids and may cue learners if needed.
- Consults (including radiologist, pediatric trauma service, pediatrician, orthopedics, social worker/CPS, and law enforcement) can be available in person or via telephone consultation.
- Optional: mother's boyfriend is belligerent.
- Optional: security.

Note: It is essential that a safe word like "time out" is predetermined during the pre-brief in case any participants are feeling unsafe during the case. Anyone saying the safe word would immediately halt the case. Instructors should discontinue the scenario/intervene quickly if they feel that any participant is in distress.

Case Narrative

Scenario Background

A 7-month-old boy presents to the ED via EMS with his father, who states that the baby has been crying inconsolably since earlier today when he picked him up from the mother's house, where he had spent the past week. The father noted leg swelling and brought the patient to the ED. The mother is on her way to the hospital.

Chief complaint:	Right leg swelling.
Patient's medical history:	Spontaneous vaginal birth, no perinatal complications, born at term, immunization up to date
Medications:	None.
Allergies:	None.
Family history:	None.
Social history:	The parents are separated, with joint legal custody. The mother lives with her boyfriend. The father lives with the grandmother.

Initial Scenario Conditions

Patient on a stretcher, crying. The father is at the bedside, visibly worried and frustrated.

Vital signs:	Temp 97.8°F (36.6°C), HR 185, RR 44, BP 120/80, SpO_2 97% on room air.
General:	Irritable and crying.
HEENT:	Anterior fontanelle flat, no bruising/abrasions. Pupils are equal, round, and reactive to light.
Neck:	Normal appearance, no stridor.

Lungs:	Bilateral breath sounds clear and symmetrical.
Heart:	Tachycardic, normal heart sounds.
Abdomen:	Soft, non-tender, non-distended, bowel sounds normal.
Genitourinary:	Normal penis and scrotum, no erythema.
Extremities:	Right thigh swelling, tenderness noted, patient does not move the extremity, dorsalis pedis palpable +2, soft compartments.
Skin:	warm, flushed, sharp demarcated lesions on the buttocks (consistent with immersion burns).

Examination findings that cannot be presented as moulage can be relayed via images on computer screen or printed handouts. Alternatively, findings can be verbally stated by the nurse when requested by the learner.

See flow diagram (Figure 11.5) for further scenario changes described.

Case Narrative, Continued

Learners should place the patient on the monitor and perform a thorough physical examination. Imaging including radiographs of the right lower extremity and a complete skeletal survey should be obtained. Pain meds should be administered.

After a time lapse of three minutes, the patient's mother will arrive providing further history: The boyfriend was watching her son last night as he usually does while she is at work. She did not notice the swelling this morning and does not know if the patient has fallen. She states, "My boyfriend has hit me many times before, but he couldn't have hurt my baby, right?"

The father will become more impatient and visibly angry, stating that the learners are taking too long to figure out what's wrong with the child. If the learner asks any questions regarding safety at home or living situation, he yells, "Are you crazy? I would never hurt my child!"

The learners should attempt to de-escalate the situation. Failure to employ appropriate de-escalation techniques will cause the father to become more aggressive (e.g., throwing things on the floor) and threaten to take the patient home. The learner should recognize the safety threat caused by the father and call for other resources such as extra nurses, security, and police.

Optional distractor: Mother's boyfriend can walk in, acting belligerent and intoxicated. He will get into a fight with the father, necessitating that the learner deal with two aggressive persons.

After de-escalating the father, radiology reports are available. This should trigger further work-up (which includes a head CT, skeletal survey, and labs). Based on the local institution's practice, activation of the pediatric trauma team or consultation of the inpatient pediatrician and orthopedist. Social worker/child protection services and law enforcement should be consulted as well. This can be facilitated by the nurse for novice learners.

The case scenario ends when the patient is admitted to an appropriate inpatient service or if the time allocated by the instructor has elapsed.

Instructor Notes

Epidemiology

- The ED is a high-risk environment for workplace violence including physical assault, verbal harassment, and threats [14].
- In a national survey, 78% of emergency medicine physicians reported at least one act of physical or verbal aggression in the previous 12 months, while 21% reported more than one episode [2].
- Most of these incidents are underreported due to fear of retaliation and lack of support from administration [3].
- Workplace violence leads to a significant decrease in ED staff productivity and job satisfaction, which contributes to early burnout [3].

Management of a Violent Person

- Use techniques of verbal de-escalation during the event [4]:
  - Respect personal space:
    - Keep at least two arms-length distance.
    - Use caution taking belongings or undressing patients.
  - Be non-confrontational and calm:
    - Consider your body language.
    - Avoid clenched fists and prolonged eye contact/staring.
    - Stand at an angle rather than directly facing the person.
  - Establish verbal contact:
    - One team member speaks at a time.
    - Introduce yourself and provide orientation and reassurance.
    - Ask their name and how they would like to be addressed:
    - Be concise.
    - Identify wants and feelings.
    - Use "free information" (from the things the patient says, their body language, etc.) to create a rapid connection.
  - Actively listen:
    - Use body language and verbal acknowledgement.
  - Agree or agree to disagree:
    - Fogging: find something about the person's position with which you can agree: the truth, principle, or odds.
    - If there is no way to honestly agree, agree to disagree.

- Offer choices and optimism:
  - Offer items for comfort (e.g., food, blankets).
  - Discuss medication administration, emphasizing safety and control.
  - Provide hope while being realistic.
- Clearly state the rules and set clear limits:
  - Establish basic working conditions as a matter of fact rather than a threat.
  - Be reasonable and respectful when setting limits.
  - Coach patient on how to stay in control using gentle confrontation with instruction, e.g. "I really want you to stop yelling; when you yell, I feel frightened and I can't pay attention to what you are saying. You could help me understand if you lowered your voice."
- *Most importantly, recognize when verbal de-escalation is not effective and further interventions (such as chemical or physical restraints) are necessary.*
- Organizational interventions [5]:
  - Educate and train all staff on dealing with an aggressive patient/visitor.
    - Develop a written plan and review periodically.
  - Institute mandatory reporting of violent events:
    - Develop a zero-tolerance policy and communicate it to all patients and visitors.
  - Develop and implement a security plan, which may include panic buttons, metal detectors, and increased security personnel.

Debriefing Plan

Plan approximately 30 minutes for discussion.

Potential Questions for Discussion

- What are the verbal de-escalation techniques to use when dealing with violent patients or family members?
- What is the policy for preventing and handling workplace violence at your ED?
- What resources are available at your institution to help you and your co-workers deal with violent patients or family members?

REFERENCES

1. May, D.D. and Grubbs, L.M. (2002). The extent, nature, and precipitating factors of nurse assault among three groups of registered nurses in a regional medical center. *J. Emerg. Nurs.* 28 (1): 11–17.
2. Behnam, M., Tillotson, R.D., Davis, S.M., and Hobbs, G.R. (2011). Violence in the emergency department: a national survey of emergency medicine residents and attending physicians. *J. Emerg. Med.* 40 (5): 565–579.

3. Gacki-Smith, J., Juarez, A.M., Boyett, L. et al. (2009). Violence against nurses working in US emergency departments. *J. Nurs. Adm.* 39 (7–8): 340–349.

4. Richmond, J.S., Berlin, J.S., Fishkind, A.B. et al. (2012). Verbal de escalation of the agitated patient: consensus statement of the American Association for Emergency Psychiatry Project BETA De-escalation workgroup. *West J. Emerg. Med.* 13 (1): 17–25.

5. American College of Emergency Physicians (2016). *Protection from Violence in the Emergency Department*. Dallas, TX: American College of Emergency Physicians.

ALCOHOL WITHDRAWAL

Educational Goals

Learning Objectives

1. Recognize the clinical features of severe alcohol withdrawal syndrome (MK, PC).
2. Demonstrate appropriate sequential management of severe alcohol withdrawal syndrome (MK, PC).
3. Identify other causes of sympathomimetic hyperactivity and altered mental status (MK).
4. Recognize the importance of obtaining a social history in all patients (MK, PC).
5. Advanced learner: demonstrate appropriate and safe management of alcohol withdrawal syndrome resistant to benzodiazepines (MK, PC).

Critical Actions Checklist

- ☐ Check a fingerstick glucose (MK, PC).
- ☐ Obtain a social history (ICS, PC).
- ☐ Order an appropriate dose of a benzodiazepines as first-line treatment of delirium tremens (MK).
- ☐ Escalate the benzodiazepines dosing appropriately in response to lack of sustained improvement/clinical deterioration (MK, PC).
- ☐ Order head CT and/or labs looking for alternate causes for altered mental status and agitation (MK).
- ☐ Perform endotracheal intubation if airway compromise occurs or when starting propofol infusion (MK, PC).
- ☐ Advanced learner: Order at least one adjunct to benzodiazepines (phenobarbital, propofol, ketamine, dexmedetomidine) after using a total of 10 mg lorazepam or 70 mg diazepam (MK, PC).
- ☐ Admit to the intensive care unit (*ICU*) (ICS, P, SBP).
- ☐ Designate a leader, maintain assigned role, and use closed-loop communication (ICS, P).

Simulation Set-Up

Environment: ED treatment area.

Mannequin: Adult male standardized patient dressed in regular clothes. No IV access in place. Diaphoresis can be simulated by spraying with a bottle of water or glycerin drops. Simulation monitor available for vital signs. Alternatively, a high-fidelity male mannequin can be used.

Props: To be displayed on plasma screen/computer screen or printed out on handouts in scenario room when participants ask for/lab returns them:

- Images (see online component for delirium tremens, Scenario 11.3 at `https://www.wiley.com/go/thoureen/simulation/workbook2e`):
  - Chest x-ray (normal) (Figure 11.6).
  - Head CT (normal) (Figure 11.7).
- Laboratory tests (see online component as above):
  - Complete blood count (Table 11.9).
  - Complete metabolic panel (Table 11.10).
  - Lactate (Table 11.11).
  - Alcohol level (Table 11.12).
  - Serum ketones (Table 11.13).
- Triage sheet (see Figure 11.8).

> Any imaging or lab work not provided can be verbally reported as normal if the learners order the study.

Available supplies:

- Basic airway and adult code cart.
- Medications:
  - Liter bags of 0.9% saline, lactated Ringer's (*LR*) solutions, "banana bag": liter bag of 0.9% saline with thiamine, folic acid, multivitamin, and magnesium sulfate.
  - Pre-labeled syringes:
    - Benzodiazepines: lorazepam, midazolam, diazepam.
    - Rapid sequence intubation medications: succinylcholine, rocuronium, midazolam, propofol, ketamine.
  - Pre-labeled IV bags:
    - Anticonvulsant/sedative infusions: phenobarbital, propofol, dexmedetomidine, ketamine, lorazepam
- Airway trainer, if a standardized patient is used (optional).

Distractor: None.

Actors

- Patient is agitated. He answers questions in abbreviated sentences, and avoids eye contact. He is intermittently wringing his hands and appears anxious. He intermittently stares at the wall behind the learners as if seeing something.

- ED nurse can administer meds/fluids. The nurse may cue learners if needed. Nurse is also inquisitive and asks advanced learners to clarify the rationale behind medical decisions and meds choices as needed.
- Patient's spouse available via telephone consultation.
- Intensivist available via telephone consultation.
- Pharmacist available via telephone consultation.

Case Narrative

Scenario Background

Forty-two-year-old man presents to the ED with "flu symptoms." Patient states that he feels bad but does not volunteer any explanation. If the learner specifically asks, the patient discloses that he is nauseated, has palpitations, feels anxious, and has vomited once. He has no symptoms of upper respiratory tract infection. He denies pain in his abdomen or chest.

Medications:	None.
Allergies:	No known drug allergies
Family history:	No significant medical Hx
Social history:	Lives with wife and works as an accountant. (If the learner specifically asks about substance use history, he reports a history of heavy alcohol use with two admissions to rehabilitation facilities. The patient was recently on a two-week vacation and relapsed on alcohol, drinking one bottle of whiskey a day. His last drink was two days ago because the vacation ended and he needed to go back to work today.)

Initial Scenario Conditions

Well-appearing man wearing regular clothes and sitting at the edge of the stretcher. He is not on a monitor and does not have IV access. Triage form with vital signs from one hour earlier are at the bedside (Figure 11.8).

Vital signs (provided only if patient is placed on the monitor): Temp 100.2°F (37.9°C) orally, HR 120, RR 22, BP 170/100, SpO$_2$ 99% on room air.

Weight:	70 kg.
Head:	Atraumatic.
Eyes:	Pupils 4 mm and reactive to light.
ENT:	No pharyngeal erythema or swelling. (If learner specifically asks, tongue fasciculations are present.)
Neck:	Supple, no lymphadenopathy or swelling.
Heart:	Tachycardic and regular, distal pulses normal.
Lungs:	Tachypneic, clear breath sounds bilaterally.
Abdomen:	Soft and non-tender. No signs of trauma. Normal bowel sounds.

Extremities: No gross deformities.

Skin: No rash or abrasions. Patient is diaphoretic.

Neurologic: Alert and oriented to place and person, but not time. Anxious, follows commands. Face is symmetrical, moves all extremities spontaneously. Ambulates with a normal gait. Stares intermittently behind the learner as if looking at something on the wall but remains responsive throughout. Fine tremors are present.

See flow diagram (Figure 11.9) for further scenario changes described.

Case Narrative, Continued

Learners should obtain a focused history. Unless learners specifically ask, the patient will not disclose alcohol-related history. Tachycardia will only transiently improve with IV fluids. A fingerstick should be obtained. Tachycardia, hypertension, confusion, and agitation will worsen over the first five minutes.

After five minutes of the scenario, if the learners have not obtained the relevant social history, they can be cued:

- For novice learners: the nurse will directly ask the patient about alcohol use as part of the nursing assessment.
- For advanced learners: the nurse can ask the learners what they think is happening, prodding them to go through a differential diagnosis.

Once the diagnosis of severe alcohol withdrawal syndrome is made, learners should order IV benzodiazepines. Failure to administer benzodiazepines after 15 minutes will lead to a seizure, after which the patient will become unresponsive and require intubation. If not intubated, the patient will have a pulseless electrical activity arrest.

For novice learners, once the patient receives a total of 10 mg of lorazepam or 70 mg of diazepam, the patient will improve. The case will end with return of ordered labs and a consultation/transfer to the ICU.

For advanced learners, there is no improvement with appropriate benzodiazepine dosing, requiring adjuncts (phenobarbital, ketamine, dexmedetomidine, propofol) and subsequent airway management. A pharmacist is available via phone consultation as well. The case ends with return of ordered labs and a consultation/transfer to the ICU.

If a standardized patient is used and the learners need to intubate the patient, the scenario is paused and an airway trainer or a mannequin is introduced for the intubation procedure.

Instructor Notes

Pathophysiology [1]

- Chronic alcohol use leads to downregulation of γ-aminobutyric acid (*GABA*) receptors and upregulation of glutaminergic receptors, such as N-methyl-D-aspartate (*NMDA*).
- Abrupt discontinuation of alcohol leaves the patient in an excitatory state (exaggerated sympathomimetic activity).

Clinical Features

- The timing and presentation of alcohol withdrawal syndrome is variable and can occur at any blood alcohol level.
- Signs and symptoms may by mild, moderate or severe and may include [2]:
  - Anxiety.
  - Tremor.
  - Insomnia.
  - Headache.
  - Palpitations.
  - Gastrointestinal disturbances.
  - Diaphoresis.
  - Hypertension.
  - Tachycardia.
  - Confusion.
  - Hyperthermia.
  - Disorientation.
  - Hallucinations.
  - Seizures:
  - Delirium tremens is the most severe form of alcohol withdrawal syndrome:
    - Characterized by alcohol withdrawal syndrome and sympathetic overdrive.
    - Around 10% of alcohol withdrawal syndrome.
- Not all patients will go through the stages of alcohol withdrawal syndrome sequentially (e.g., a seizure may be the first presentation) [1, 3].

Diagnosis

- Primarily clinical using the following diagnostic criteria [3]:
  - ≥2 of the following symptoms occurring within hours to days of the sudden cessation (or marked decrease) of heavy or prolonged alcohol consumption:
    - Autonomic hyperactivity (tachycardia, diaphoresis, hypertension, elevated body temperature).

- Increased hand tremor.
- Insomnia.
- Nausea or vomiting.
- Transient hallucinations (auditory, visual, or tactile).
- Psychomotor agitation.
- Anxiety.
- Seizures (generalized, tonic–clonic).
- Symptoms are not the result of another medical condition
- Exclude other causes of altered mental status such as hypoglycemia, Wernicke encephalopathy, meningitis/encephalitis, alcoholic ketoacidosis, sepsis.

Management

- Several tools are available to "quantify" the severity of alcohol withdrawal syndrome, such as Clinical Institute Withdrawal Assessment (*CIWA*) [4]:
  - They are not meant to diagnose alcohol withdrawal syndrome.
  - They are helpful in treating mild but not severe alcohol withdrawal syndrome.
- Patients in severe alcohol withdrawal syndrome should be reassessed every 15–30 minutes.
- Medications:
  - Benzodiazepines [5]:
    - Lorazepam 2 mg IV, double the dose every 15 minutes up to 20 mg per dose *or* diazepam 10 mg IV, increase by 10 mg every 10–20 minutes.
    - Benzodiazepine-resistant alcohol withdrawal syndrome is defined as requiring [6] > 10 mg lorazepam in one hour *or* > 40 mg lorazepam in four hours *or* > 200 mg diazepam in three hours.
    - The most common mistake is underdosing.
  - Phenobarbital [7]:
    - Monotherapy dosing: 10 mg/kg over 30 minutes (max. 650 mg).
    - As adjunct (with benzodiazepines): 75 mg or 130 mg IV.
    - Maximum dose is 30 mg/kg; lower if patient already received large dose of benzodiazepine.
    - Time of onset is 20–40 minutes.
    - Avoid redosing prematurely.
  - Pharmacological adjuncts for patients with benzodiazepine-resistant alcohol withdrawal syndrome:
    - Ketamine [8]:
      - NMDA antagonist.
      - Dose: infusion 0.2 mg/kg/hour. Consider a bolus of 0.3 mg/kg.
    - Dexmedetomidine [9]:

- Alpha-2 agonist (reduces sympathetic output).
- Weak evidence for benefit.
- Dose: 0.2–1.2 µg/kg/hour.
- Propofol [4]:
  - GABA agonist and NMDA antagonist.
  - Patients are typically intubated.
  - Dose: 5–80 µg/kg/minute.
- No role:
  - Magnesium (except for correction of hypomagnesemia) [10].
  - Antipsychotics.
  - Clonidine.
  - Beta-blockers.
  - Baclofen.
  - Gabapentin.
- End point of treatment:
  - Calm and cooperative or mildly sedated patient.
  - Normal vitals.
  - Minimal/no tremor.

Disposition

- All patients with severe alcohol withdrawal syndrome must be admitted to the hospital, either to the ICU or a monitored floor, depending on the severity of the case.

Debriefing Plan

Plan approximately 30 minutes for discussion.

Potential Questions for Discussion

- How is alcohol withdrawal syndrome diagnosed?
- How do you dose benzodiazepines in alcohol withdrawal syndrome? What is the maximum dose?
- What additional medications can be used for benzodiazepines refractory alcohol withdrawal syndrome?
- What is the role of beta-blockers in treating severe alcohol withdrawal syndrome? How about antipsychotics?
- What is the role of algorithms such as CIWA in treatment of alcohol withdrawal syndrome?
- What is the appropriate disposition of a patient with severe alcohol withdrawal syndrome?

REFERENCES FOR ALCOHOL WITHDRAWAL

1. Olmedo, R. and Hoffman, R.S. (2000). Withdrawal syndromes. *Emerg. Med. Clin. North Am.* 18 (2): 273–288.

2. Muncie, H.L., Yasinian, Y., and Oge', L. (2013). Outpatient management of alcohol withdrawal syndrome. *Am. Fam. Phys.* 88 (9): 589–595.

3. American Psychiatric Association (2013). Substance-related and addictive disorders. In: *Diagnostic and Statistical Manual of Mental Disorders*, 5e, 481–591. Washington, DC: American Psychiatric Association.

4. Sullivan, J.T., Sykora, K., Schneiderman, J. et al. (1989). Assessment of alcohol withdrawal: the revised clinical institute withdrawal assessment for alcohol scale (CIWA-Ar). *Br. J. Addict.* 84 (11): 1353–1357.

5. Amato, L., Minozzi, S., Vecchi, S., and Davoli, M. (2010). Benzodiazepines for alcohol withdrawal. *Cochrane Database Syst. Rev.* 3: CD005063.

6. Brotherton, A.L., Hamilton, E.P., Kloss., H.,.G., and Hammond, D.A. (2016). Propofol for treatment of refractory alcohol withdrawal syndrome: a review of the literature. *Pharmacotherapy.* 36 (4): 433–442.

7. Rosenson, J., Clements, C., Simon, B. et al. (2013). Phenobarbital for acute alcohol withdrawal: a prospective randomized double-blind placebo-controlled study. *J. Emerg. Med.* 44 (3): 592–598.e2.

8. Pizon, A.F., Lynch, M.J., Benedict, N.J. et al. (2018). Adjunct ketamine use in the management of severe ethanol withdrawal. *Crit. Care Med.* 46 (8): e768–e771.

9. Muzyk, A.J., Kerns, S., Brudney, S., and Gagliardi, J.P. (2013). Dexmedetomidine for the treatment of alcohol withdrawal syndrome: rationale and current status of research. *CNS Drugs.* 27 (11): 913–920.

10. Wilson, A. and Vulcano, B. (1984). A double-blind, placebo-controlled trial of magnesium sulfate in the ethanol withdrawal syndrome. *Alcohol Clin. Exp. Res.* 8 (6): 542–545.

SELECTED READINGS FOR ALCOHOL WITHDRAWAL

Hughes, D (2016). Benzodiazepine-refractory alcohol withdrawal. *REBEL EM* (28 April 2016) (blog post). https://rebelem.com/benzodiazepine-refractory-alcohol-withdrawal (accessed 7 September 2021).

Long, D., Long, B., and Koyfman, A. (2017). The emergency medicine management of severe alcohol withdrawal. *Am. J. Emerg. Med.* 35 (7): 1005–1011. https://doi.org/10.1016/j.ajem.2017.02.002.

APPENDIX

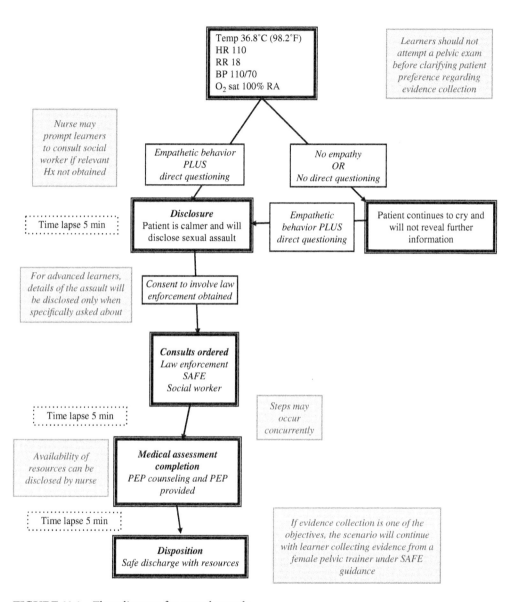

FIGURE 11.1   Flow diagram for sexual assault.

Radiology Results

XR Chest 2 views

Impression:
4th, 5th posterior rib healing fractures. No infiltrate. No pneumothorax. Injury pattern is consistent with non-accidental injury.

FIGURE 11.2   Chest x-ray radiology read.

Radiology Results:

XR femur 2 views Right

Impression:
Displaced spiral mid shaft femur fracture with surrounding soft tissue swelling. Injury pattern is consistent with non-accidental injury.

FIGURE 11.3   Right femur x-ray radiology read.

Radiology results

CT head without contrast:

No acute intracranial hemorrhage or lesions noted.

FIGURE 11.4   Computed tomography of the head radiology read.

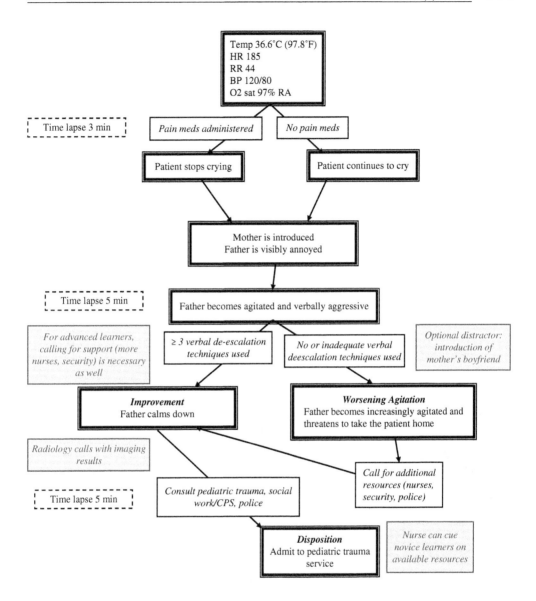

FIGURE 11.5 Flow diagram for non-accidental trauma with aggressive family member.

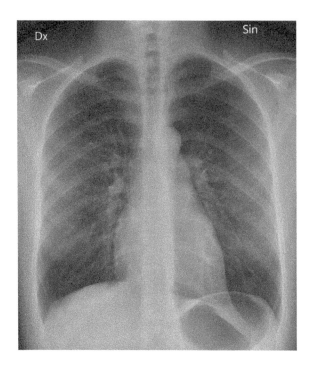

FIGURE 11.6   Chest x-ray (normal).

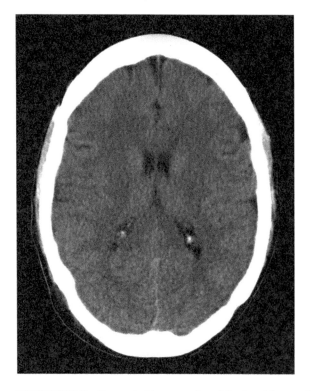

FIGURE 11.7   Computed tomography of the head (normal).

Triage

Date
Patient Name: Omar Adil

Vitals Signs
Temp 37.9° C orally (100.2° F)
HR 120
RR 22
BP 170/100
O_2 sat 99% on room air

Weight is 70 kg

FIGURE 11.8   Triage sheet at presentation for delirium tremens.

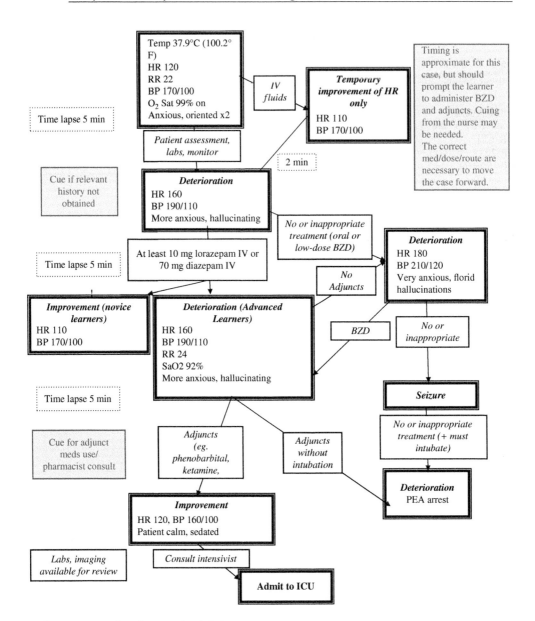

FIGURE 11.9   Flow diagram for delirium tremens.

TABLE 11.1   Complete blood count.

Test	Value	Reference range
White blood cells ($10^3/\mu l$)	10.8	4.5–11
Hemoglobin (g/dl)	14.4	11.9–15.7
Hematocrit (%)	42.2	35–45
Platelets ($10^3/\mu l$)	396	153–367

TABLE 11.2   Complete metabolic panel.

Test	Value	Reference range
Sodium (mmol/l)	139	135–145
Potassium (mmol/l)	4.0	3.5–5
Chloride (mmol/l)	101	98–107
Bicarbonate (mmol/l)	25	21–30
Blood urea nitrogen (mg/dl)	22	7–17
Creatinine (mg/dl)	0.68	0.7–1.5
Glucose (mg/dl)	103	74–106
Calcium (mg/dl)	9.6	8.4–10.2
Magnesium (mg/dl)	2.0	1.6–2.3
Phosphate (mg/dl)	4.1	2.5–4.5
Alkaline phosphatase (iu/l)	109	38–126
alanine aminotransferase (iu/l)	22	0–34
aspartate aminotransferase (iu/l)	40	14–36
Albumin (g/dl)	4.8	3.5–5

TABLE 11.3   Pregnancy test.

Test	Result
hCG	Negative

TABLE 11.4   HIV antibody test.

Test	Result
HIV antibody	Pending

TABLE 11.5 Rapid plasma reagin.

Test	Result
Rapid plasma reagin	Pending

TABLE 11.6 Pregnancy and sexually transmitted infection prophylaxis [1, 9, 10].

Condition	Prophylaxis
Pregnancy	One of the following: • Levonorgestrel, 1.5 mg once or 0.75 mg at 1 and 12 hours • Combined estrogen and progestin (100 µg ethinyl estradiol plus 0.50 mg levonorgestrel) at 1 and 12 hours • Ulipristal acetate, 30 mg orally, single dose
Gonorrhea	Ceftriaxone, 250 mg IM, single dose or Cefixime, 400 mg orally, single dose
Chlamydia	Azithromycin, 1 g orally, single dose or Doxycycline, 100 mg orally, twice a day for 7 days
Trichomonas and bacterial vaginosis	Metronidazole, 2 g orally, single dose

TABLE 11.7 Complete blood count.

Test	Value	Reference range
White blood cells (10^3/µl)	8.9	4.5–11
Hemoglobin (g/dl)	12.2	11.9–15.7
Hematocrit (%)	36.6	35–45
Platelets (10^3/µl)	357	153–367
Segmented neutrophils (%)	12	40–60
Lymphocytes (%)	59	20–40

TABLE 11.8 Complete metabolic panel.

Test	Value	Reference range
Sodium (mmol/l)	139	135–145
Potassium (mmol/l)	4.3	3.5–5
Chloride (mmol/l)	106	98–107
Bicarbonate (mmol/l)	22	21–30
Blood urea nitrogen (mg/dl)	12	7–17
Creatinine (mg/dl)	0.33	0.7–1.5
Glucose (mg/dl)	182	74–106
Calcium (mg/dl)	9.4	8.4–10.2
Magnesium (mg/dl)	2.0	1.6–2.3
Phosphate (mg/dl)	4.3	2.5–4.5
Alkaline phosphatase (iu/l)	140	38–126
alanine aminotransferase (iu/l)	29	0–34
aspartate aminotransferase (iu/l)	47	14–36
Albumin (g/dl)	4.0	3.5–5

TABLE 11.9 Complete blood count.

Test	Value	Reference range
White blood cells ($10^3/\mu l$)	8.7	4.5–11
Hemoglobin (g/dl)	11.8	11.9–15.7
Hematocrit (%)	35.4	35–45
Platelets ($10^3/\mu l$)	397	153–367
Segmented neutrophils (%)	12	40–60
Lymphocytes (%)	69	20–40

TABLE 11.10   Complete metabolic panel.

Test	Value	Reference range
Sodlum (mmol/l)	140	135–145
Potassium (mmol/l)	3.1	3.5–5
Chloride (mmol/l)	106	98–107
Bicarbonate (mmol/l)	20	21–30
Blood urea nitrogen (mg/dl)	16	7–17
Creatinine (mg/dl)	0.83	0.7–1.5
Glucose (mg/dl)	182	74–106
Calcium (mg/dl)	9.5	8.4–10.2
Magnesium (mg/dl)	1.2	1.6–2.3
Phosphate (mg/dl)	2.2	2.5–4.5
Alkaline phosphatase (iu/l)	210	38–126
alanine aminotransferase (iu/l)	29	0–34
aspartate aminotransferase (iu/l)	47	14–36
Albumin (g/dl)	3.9	3.5–5

TABLE 11.11   Lactate level.

Test	Value	Reference range
Lactate (mmol/l)	3.1	0–2

TABLE 11.12   Alcohol level.

Test	Value
Ethanol (mg/dl)	60

TABLE 11.13   Serum ketones.

Test	Result
Serum ketones	Positive

CHAPTER 12

Renal and Urogenital Emergencies

Rupal Jain, Diane Kuhn, and Sarah B. Dubbs

Department of Emergency Medicine, University of Maryland School of Medicine, Baltimore, MD, USA

ACUTE KIDNEY INJURY

Educational Goals

Learning Objectives

1. Demonstrate effective communication skills in obtaining further information from the emergency medical services (EMS) and the patient's family (PC, ICS).
2. Recognize wide complex bradycardia secondary to hyperkalemia and initiate appropriate management (MK, PC).
3. Identify etiology of acute kidney injury (*AKI*) (MK, PC).
4. Recognize indications for emergent dialysis and consult nephrology (MK, PC).
5. Evaluate response to treatment of hyperkalemia (MK, PC).
6. Recognize and avoid iatrogenic causes of kidney injury (MK, PC).

Emergency Medicine Simulation Workbook: A Tool for Bringing the Curriculum to Life, Second Edition. Edited by Traci L. Thoureen and Sara B. Scott.
© 2022 John Wiley & Sons Ltd. Published 2022 by John Wiley & Sons Ltd.
Companion website: www.wiley.com/go/thoureen/simulation/workbook2e

Critical Actions Checklist

- ☐ Obtain electrocardiogram (ECG) (PC).
- ☐ Administer medications for suspected hyperkalemia (MK, PC).
- ☐ Recognize AKI based on laboratories (MK, PC).
- ☐ Initiate fluid resuscitation (PC).
- ☐ Assess for urinary tract obstruction with post-void residual or renal/bladder ultrasound (MK).
- ☐ Place a foley catheter for relief of urinary obstruction (PC).
- ☐ Consult nephrology (ICS, P, SBP).

Simulation Set-up

Environment: Emergency department (ED) resuscitation.

Mannequin: Male simulator mannequin, sitting upright, wearing a patient gown, with an emesis basin full of vomitus. Moistened oatmeal can be used to simulate vomit. If the mannequin does not permit foley catheter placement, a genitourinary task trainer will also be needed.

Props: To be displayed on plasma screen/computer screen or printed out on hand-outs in scenario room when asked for/return from laboratory:

- Images (see online component for AKI Scenario 12.1 at https://www.wiley.com/go/thoureen/simulation/workbook2e):
  - ECG: sinus rhythm with widening of QRS interval (Figure 12.1)
  - Chest x-ray demonstrating mild pulmonary edema (Figure 12.2)
  - ECG of stabilized patient demonstrating resolution of QRS prolongation (Figure 12.3)
- Laboratory tests (see online component as above):
  - Complete blood count (Table 12.1)
  - Complete metabolic panel (Table 12.2)
  - Lactate (Table 12.3)
  - Troponin (Table 12.4)
  - Fingerstick glucose (Table 12.5)
  - Venous blood gas (Table 12.6)

> Any imaging or lab work not provided (such as computed tomography of the head or urine drug screen) can be verbally reported as normal if the learners order the study.

Available supplies:

- Adult code cart with pacer/defibrillation pads and advanced airway supplies.
- Medications:
  - Liter bags of 0.9% saline and PlasmaLyte®.
  - Pre-labeled syringes:
    - Regular insulin.
    - 50% dextrose.
    - Rapid sequence intubation medications (paralytic and induction medication of choice for your institution).
    - Calcium gluconate and/or calcium chloride.
- Foley catheter.
- Emesis basin.
- Nebulizer delivery device (e.g., face mask).
- Coudé catheter (optional).

Distractor: none

Actors

- EMS personnel.
- Patient voice is male. Patient should sound confused and lethargic. He is not able to appropriately follow commands or answer questions.
- ED nurse can administer medications/fluids. The nurse does have medical knowledge and may cue learners if needed.
- Nephrology and medical admitting service available via telephone consultation.

Case Narrative

Scenario Background

A 66-year-old man presents with altered mental status and chief complaint of nausea/vomiting. He arrives from home via ambulance. Per EMS, over the past few days the patient has had intermittent confusion, dizziness, and generalized weakness.

Chief complaint: Nausea/vomiting and confusion.
Patient's medical history: Type II diabetes, hypertension, glaucoma, fatty liver disease, benign prostatic hypertrophy, coronary artery disease.
Medications: Metformin, lisinopril, aspirin, amlodipine.
Allergies: No known drug allergies.
Family history: Unknown.
Social history: Unknown.

Initial Scenario Conditions

Elderly man on EMS stretcher attached to cardiac monitor. Patient is moaning, breathing rapidly. He is holding an emesis basin containing nonbloody, nonbilious emesis.

> Case may start with EMS receiving this case "on scene" as presented and performing their objectives to initiate treatment and transport, including obtaining the first set of vital signs, finger stick blood glucose, and calculation of GCS. Identification of bradycardia should trigger the essential next step of placing the patient on cardiac monitor and obtaining 12-lead ECG. Alternatively, case background may be presented prior to case as an EMS medical consult or by EMS on arrival.

Vital signs: Temp 97.9°F (36.6°C), HR 80, RR 26, BP 144/96, SpO_2 97% on room air.

Head: Head atraumatic.

Eyes: Pupils 4 mm and reactive to light.

Neck: No jugular vein distention.

Heart: Regular rate and rhythm, no murmur.

Lungs: Tachypneic, shallow respirations. Lungs clear.

Abdomen: No surgical incisions. Soft. Distension and tenderness in the suprapubic region.

Genitourinary: No paraphimosis or concerning edema.

Extremities: Mild peripheral edema. No gross deformities.

Skin: Warm, dry, no signs of trauma.

Neurologic: Eyes open. Incomprehensible words. Does not follow commands. Localizes to pain. (Glasgow Coma Scale score 11).

> Physical exam findings not available on your mannequin can be reported verbally if asked for by learners; for example, if you are unable to simulate bladder distension you can verbally report a firm mass in the suprapubic region.

See flow diagram Figure 12.4 for further scenario changes described.

Case Narrative, Continued

Learners of all levels should initially obtain a report from EMS. Altered mental status should prompt IV placement, cardiac monitoring, and ECG. Failure to obtain ECG and initiate empiric calcium for a wide complex rhythm will lead to progressive bradycardia and the patient will go into cardiac arrest. If just atropine or epinephrine are administered (whether pre-arrest or during the code), there will be no improvement in status.

After administration of calcium, ECG, and cardiac monitor will demonstrate narrowing of the QRS. There is an initial period of stabilization. During this time, any ordered imaging/labs return.

All learners should identify AKI, acidosis, and hyperkalemia. Therapy for hyperkalemia should include insulin and glucose and may include continuous albuterol and bicarbonate. If hyperkalemia is untreated, the patient will decompensate into cardiac arrest.

The advanced learner should evaluate the cause of AKI. Workup should include bladder ultrasound or empiric foley catheter placement to evaluate for oliguria/anuria or postrenal/obstructive etiologies of AKI. Results indicate urinary retention.

If not already done, a urinary catheter should be placed to relieve obstruction. For the advanced learner, if desired as a learning objective, a difficult foley catheter placement can prompt placement of a coudé catheter.

If obstruction is not recognized as the cause of the patient's AKI, the learner may be prompted to obtain bladder ultrasound by the nurse stating there has been no urine output, or by nephrology questioning why the patient has AKI.

The case ends when the patient is stabilized, nephrology has been consulted due to concern for AKI, and the patient has been admitted to a monitored unit.

Instructor Notes

Pathophysiology

- Etiologies:
  - Prerenal – related to renal hypoperfusion:
    - Hypovolemic state:
    - Hemorrhage.
    - Dehydration.
    - Increased renal venous pressures:
    - Abdominal compartment syndrome.
  - Intrinsic:
    - Renal vascular pathologies.
    - Tubulointerstitial disease
    - Rhabdomyolysis
    - Common nephrotoxic medications
      - Antibiotics (aminoglycosides, vancomycin).
      - Metformin.
      - Non-steroidal anti-inflammatories.
    - Glomerular disease:
      - Postrenal: obstruction of urinary outflow.

Clinical Features

- Often asymptomatic or mild symptoms such as nausea, weakness, confusion.
- Common clinical features with more severe injury and renal failure may include:
  - Oliguria or anuria.
  - Refractory hypertension.
  - Edema.

Diagnosis

- Laboratory:
  - Elevated creatine or reduced glomerular filtration rate.
  - Possible associated abnormalities:
    - Hyperkalemia.
    - Metabolic acidosis.
    - Uremia.
  - Urinalysis:
    - Muddy brown casts/renal tubular casts = acute tubular necrosis.
    - Red blood cells, red blood cell casts = glomerular disease.
    - White blood cells, white blood cell casts = pyelonephritis or acute interstitial nephritis.
  - Urine osmolality and urine electrolytes.
- Imaging:
  - Ultrasound of the urinary system (kidneys and bladder).
  - Assess for hydronephrosis or distended bladder.

Management

- Initial resuscitation:
Assess and manage ABCs.
  - Obtain EKG for evaluation of significant hyperkalemia
    - Peaked T waves.
    - ST depression or elevation.
    - Bradycardia or other arrhythmias.
    - QRS widening and PR lengthening.
    - Flattening or loss of P waves.
  - Treat hyperkalemia-related ECG abnormalities>
    - Stabilize myocardium:
      - Calcium gluconate or calcium chloride.

- Shift potassium intracellularly:
  - Insulin and glucose.
  - β-agonist (e.g., albuterol)
  - Sodium bicarbonate:
    - Remove potassium
    - Loop diuretics (e.g., furosemide)
    - Potassium binders (e.g., patiromer, sodium zirconium cyclosilicate).
    - Dialysis.
- Interventions specific to etiology of AKI:
  - Prerenal:
    - Volume resuscitate or relieve intra-abdominal pressure.
  - Intrinsic:
    - Identify nephrotoxic insult:
    - Check creatine phosphokinase.
    - Avoid nephrotoxic medications.
  - Postrenal:
    - Relieve urinary tract obstruction.
- Indications for emergent dialysis:
  - Severe acidemia refractory to medical management.
  - Significant hyperkalemia.
  - Presence of nephrotoxic, dialyzable substance.
  - Volume overload with respiratory compromise.
  - Symptomatic uremia.

Debriefing Plan

Plan for approximately 30 minutes for discussion.

Potential Questions for Discussion

- What is the approach to AKI?
- What are common etiologies of AKI, and what laboratory values or imaging studies can you use to distinguish between these etiologies?
- What are typical features of hyperkalemia on ECG?
- What is the management of severe hyperkalemia?
- What are the indications for emergent dialysis?
- What are some examples of medications that should be avoided in patients with AKI?

SELECTED READING FOR ACUTE KIDNEY INJURY

Hertzberg, D., Rydén, L., Pickering, J.W. et al. (2017). Acute kidney injury-an overview of diagnostic methods and clinical management. *Clin. Kidney J.* 10 (3): 323–331.

Long, B., Warix, J.R., and Koyfman, A. (2018). Controversies in the management of hyperkalemia. *J. Emerg. Med.* 55: 192.

Mehta, R.L., Kellum, J.A., Shah, S.V. et al. (2007). Acute kidney injury network: report of an initiative to improve outcomes in acute kidney injury. *Crit. Care* 11 (2): R31.

KDIGO Acute Kidney Injury Work Group (2012). KDIGO clinical practice guidelines for acute kidney injury. *Kidney Int.* 2 (Suppl 1): 1–138.

FOURNIER'S GANGRENE

Educational Goals

Learning Objectives

1. Demonstrate effective communication skills to obtain further information from the patient and their family (PC, ICS).
2. Perform a full clinical exam, including skin exam, in the setting of sepsis of unclear etiology (MK, PC).
3. Identify clinical features concerning for necrotizing soft tissue infection (MK, PC).
4. Demonstrate application of standard sepsis protocols (MK, PC).
5. Select appropriate antibiotic coverage for necrotizing skin infection, including empiric coverage for toxin-releasing bacteria (MK, PC).
6. Demonstrate effective communication with a surgical consultant (PC, ICS).

Critical Actions Checklist

☐ Activate sepsis protocol including:
- Administration of 30 cc/kg of crystalloid fluid.
- Ordering laboratory tests that include lactate.
- Blood cultures.
- Initiation of broad spectrum antibiotics (PC, MK).

☐ Perform a full skin exam (MK, PC).
☐ Administer clindamycin, in addition to broad antibiotic coverage (MK, PC).
☐ Consult surgical specialist (ICS, P, SBP).

Simulation Set-up

Environment: ED resuscitation room.

Mannequin: Male simulator mannequin, with genital/perineum/right-thigh moulage. Reddish violet and skin-toned make-up can be applied to mimic some mild superficial skin changes, or similar colored modeling clay or dough can be applied and made to include a few bullous lesions. The patient should be dressed in a hospital gown with a sheet overtop.

Props: To be displayed on a plasma screen/computer screen or printed out on handouts in scenario room when asked for/return from lab:

- Images (see online component for Fournier's gangrene, Scenario 12.2 at https://www.wiley.com/go/thoureen/simulation/workbook2e):
  - Chest x-ray (normal) (Figure 12.5).
  - ECG: Sinus tachycardia (Figure 12.6).
  - Computed tomography (CT) of the abdomen/pelvis (one slice) showing scrotal and perineal subcutaneous air (Figure 12.7).

- Laboratory tests (see online component as above):
  - Complete blood count (Table 12.7).
  - Complete metabolic panel (Table 12.8).
  - Lactate (Table 12.9).
  - C-reactive protein (Table 12.10).
  - Troponin (Table 12.11).
  - Venous blood gas (Table 12.12).

Available supplies:

- Basic airway and code cart.
- Medications:
  - Liter bags of 0.9% saline and lactated Ringer's solution (*LR*).
  - Pre-labeled IV bags:
    - Antibiotic including: meropenem, piperacillin-tazobactam, vancomycin, clindamycin.
    - Sedative of choice for your institution.
  - Pre-labeled syringes:
    - Rapid sequence intubation medications (paralytic and induction medication of choice for your institution).
    - Analgesic medication (e.g., fentanyl, morphine).
- Video-assisted laryngoscope, bedside ultrasound machine (optional).
Distractor: None.

Actors

- Patient voice is male. Patient should sound tired. He is able to respond to questions, but is unclear about his medical issues. He reports pain over the lower abdomen, right hip, and upper right thigh.
- Daughter can provide relevant medical history.
- ED nurse can administer medications/fluids. The nurse does have some medical knowledge and may cue learners if needed.
- Surgical consultant available by telephone or transfer line.

Case Narrative

Scenario Background

A 57-year-old man presents with abdominal pain and fever. He is brought in by his daughter who states that he had been feeling "unwell" over the past two days, but got significantly worse today. She took his temperature with a forehead thermometer, which read 101.2°F (38.4°C). The patient reports that he has been having some lower abdominal pain over the past day or two, but cannot describe it further.

Chief complaint: "I feel sick".
Patient's medical history: Type II diabetes, obesity, hyperlipidemia.
Medications: Metformin, atorvastatin.
Allergies: No known drug allergies.
Family history: Denies.
Social history: Half pack/day, smoker for 30 years, social alcohol use.

Initial Scenario Conditions

Obese man lying in bed looking uncomfortable and mildly diaphoretic.

Vital signs: Temp 103.5°F (39.7°C), HR 118, RR 16, BP 105/70, SpO$_2$ 98% on room air.
Head: Head is atraumatic.
Eyes: Pupils 3 mm and reactive to light.
Neck: No jugular vein distension.
Heart: Tachycardic and regular, symmetric 2+ radial pulses.
Lungs: Clear bilaterally.
Abdomen: No apparent surgical incisions. Obese but not rigid. Patient exhibits significant tenderness to palpation of the lower abdomen, despite not having peritoneal signs.
Genitourinary: See below for skin findings in the genital area.
Extremities: No gross deformities or peripheral edema.
Skin: Patient has a purpuric rash that is expanding over the perineum and genital area to the upper right thigh. Several individual bullae are present. The patient is unaware of this rash.
Neurologic: Drowsy but oriented, no focal deficits

> Genital exam and skin findings should only be reported to learners if they do a complete skin exam, including removing the patient's sheet/gown.

See flow diagram (Figure 12.8) for further scenario changes described.

Case Narrative, Continued

Learners of all levels should initially request vitals and obtain as much history from patient and daughter as possible. Learners should recognize potential sepsis and initiate resuscitation following appropriate sepsis protocol, including early fluid resuscitation, broad-spectrum antibiotics, lactate level, and blood cultures.

The patient and his daughter are unaware of the patient's rash. Early learners may need prompting to conduct a complete secondary exam after initial resuscitation has been established. If learners do not completely expose the patient, nursing, or family member may prompt the learner with remarks about having noticed a rash. Antibiotics should be initiated for Fournier's gangrene. If antibiotics do not include methicillin-resistant *Staphylococcus aureus* (MRSA) coverage, β-lactam inhibitor and clindamycin, the patient will further deteriorate, becoming hypotensive.

Appropriate imaging studies should be ordered. Learners of all levels should recognize the high acuity and need for emergent surgical intervention in the case, and should escalate care by contacting a surgical service.

For advanced learners, a deterioration in mental status and vital signs will prompt need for airway intervention and blood pressure support prior to transfer of the patient to definitive management. Learners will need to volume resuscitate, initiate vasopressors and intubate the patient. Learners should also be asked to provide ventilator setting recommendations.

The case ends when the patient is stabilized and goes to the operating room or transfer to a specialty surgical center has been arranged.

Instructor Notes

Pathophysiology

- Infection of the deep soft tissues spreading along the muscle fascia due to poor blood supply.
  - Polymicrobial: typically caused by both aerobic and anaerobic bacteria.
- Thrombosis of small subcutaneous vessels results in gangrene of skin.

Epidemiology and Risk Factors

- Uncommon disease: < 2000/year in the United States.
- Many studies show a slight predominance in male patients:
- Increased risk in patients with:
  - Diabetes.
  - Alcoholism.
  - Peripheral vascular disease.
  - Immunocompromised state.

Clinical Features

- Pain out of proportion to exam findings.
- Signs of sepsis.
- Skin findings:
  - Bullae formation.
  - Purpuric rash.
  - Crepitus.
  - Skin necrosis.
- Motor or sensory deficits are late signs.

Diagnosis

- Primarily clinical, based on risk factors and clinical features
  - Commonly misdiagnosed as cellulitis or abscesses
- Laboratory tests may be useful for risk stratification:

  Laboratory risk indicator for necrotizing fasciitis (*LRINEC*) score for risk stratification [1]:
  - Score ≥ 6 is highly concerning for possible necrotizing soft-tissue infection ($> 90\%$ positive predictive value).
  - Components of LRINEC score are shown in Table 12.13.
- CT imaging may be helpful.
  - Imaging cannot rule out necrotizing fasciitis.
  - Common CT characteristics are:
    - Gas tracking along fascia.
    - Fascial thickening or fat stranding.
    - Abscesses.
- Blood cultures should be obtained.

Management

- Resuscitation:
  - Manage ABCs.
  - Treat sepsis following established guidelines.
  - Early initiation of norepinephrine to maintain a goal mean arterial pressure of $\geq 65\,\text{mmHg}$.
- Antibiotics:
  - Vancomycin (MRSA coverage).
  - Piperacillin-tazobactam or a carbapenem (β-lactamase inhibitor).
  - Clindamycin (activity against toxins released by streptococci and staphylococci)
- Surgical consultation:
  - If clinical suspicion is high (LRINEC ≥ 6).
  - Early consult and intervention is the most important prognostic indicator.

Debriefing Plan

Plan for approximately 30 minutes for discussion.

Potential Questions for Discussion

- What is the approach to treating sepsis?
- What are diagnostic features of Fournier's gangrene and other necrotizing skin infections?

- How do you risk stratify patients with necrotizing fasciitis?
- What antibiotic(s) should be selected for the treatment of necrotizing fasciitis?
- What is considered the definitive treatment for necrotizing fasciitis?

REFERENCE FOR FOURNIER'S GANGRENE

1. Wong, C.-H., Khin, Heng, L.-W. et al. (2004). The LRINEC (laboratory risk indicator for necrotizing fasciitis) score: a tool for distinguishing necrotizing fasciitis from other soft tissue infections. *Crit. Care Med.* 32 (7): 1535–1541.

SELECTED READINGS FOR FOURNIER'S GANGRENE

Hagedorn, J. and Wessells, H. (2017). A contemporary update on Fournier's gangrene. *Nat. Rev. Urol.* 14: 205–214.

Montrief, T., Long, B., Koyfman, A., and Auerbach, J. (2019). Fournier gangrene: a review for emergency clinicians. *J. Emerg. Med.* 57 (4): 488–500.

Bonne, S.L. and Kadri, S.S. (2017). Evaluation and management of necrotizing soft tissue infections. *Infect. Dis. Clin. North Am.* 31 (3): 497–511.

Levenson, R.B., Singh, A.K., and Novelline, R.A. (2008). Fournier gangrene: role of imaging. *Radiographics* 28: 519–528.

Eke, N. (2000). Fournier's gangrene: a review of 1726 cases. *Br. J. Surg.* 87: 718–728.

Wong, C.-H., Chang, H.-C., Pasupathy, S. et al. (2003). Necrotizing fasciitis: clinical presentation, microbiology, and determinants of mortality. *J. Bone Joint Surg.* 85 (8): 1454–1460.

PEDIATRIC PRIAPISM

Educational Goals

Learning Objectives

1. Recognize priapism and initiate IV access, analgesics and hydration (MK, PC).
2. Discuss the indications for intracavernosal aspiration and irrigation, and list important potential complications when obtaining consent (MK, PC).
3. Explain or demonstrate intracavernosal aspiration and irrigation (MK, PC).
4. Demonstrate appropriate ED management of sickle cell disease (*SCD*) (MK, ICS, P, SBP).
5. Demonstrate effective and empathetic communication with patient's guardian (ICS).
6. Demonstrate appropriate consultation with pediatric urologist and hematologist (PC, ICS, P).

Critical Actions Checklist

☐ Obtain IV access and IV fluids. (PC).
☐ Administer analgesia (PC).
☐ Ensure that the patient is nil by mouth (PC).
☐ Obtain pediatric urologic consultation (ICS, P, SBP).
☐ Obtain informed consent for intracavernosal aspiration and irrigation (MK, PC).
☐ Perform intracavernosal aspiration and irrigation (MK, PC).
☐ Place patient on cardiac monitor prior to local injection of α-agonist (MK, PC).
☐ Obtain pediatric hematology consultation for consideration of exchange transfusion (ICS, P, SBP).
☐ Evaluate response to therapy (PC).

Critical actions can be changed to address the educational needs of the learner. For example: The novice learner may require significant assistance from a urology consultant who is "in house" and arrives at bedside for the procedure, whereas the advanced learner may only have urology available by telephone.

Simulation Set-up

Environment: ED treatment room.

Mannequin: Male pediatric simulator mannequin (elementary-aged size), wearing a patient gown. Optional: erect penile task trainer can be constructed [1].

Props: To be displayed on plasma display/computer screen or printed out on handouts in scenario room when asked for/return from laboratory:

- Laboratory tests (see online component for priapism, Scenario 12.3 at https://www.wiley.com/go/thoureen/simulation/workbook2e):
  - Complete blood count (Table 12.14).
  - Complete metabolic panel (Table 12.15).
  - Reticulocyte percentage (Table 12.16).
  - Corporal blood gas (Table 12.17).

Available Supplies

- 23- or 21-gauge butterfly needle, 10 ml syringe.
- Syringe and small gauge needle for local anesthetic injection.
- Medications:
  - Liter bags of 0.9% saline and dextrose containing maintenance fluids.
  - Pre-labeled syringes:
    - Analgesic medications such as fentanyl or morphine.
    - Lidocaine without epinephrine for local injection.
    - Terbutaline.
    - Phenylephrine.
- Penile task trainer (optional) [1].

Distractor: Frantic, concerned mother.

Actors

- Patient has a male pediatric voice. Patient should sound scared, shy, and uncomfortable.
- Mother is upset, somewhat agitated, speaking with a raised voice.
- ED nurse can administer medications/fluids. The nurse does have some medical knowledge and may cue learners if needed.
- Pediatric urology may be available in person (junior learners) or by telephone (advanced learners).
- Hematology available via telephone consultation.

Case Narrative

Scenario Background

A 6-year-old boy presents with apparent discomfort. He arrives with mom via EMS. The boy appears shy, providing little history. Mother provides additional information that the patient has been complaining of genital pain over the past five hours. No prior history of the same.

Chief complaint: penile pain.
Patient's medical history: SCD.
Medications: Hydroxyurea, l-glutamine.
Allergies: Penicillin.
Family history: Non-contributory.
Social history: Non-contributory.

Initial Scenario Conditions

Young boy brought in on EMS stretcher, appearing uncomfortable. Patient is moaning.

Case may start with EMS receiving this case on scene as presented, and performing their objectives to initiate treatment and transport, including obtaining the first set of vital signs, IV access and weight-based administration of analgesic. Alternatively, case background may be presented prior to case as an EMS medical consult or by EMS on arrival.

Vital signs: Temp 97.9°F (36.6°C), HR 121, RR 24, BP 105/60, SpO_2 99% on room air.
Weight: 16 kg.
Head: Head is atraumatic.
Eyes: Pupils 4 mm and reactive to light.
Neck: No jugular vein distension.
Heart: Slightly tachycardic and regular.
Lungs: Lungs clear bilaterally.
Abdomen: No apparent surgical incisions. Soft, nondistended. Mild suprapubic tenderness.
Genitourinary: Tumescent penis without signs of trauma. No paraphimosis or concerning scrotal edema or tenderness.
Extremities: Normal.
Skin: Warm, dry.
Neurologic: Eyes open. Answers questions appropriately and follows commands.

Physical exam findings not available on your mannequin can be reported verbally if asked for by learners; for example, if your mannequin cannot simulate the described genitourinary exam, you can verbally report the findings when requested.

See flow diagram (Figure 12.9) for further scenario changes described.

Case Narrative, Continued

Learners of all levels (EMS, students, and postgraduate learners) should promptly evaluate the patient. If EMS has not already initiated care, learners should request IV access and order analgesics.

Identification of priapism in the setting of known SCD should prompt ordering of blood work. Failure to obtain prompt urology consultation will result in increased aggravation of the patient's mother and she will express concern for future erectile dysfunction/impotence.

After urology is consulted, intracavernosal aspiration and irrigation should be performed. The beginner learners may require significant assistance from a urology consultant, who is present to teach the procedure. Advanced learners only have urology consultation available by telephone.

All learners will need to obtain informed consent for the procedure from the patient's mother. It is important that the learners discuss both the risks and benefits of the procedure.

Advanced learners should consider options for additional procedural pain control such as regional block with pudendal nerve block, penile ring block, and/or procedural sedation. The learners should perform (or describe) aspiration of the corpus cavernosum and obtain corporal venous blood gas prior to injection of phenylephrine. Phenylephrine may need to be diluted to a final concentration of 100 µg/ml prior to injecting in the corpus cavernosum. The patient should be placed on a cardiac monitor with reassessment of blood pressure if not already done so for procedural sedation.

Following phenylephrine injection, the patient will have hypertension and reflex bradycardia. If the patient was not previously placed on the cardiac monitor, the patient will complain that he feels "dizzy" following the procedure. The vital signs will normalize after one minute without intervention.

Additional laboratories are available once the procedure is complete. The learner should reassess and treat for pain and recurrent tumescence.

The case ends when the penis has been detumesced, pediatric hematology has been consulted and the patient is admitted to the hospital. Hematologist may request the learners' interpretation of corporal blood gas as either low-flow priapism or high-flow priapism.

Instructor Notes

Pathophysiology

- Priapism is defined as a painful, prolonged (> 4 hours) erection of the penis in the absence of sexual arousal.
- Etiology in children [2]:
  - SCD (65%).
  - Leukemia (10%).
  - Trauma (10%).
  - Idiopathic (10%).
  - Pharmacologically induced (5%).
- Types of priapism:

- Low-flow priapism (ischemic):
  - Most common.
  - Secondary to poor venous outflow.
  - Leads to ischemia and thrombosis due to stagnant and hypoxic blood leading to fibrosis, disfigurement, and erectile dysfunction.
  - Sickle cell anemia is the most common cause in children.
- High-flow priapism (non-ischemic):
  - Rare.
  - Secondary to arterial laceration with uncontrolled inflow of oxygenated arterial blood.
  - Ischemia and erectile dysfunction are uncommon sequelae.

Clinical Features

- Prolonged tumescence of the penis in absence of sexual arousal.
- May be associated with or without pain depending on etiology of priapism.

Diagnosis

- Based on history and physical examination
- Laboratory tests:
- Intracavernosal blood gas analysis may help differentiate ischemic versus non ischemic etiologies.
- Imaging studies:
- Duplex ultrasound (if available) may help differentiate ischemic versus non ischemic etiologies.

Management

- Initial management:
  - Pain control with analgesics.
  - IV fluids.
  - Evaluate and monitor for urinary retention.
  - Evaluation for specific etiologies (e.g., laboratory evaluation for SCD).
- Regional anesthesia:
  - Pudendal nerve block.
  - Penile ring block.
- Intracavernosal aspiration and irrigation:

- Corpus cavernosum is drained using butterfly or hollow bore needle placed laterally at the 2- or 10-o'clock position at a 45-degree angle.
- Avoid dorsal neurovascular bundle and ventral urethra.
- 3–5 ml aliquots of blood should be removed until bright red blood returns.
- Do not exceed 10% of blood volume.
- Aspiration bilaterally is unnecessary as the corpus cavernosa are connected by shunts.
- Follow with irrigation with warm saline.
- Intracorporal injection of alpha-adrenergic agonist:
  - If refractory to aspiration/irrigation or recurrence of tumescence.
  - Place on cardiac monitor with frequent assessment of blood pressure.
  - Phenylephrine (in boys aged ≥11 years).
    - Diluted to a final concentration of 100 µg/ml and injected in 1 ml aliquots every 5–10 minutes in the corpus cavernosum (up to 10 times).
  - Epinephrine (in boys aged <10 years):
    - Diluted to a final concentration of 1 µg/ml and injected in 10 ml aliquots if over the age of two years, and in 2.5–5 ml aliquots if under age of two years, every 10 minutes (up to four times).
- Wrap elastic bandage around penis once detumescence is achieved.
- Consider exchange transfusion (red blood cell apheresis) if priapism secondary to SCD and refractory to surgical and medical management.

Debriefing Plan

Plan for approximately 30 minutes for discussion.

Potential Questions for Discussion

- What is the approach to priapism in a pediatric patient with SCD?
- Why is priapism a time-sensitive and critical diagnosis?
- What are the key features of informed consent for this intracavernosal aspiration and intracorporal injection?
- What are the steps of performing a penile ring block or pudendal nerve block?
- What are the steps of intracavernosal aspiration and irrigation?
- What further treatment for priapism should be considered in patients with SCD who are refractory to initial management?

REFERENCES FOR PEDIATRIC PRIAPISM

1. Eyre, A. and Dobiesz, V. (2021). Design and implementation of a low-cost priapism reduction task trainer. *J. Educ. Teach. Emerg. Med.* 6(1) https://doi.org/10.21980/J8K64F.

2. Donaldson, J.F., Rees, R.W., and Steinbrecker, H.A. (2014). Priapism in children: a comprehensive review and clinical guideline. *J. Pediatr. Urol.* 10 (1): 11–24.

SELECTED READING FOR PEDIATRIC PRIAPISM

Miller, S.T., Rao, S.P., Dunn, E.K., and Glassberg, K.I. (1995). Priapism in children with sickle cell disease. *J. Urol.* 154: 844–847.

Ramos-Fernandez, M.R., Medero-Colon, R., and Mendez-Carreno, L. (2013). Critical urologic skills and procedures in the emergency department. *Emerg. Med. Clin. North Am.* 31: 237–260.

APPENDIX

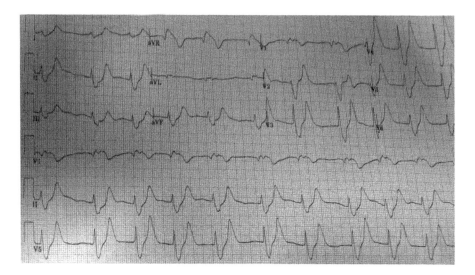

FIGURE 12.1 Electrocardiogram demonstrating peaked T waves of hyperkalemia.

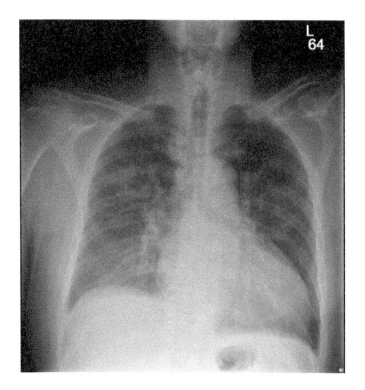

FIGURE 12.2 Chest x-ray demonstrating mild pulmonary edema.

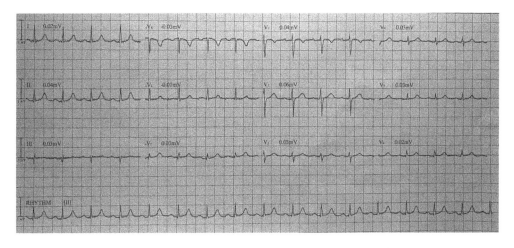

FIGURE 12.3 Normalized electrocardiogram demonstrating resolution of peaked T waves.

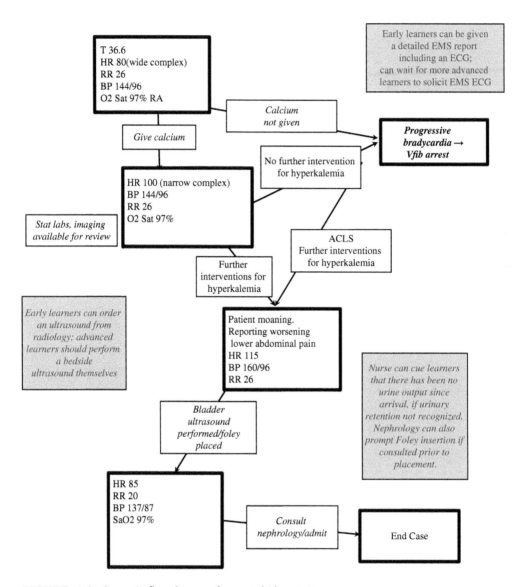

FIGURE 12.4　Scenario flow diagram for acute kidney injury.

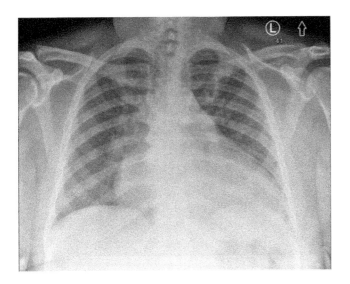

FIGURE 12.5 Chest x-ray (normal).

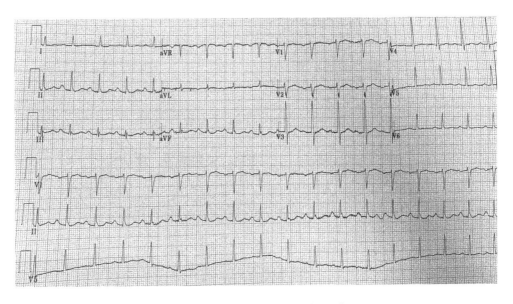

FIGURE 12.6 Electrocardiogram demonstrating sinus tachycardia.

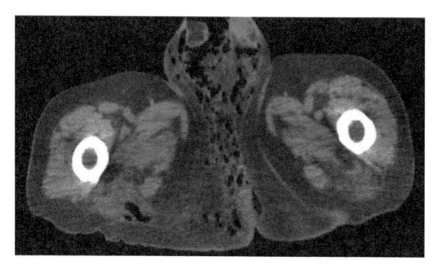

FIGURE 12.7   Computed tomography of the abdomen/pelvis demonstrating scrotal and perineal subcutaneous air.

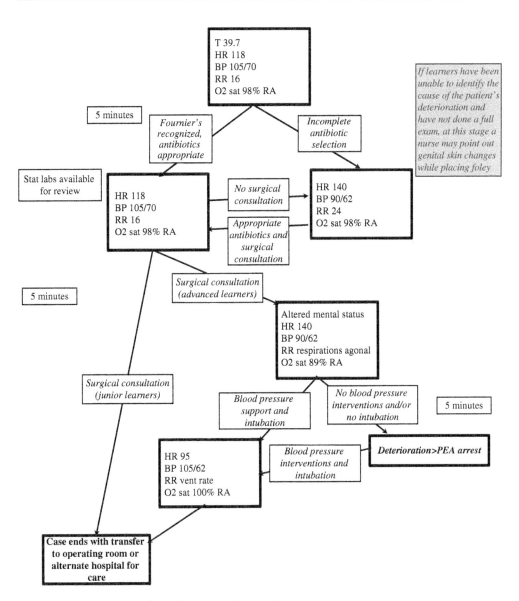

FIGURE 12.8 Scenario flow diagram for Fournier's gangrene.

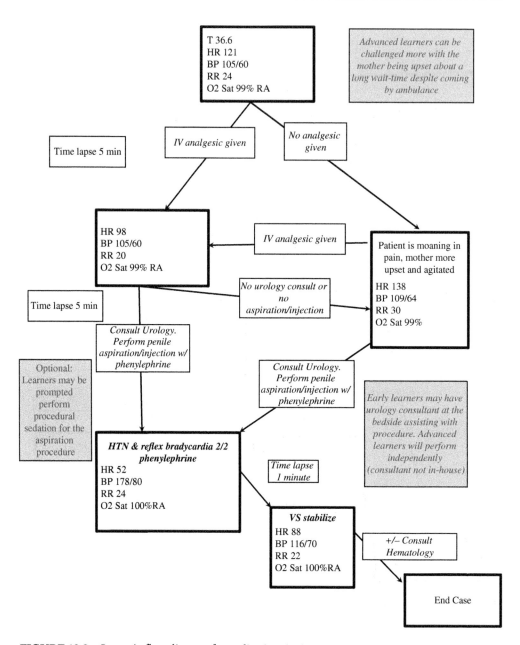

FIGURE 12.9   Scenario flow diagram for pediatric priapism.

TABLE 12.1 Complete blood count.

Test	Value	Reference range
White blood cells (k/µl)	6.3	4.5–11.5
Hemoglobin (g/dl)	10.2	14.0–18.0
Hematocrit (%)	27.4	40–54
Platelets (k/µl)	364	150–450

TABLE 12.2 Complete metabolic panel.

Test	Value	Reference range
Sodium (mmol/l)	132	135–145
Potassium (mmol/l)	8.1	3.5–5.1
Chloride (mmol/l)	101	98–106
CO_2 (mmol/l)	16	24–31
Glucose (mg/dl)	99	70–110
Blood urea nitrogen (mg/dl)	24	10–20
Creatinine (mg/dl)	3.6	0.7–1.3
Total protein (g/dl)	9.2	5.6–8.4
Albumin (g/dl)	3.9	3.4–5.4
Aspartate aminotransferase (iu/l)	23	0–35
Alanine transaminase (iu/l)	17	0–35
Total bilirubin (mg/dl)	0.8	0.3–1.2
Alkaline phosphatase (iu/l)	80	25–115

TABLE 12.3 Lactate.

Test	Value	Reference range
Lactate (mmol/l)	2.6	0.6–1.8

TABLE 12.4 Troponin.

Test	Value	Reference range
Troponin (ng/ml)	0.04	0–0.04

TABLE 12.5 Fingerstick glucose.

Test	Value	Reference range
Fingerstick glucose (mg/dl)	93	70–110

TABLE 12.6 Venous blood gas.

Test	Value	Reference range
pH	7.29	7.31–7.41
pCO_2 (mmHg)	33	41–51
Bicarbonate (mmol/l)	16	23–29
pO_2 (mmHg)	32	30–40

TABLE 12.7 Complete blood count.

Test	Value	Reference range
White blood cells (k/μl)	18.3	4.5–11.5
Hemoglobin (g/dl)	11.2	14.0–18.0
Hematocrit (%)	28.4	40–54
Platelets (k/μl)	231	150–450

TABLE 12.8 Complete metabolic panel.

Test	Value	Reference range
Sodium (mmol/l)	124	135–145
Potassium (mmol/l)	5.1	3.5–5.1
Chloride (mmol/l)	101	98–106
CO_2 (mmol/l)	19	24–31
Glucose (mg/dl)	541	70–110
Blood urea nitrogen (mg/dl)	24	10–20
Creatinine (mg/dl)	2.2	0.7–1.3
Total protein (g/dl)	9.2	5.6–8.4
Albumin (g/dl)	3.9	3.4–5.4
Aspartate aminotransferase (iu/l)	24	0–35

TABLE 12.8   (Continued)

Test	Value	Reference range
Alanine transaminase (iu/l)	13	0–35
Total bilirubin (mg/dl)	0.9	0.3–1.2
Alkaline phosphatase (iu/l)	84	25–115

TABLE 12.9   Lactate level.

Test	Value	Reference range
Lactate (mmol/l)	4.6	0.6–1.8

TABLE 12.10   C-reactive protein.

Test	Value	Reference range
C-reactive protein (mg/l)	3.9	0.0–1.0

TABLE 12.11   Troponin.

Test	Value	Reference range
Troponin (ng/ml)	< 0.02	0–0.04

TABLE 12.12   Venous blood gas.

Test	Value	Reference range
pH	7.18	7.31–7.41
pCO_2 (mmHg)	40	41–51
Bicarbonate (mmol/l)	14	23–29
pO_2 (mmHg)	32	30–40

TABLE 12.13 Components of laboratory risk indicator for necrotizing fasciitis score.

Test	Value	Score
C-reactive protein (mg/dl)	< 15	0
	≥ 15	4
White blood cell count (× 10,000/μl)	<15	0
	15–25	1
	25	2
Hemoglobin (g/dl)	> 13.5	0
	11–13.5	1
	< 11	2
Sodium (mEq/l)	≥ 135	02
	< 135	
Creatinine (mg/dl)	≤ 1.6	0
	> 1.6	2
Glucose (mg/dl)	≤ 180	0
	> 180	1

TABLE 12.14 Complete blood count.

Test	Value	Reference range
White blood cells (k/μl)	4.3	4.5–11.5
Hemoglobin (g/dl)	7.2	14.0–18.0
Hematocrit (%)	21.4	40–54
Platelets (k/μl)	101	150–450

TABLE 12.15   Complete metabolic panel.

Test	Value	Reference range
Sodium (mmol/l)	141	135–145
Potassium (mmol/l)	4.1	3.5–5.1
Chloride (mmol/l)	101	98–106
CO_2 (mmol/l)	21	24–31
Glucose (mg/dl)	108	70–110
Blood urea nitrogen (mg/dl)	9	10–20
Creatinine (mg/dl)	0.9	0.7–1.3
Total protein (g/dl)	7.2	5.6–8.4
Albumin (g/dl)	3.6	3.4–5.4
Aspartate aminotransferase (iu/l)	22	0–35
Alanine transaminase (iu/l)	15	0–35
Total bilirubin (mg/dl)	2.1	0.3–1.2
Alkaline phosphatase (iu/l)	81	25–115

TABLE 12.16   Reticulocytes.

Test	Value	Reference range
Reticulocytes (%)	6.8	0.5–1.5

TABLE 12.17   Corporal blood gas.

Test	Value	Reference range
pH	7.18	7.31–7.41
pCO_2 (mmHg)	68	41–51
Bicarbonate (mmol/l)	20	23–29
pO_2 (mmHg)	18	30–40

CHAPTER 13

Thoracic and Respiratory Emergencies

Michael Billet

Department of Emergency Medicine, University of Maryland, Baltimore, MD, USA

CHRONIC OBSTRUCTIVE PULMONARY DISEASE

Educational Goals

Learning Objectives

1. Recognize exam findings and historical features suggesting acute exacerbation of chronic obstructive pulmonary disease (COPD) (MK, PC).
2. Demonstrate knowledge of pharmacologic agents to treat exacerbation of COPD (MK, PC).
3. Identify and manage respiratory decompensation caused by acute exacerbation of COPD (PC).
4. Demonstrate knowledge of preferred agents for intubation in the setting of acute exacerbation of COPD (MK, PC).

Critical Actions Checklist

☐ Place the patient on continuous pulse oximetry and cardiac monitoring (PC).
☐ Treat hypoxemia with supplemental oxygen (PC).

Emergency Medicine Simulation Workbook: A Tool for Bringing the Curriculum to Life,
Second Edition. Edited by Traci L. Thoureen and Sara B. Scott.
© 2022 John Wiley & Sons Ltd. Published 2022 by John Wiley & Sons Ltd.
Companion website: www.wiley.com/go/thoureen/simulation/workbook2e

☐ Initiate bronchodilator therapy with an inhaled beta agonist and anticholinergic agent (PC, MK).

☐ Initiate parenteral steroid therapy (PC, MK).

☐ Initiate non-invasive positive pressure ventilation (NIPPV) or endotracheal intubation for respiratory decompensation (PC).

☐ Consult critical care specialist and admit to medical intensive care (SBP, ICS).

> Critical actions can be changed to address the educational needs of the learner. For example, in the prehospital setting, choice of pharmacotherapy may be limited by local emergency medical services (EMS) protocols or available resources.

Simulation Set-Up

Environment: Emergency department (ED)/resuscitation area. May also start on scene and transition to a hospital setting.

Mannequin: Male or female simulator mannequin, moulaged to appear elderly, in hospital bed, wearing a hospital gown. Intravenous (IV) access can be present or absent depending on the needs of the learners.

Props: To be displayed on screen or given as handouts when asked for/returned from laboratory:

- Images (see online component for exacerbation of COPD, Scenario 13.1 at https://www.wiley.com/go/thoureen/simulation/workbook2e)
  - Electrocardiogram (ECG) showing sinus tachycardia (Figure 13.1).
  - Chest x-ray showing no acute findings (Figure 13.2)
  - Post-intubation x-ray showing appropriate endotracheal tube placement (Figure 13.3).
- Laboratory tests (see online component as above):
  - Complete blood count (Table 13.1)
  - Basic metabolic panel (Table 13.2)
  - Arterial blood gas (Table 13.3)
  - Troponin (Table 13.4)
  - B-type natriuretic peptide (Table 13.5).

Available supplies:

- Basic airway equipment, including equipment for intubation.
- Code cart.
- Non-invasive positive pressure device (e.g., continuous/bi-level positive airway pressure (CPAP/BiPAP) mask, high-flow nasal cannula).

- Nebulizer delivery device.
- Medications:
  - Liter bags of 0.9% and lactated Ringer's solution (LR).
  - Pre-labeled syringes:
    - Methylprednisolone or dexamethasone.
    - Rapid sequence intubation (RSI) medication (paralytic and induction medication of choice for your institution).
- Optional: Fiberoptic/video-assisted laryngoscope.

Distractor: None.

Actors

- EMS may be an actor or another learner, if a prehospital component is part of the scenario.
- If the scenario begins on scene, an actor can portray the patient's family and provide a limited history of present illness and medical history.
- Patient voice can be male or female. Patient can interact with learners but should be sleepy throughout the interaction and should provide only minimal history.
- ED nurse can administer medications or start respiratory therapies. The nurse can cue learners if needed.
- Intensivist, available via telephone.

Case Narrative

Scenario Background

A 70 year-old patient brought in by EMS from home for three days of worsening dyspnea. Patient has a history of COPD and his family has noted increased cough and sputum production. They have been minimally responsive to home bronchodilator therapy.

Chief complaint: Shortness of breath.
Patient's medical history: Hypertension, type 2 diabetes, COPD.
Medications: Lisinopril, metformin, albuterol metered-dose inhaler.
Allergies: No known drug allergies.
Family history: Non-contributory.
Social history: Prior tobacco use.

Initial Scenario Conditions

Older patient sitting-up in hospital bed or stretcher with significant respiratory distress.

> Case may start with EMS receiving this case on scene as presented and performing their objectives to initiate treatment and transport, including initial assessment and treatment of the patient. Alternatively, case background may be presented prior to case as an EMS medical consult or by EMS on arrival.

Vital signs: Temp 98.8°F (37.1°C), HR 110, BP 140/70, RR 30, SpO$_2$ 84% on room air.
Head: Normocephalic and atraumatic.
Eyes: Half-open, pupils 4mm and reactive to light.
Heart: Tachycardic, regular, distal pulses normal.
Lungs: Tachypneic, shallow respirations, coarse breath sounds with wheezing. Not able to complete full sentences.
Abdomen: Normal bowel sounds.
Extremities: No gross deformities, no edema.
Neurologic: Oriented to self and basic situation, drowsy with decreased responsiveness.

See flow diagram (Figure 13.4) for further scenario changes described.

Case Narrative, Continued

Learners of all levels should attempt to obtain a history from the patient, EMS and the patient's family, establish IV access, administer supplemental oxygen to correct hypoxemia, and start treatment with inhaled bronchodilators. Oxygen and bronchodilators will improve vitals, but will not significantly improve work of breathing or mental status. Learners will need to recognize this and respond with NIPPV or intubation.

In addition to management, workup should confirm diagnosis and exclude alternate cardiopulmonary processes. Failure to address respiratory distress in a timely manner will lead to decompensation.

For advanced learners, the need for intubation is built into the case. This can provide an opportunity to address pre-oxygenation and ventilator management, both of which are affected by the pathophysiology of COPD. Specifically, patients should be aggressively preoxygenated, and ventilator settings should be tailored to avoid barotrauma. Although steroids and antibiotics will not acutely reverse symptoms, they should be administered as early as possible.

The case ends when the patient is stabilized and has been hospitalized to an intensive care setting.

Instructor Notes

Pathophysiology

- Chronic, progressive inflammation leads to decreased elasticity of lung tissue and obstruction, impairing the ability to completely exhale.

Clinical Features

- Acute exacerbations characterized by worsening dyspnea and cough with increased sputum production.
- Can be caused by infection, pollution/smoke exposure, changing weather, or due to another cardiopulmonary process.
- Signs may include:
  - Wheezing.
  - Increased work of breathing.
  - Accessory muscle use.
  - Pursed-lip breathing.
- Impaired oxygenation and ventilation can lead to altered mental status and respiratory depression.

Diagnosis

- Primarily clinical.
- Targeted workup to rule out alternate cardiopulmonary process (e.g., ECG, chest x-ray).
- Blood gas to identify hypercapnia and quantify severity.

Management

- Airway/Breathing
  - Supplemental oxygen to keep SpO_2 88–92%:
    - Risk of decreasing respiratory drive in hypoxia-sensitive patients [1].
  - NIPPV preferred to intubation, unless specifically contraindicated.
  - Intubation carries a high mortality with COPD:
    - Baseline hypercapnia leads to acidosis with even brief interruption in breathing (i.e., RSI).
    - Impaired clearing of secretions while intubated.
    - If intubation is necessary, use NIPPV to preoxygenate/hyperventilate before intubation.
- Medications:
  - Inhaled bronchodilators:
    - Albuterol (repeat as needed).
    - Can also be administered through compatible NIPPV device or ventilator.
    - Ipratropium.
  - Steroids
    - Prednisone 60 mg orally, dexamethasone 10 mg IV, and methylprednisolone 50 mg IV are roughly equivalent in terms of potency.
    - Methylprednisolone 125 mg is often given due to convenience and availability; however, this dose is more than double what is needed and may lead to adverse effects [2].

- Effects not seen until hours or days later.
- Antibiotics:
  - Azithromycin has been shown to have a mortality benefit for inpatients hospitalized for COPD [3].
  - Additional antibiotics may be needed if pneumonia or other acute infection is present.
- Other agents:
  - Magnesium, epinephrine, and methylxanthines have little to no benefit in COPD, unlike with asthma exacerbation [4].

Debriefing Plan

Plan for around 15 minutes for discussion.

Potential Questions for Discussion

- What exam findings can help differentiate COPD from other cardiopulmonary emergencies?
- What are some key differences between COPD and asthma?
- What are options for steroids? What if the patient is able/unable to take oral medications?
- Are antibiotics useful even in exacerbations without any other signs of infection?

REFERENCES FOR CHRONIC OBSTRUCTIVE PULMONARY DISEASE

1 Brill, S.E. and Wedzicha, J.A. (2014). Oxygen therapy in acute exacerbations of chronic obstructive pulmonary disease. *Int. J. Chron. Obstruct. Pulmon. Dis.* 9: 1241–1252.

2 Woods, J.A., Wheeler, J.S., Finch, C.K., and Pinner, N.A. (2014). Corticosteroids in the treatment of acute exacerbations of chronic obstructive pulmonary disease. *Int. J. Chron. Obstruct. Pulmon. Dis.* 9: 421–430.

3 Vermeersch, K., Gabrovska, M., Aumann, J. et al. (2019). Azithromycin during acute chronic obstructive pulmonary disease exacerbations requiring hospitalization (BACE): a multicenter, randomized, double-blind, placebo-controlled trial. *Am. J. Respir. Crit. Care Med.* 200 (7): 857–868.

4 Barr, R.G., Rowe, B.H., and Camargo, C.A. (2003). Methylxanthines for exacerbations of chronic obstructive pulmonary disease. *Cochrane Database Syst. Rev.* (2): CD002168.

SELECTED READING FOR CHRONIC OBSTRUCTIVE PULMONARY DISEASE

Ko, F.W., Chan, K.P., Hui, D.S. et al. (2016). Acute exacerbation of COPD. *Respirology.* 21 (7): 1152–1165.

ACUTE RESPIRATORY DISTRESS SYNDROME

Educational Goals

Learning Objectives

1. Recognize exam findings, vital sign abnormalities, and historical features suggesting acute respiratory distress syndrome (ARDS) (MK, PC).
2. Demonstrate knowledge of the pathophysiology of ARDS (MK, PC).
3. Manage ARDS, with a focus on ventilator management (PC).
4. Demonstrate appropriate consultation with intensivist (PC, ICS).

Critical Actions Checklist

☐ Place the patient on continuous pulse oximetry and cardiac monitoring (PC).
☐ Treat hypoxemia with supplemental oxygen (PC).
☐ Rapidly initiate NIPPV for respiratory distress (PC).
☐ Initiate lung-protective ventilator settings (PC).
☐ Admit the patient to the intensive care unit (ICU) (SBP).

Simulation Set-Up

Environment: ED/resuscitation area.

Mannequin: Male simulator mannequin, seated upright in hospital bed, wearing gown. IV access can be present or absent depending on the needs of learners.

Props: To be displayed on screen or given as handouts when asked for/returned from the laboratory:

- Images (see online component for ARDS, Scenario 13.2 https://www.wiley.com/go/thoureen/simulation/workbook2e)
  - Cardiac ultrasound showing normal ejection fraction (Video 13.1).
  - Thoracic ultrasound showing B-lines in multiple lung fields (Video 13.2).
  - ECG showing sinus tachycardia (Figure 13.1).
  - Chest x-ray showing diffuse ground glass opacities and interstitial edema (Figure 13.5).
  - Post-intubation x-ray showing appropriate endotracheal tube placement (Figure 13.6).
- Laboratory tests (see online component as above):
  - Complete blood count (Table 13.6).
  - Basic metabolic panel (Table 13.7).

- Troponin (Table 13.8).
- B-type natriuretic peptides (Table 13.9).
- Arterial blood gas (Table 13.10).

Available Supplies

- Basic airway equipment, including equipment for intubation.
- Code cart.
- Non-invasive positive pressure device (e.g., CPAP/BiPAP mask, high-flow nasal cannula).
- Medications:
  - Pre-labeled syringes:
    - Antibiotics (e.g., ceftriaxone, vancomycin, piperacillin-tazobactam).
    - Furosemide.
    - RSI medication (paralytic and induction medication of choice for your institution).
- Fiberoptic/video assisted laryngoscope, cricothyroidotomy tray (optional).

Distractor: None.

Actors

- EMS provides handoff and history that was obtained from the family on scene.
- Patient is obtunded and does not provide any history.
- ED nurse can administer medications or start respiratory therapies. The nurse can cue learners if needed.
- Intensivist available via telephone but should provide limited insight into management.

Case Narrative

Scenario Background

A 55 year-old man is brought in by EMS from home for one week of flu-like illness, subjective fevers, and general malaise. Reportedly, the family stated that he has been complaining of worsening dyspnea for the past day, which acutely worsened in the hours prior to arrival. Prehospital vitals notable for hypoxia despite supplemental oxygen.

Chief complaint: fever, weakness.
Patient's medical history: Diabetes, hypertension.
Medications: Lisinopril, metformin.
Allergies: No known drug allergies.
Family history: Unable to obtain.
Social history: Unable to obtain.

Initial Scenario Conditions

Adult patient in hospital bed or stretcher.
Vital signs: Temp 99.9 °F (37.7 °C), HR 110, RR 30, BP 150/90, SpO$_2$ 66% on room air.
Head: Normocephalic and atraumatic
Eyes: Half-open, pupils 4 mm and reactive to light
Heart: Tachycardic and regular, normal distal pulses. No jugular vein disten-
              sion (if asked).
Lungs: Tachypneic, shallow respirations, crackles in all fields.
Abdomen: Normal bowel sounds.
Extremities: No gross deformities. No leg edema (if asked).
Neurologic: Unable to answer orientation questions, not interactive with exam or
              questioning.
Skin: Diaphoretic.

See flow diagram (Figure 13.7) for further scenario changes described.

Case Narrative, Continued

Learners of all levels should perform an examination with attention given to pulmonary auscultation and assessment of mental status. All learners should rapidly establish IV access and administer supplemental oxygen at the highest available rate to correct hypoxemia.

As soon as the diagnosis is suspected, aggressive management should be initiated to correct the patient's respiratory failure. NIPPV may be used to optimize respiratory status, but intubation will be required due to altered mental status and refractory hypoxia. If intubation is attempted prior to correction of hypoxia, the patient will have a pulseless electrical activity arrest.

In addition to management, workup should attempt to confirm the diagnosis, assess for a cause of ARDS, and exclude alternate cardiopulmonary processes. Labs will not be available in the initial period of stabilization and learners should not wait for results (e.g., arterial blood gases) to initiate treatment.

The case ends when the patient has been intubated with appropriate ventilator settings and has been admitted to the ICU.

Instructor Notes

Pathophysiology

- Inflammation leads to vascular permeability in the lungs, causing decreased lung compliance, impaired gas exchange, ventilation/perfusion mismatch, and ultimately respiratory failure.
- Underlying inflammation can be caused by sepsis, trauma, pancreatitis, aspiration, pneumonitis, or any process leading to an excessive inflammatory response.

Clinical Features

- Typical signs include tachypnea, profoundly/persistently hypoxia, and respiratory distress.
- Shares clinical features with pulmonary infections and left-sided heart failure, although patients will usually be euvolemic.
- Mortality is high (30–50%) even with aggressive management [1].

Diagnosis

- Bilateral opacities on chest imaging, plus acute respiratory failure, plus PaO_2/FiO_2 less than 300 mmHg.
- Must not be explained by heart failure or fluid overload [2].

Management

- Airway/breathing:
  - NIPPV can be used to optimize the patient's oxygenation, but intubation will be required in ARDS.
  - Intubation should be done by the most experienced provider with pre-oxygenation and apneic oxygenation:
  - Ventilator settings should be "lung protective"
    - Low tidal volumes (6–8 ml/kg of ideal body weight).
    - Hypercapnia may be unavoidable.
    - Minimum positive end-expiratory pressure (PEEP) of 5 cm H_2O.
    - Titrate PEEP and FiO_2 to pulse oximetry or blood gas analysis.
    - Plateau pressures less than 30 cm water to avoid barotrauma.
  - Placing the patient in the prone position while intubated shows benefit:
    - Thought to improve oxygenation by shifting blood to areas with less atelectasis.
    - Cumbersome and requires multiple experienced providers (physician, nursing, and respiratory therapist).

- Medications:
  - Avoid aggressive fluid resuscitation.
  - Supportive care and treatment of the underlying cause.
  - Diuretics may be useful if volume overloaded.
  - Anti-inflammatory medications (e.g., steroids, vitamin C) and therapies intended to improve lung compliance (e.g., surfactants, N-acetylcysteine) have not been shown to improve mortality rate or time on a ventilator [3].

Debriefing Plan

Plan for approximately 20 minutes for discussion.

Potential Questions for Discussion

- What are potential precipitants for ARDS?
- How do you distinguish ARDS from pulmonary infections and cardiogenic pulmonary edema?
- What preparations should be made prior to intubating a hypoxic patient with ARDS?
- In a patient with ARDS due to sepsis, how should fluid resuscitation be approached?

REFERENCES FOR ACUTE RESPIRATORY DISTRESS SYNDROME

1 Fan, E., Brodie, D., and Slutsky, A.S. (2018). Acute respiratory distress syndrome: advances in diagnosis and treatment. *JAMA*. 319 (7): 698–710.
2 Ranieri, V.M., Rubenfeld, G.D., Thompson, B.T. et al. (2012). Acute respiratory distress syndrome: the Berlin definition. *JAMA*. 307 (23): 2526–2533.
3 Lewis, S.R., Pritchard, M.W., Thomas, C.M., and Smith, A.F. (2019). Pharmacological agents for adults with acute respiratory distress syndrome. *Cochrane Database Syst. Rev.* 7: CD004477.

EPIGLOTTITIS

Educational Goals

Learning Objectives

1. Recognize exam findings and historical features suggesting epiglottitis in a child (MK, PC).
2. Demonstrate appropriate preparation for deterioration in a patient with epiglottitis (PC, PBLI).
3. Perform advanced airway control in a pediatric patient (MK, PC).
4. Demonstrate effective team-based communication skills (ICS).

Critical Actions Checklist

☐ Diagnose epiglottitis (MK).
☐ Consult otolaryngology/anesthesia for difficult airway management (PC, SBP).
☐ Prepare for a difficult airway (PC).
☐ Communicate the need to avoid unnecessary agitation or excessive examination with other care team members (PC, ICS).
☐ Admit or transfer to pediatric intensive care (PC, SBP).

Simulation Set-Up

Environment: ED/resuscitation area.

Mannequin: Female, elementary-aged, simulator mannequin, in hospital bed wearing gown. No IV access.

Props: To be displayed on screen or given as handouts when asked for/returned from laboratory:
- Images (see online component for epiglottitis, Scenario 13.3 at https://www.wiley.com/go/thoureen/simulation/workbook2e):
- Lateral neck x-ray showing epiglottitis/thumbprint sign (Figure 13.8).
- Chest x-ray (normal) (Figure 13.9).
- Post-intubation chest x-ray showing appropriate endotracheal tube placement (Figure 13.10).

Available supplies:

- Pediatric code cart and basic airway supplies.
- Nebulizer mask.
- Medications:
  - Liter bags of 0.9% saline and LR.
  - Pre-labeled syringes:
    - Dexamethasone 4 mg vial.
    - RSI medication (paralytic and induction medication of choice for your institution).
- Fiberoptic/video assisted laryngoscope, cricothyroidotomy tray, transtracheal jet ventilation supplies (14 g angiocatheter, oxygen tubing, 3-0 endotracheal tube adapter), and supraglottic airway device (optional).

Distractor: Parent can be present to provide history, and should be concerned about their child's condition, emphasizing that she is not acting normally. They should be hesitant to let the learner examine the child, requiring reassurance and demonstration of interpersonal skills.

Actors

- Parent gives medical history; can be available over the phone if an additional actor is unavailable.
- Patient groans and has stridor, but does not speak. If the learner attempts to do an exam of oropharynx, the patient will start coughing violently causing desaturation.
- ED nurse can administer medications or start respiratory therapies. The nurse can cue learners if needed.
- Anesthesiologist or otolaryngologist available via telephone.

Case Narrative

Scenario Background

A six-year-old girl is brought in by a parent for trouble with breathing. Symptoms started this morning as malaise, headache, and a non-productive cough, and have gotten worse throughout the day. Parent became concerned as the child is no longer drinking fluids. If asked, siblings have had flu-like illness for the past several days

Chief complaint: Difficulty breathing.

Patient's medical history: No chronic medical issues. Born at full term. Has not received any childhood vaccines (only offer this information if prompted).

Medications: None.

Allergies:	No known drug allergies.
Family history:	Non-contributory.
Social history:	Lives at home with both parents and two younger siblings.

Initial Scenario Conditions

Pediatric patient seated upright/leaning forward in hospital bed or stretcher.

Vital signs:	Temp 102.4°F (39.1°C), HR 130, RR 30, BP 90/60, SpO$_2$ 96% on room air.
Head:	Normocephalic and atraumatic.
Eyes:	Half-open, pupils 5 mm and reactive to light.
Neck:	Stridor.
Heart:	Tachycardic and regular, no abnormal sounds, no central or peripheral cyanosis.
Lungs:	Tachypneic, shallow respirations. Increased work of breathing if asked.
Abdomen:	Normal bowel sounds.
Extremities:	No gross deformities.
Neurologic:	Groans with questioning, minimally interacts with exam.
Skin:	Pale and clammy.

See flow diagram (Figure 13.11) for further scenario changes described.

Case Narrative, Continued

Stridor should be recognized early and the diagnosis of epiglottitis should be verbalized (nurse, parent, or consultant can prompt this if needed). As this child is in respiratory distress, care should be taken to keep the child comfortable and avoid painful procedures or invasive examination of the oropharynx. IV access should only be attempted if the need for intubation is imminent, or if the child can remain calm throughout the procedure. Ideally, this would be done by an experienced practitioner (e.g., pediatric nurse), and the parent should be involved to keep the child as calm as possible.

If the learner attempts an oropharynx exam early, the patient will cough and desaturate, dissuading them from the exam. Learners should recognize the need to control a difficult airway and involve anesthesiology, otolaryngology, or both depending on institutional practice patterns. Risks–benefits of controlling the airway in the ED versus transferring to an operative setting will be at the discretion of the learner; this can be prompted by the consultant for an additional level of complexity. In either case, learners should remain with the child at all times and have difficult airway supplies available.

For advanced learners, the child can deteriorate, or specialists will not be immediately available, necessitating intubation. "Awake" fiberoptic intubation with minimal sedation is the preferred method. In the event of a failed airway, supraglottic devices will not be effective. Transtracheal jet ventilation can be used as a rescue therapy until specialist assistance is present. The case ends when the airway is controlled, or the child has been transferred to an operating room.

Instructor Notes

Pathophysiology

- Infection causes inflammation of the epiglottis leading to upper airway obstruction and respiratory failure.
- *Staphylococcus* and *Streptococcus* are most common infectious etiologies.
- Prior to vaccination, the most common causative organism was *Haemophilus influenzae* type B.

Clinical Features

- Rapid onset of symptoms progressing from sore throat to stridor and respiratory distress over hours.
- Classically, patient will be seated upright with head held in the "sniffing position."
- May also have symptoms of fever, headache, and general malaise.

Diagnosis

- Clinical diagnosis based on stridor and ill-appearance of children
- Lateral neck x-ray may show a "thumbprint sign" of an edematous epiglottis:
  - Only obtain if the child is more stable or the diagnosis is unclear.
- Direct visualization of the epiglottis is the gold standard:
  - Only attempt with a plan for airway control in place.

Management

- Airway/breathing:
  - Intubation is challenging:
    - Early involvement of anesthesiology, otolaryngology, or both is critical.
    - Preferred method of airway control is "awake" fiberoptic intubation with surgical backup immediately available.
    - Paralytics should only be given once securing the airway is nearly guaranteed, as their use commits you to intubating or a surgical airway.
    - Care must be taken to avoid agitating the child or aggressively examining the airway.
  - Rescue devices:
    - Supraglottic devices will not be able to overcome the obstruction.
    - Cricothyroidotomy is technically difficult and associated with short and long-term complications below age 10–12 years [1].
    - Transtracheal jet ventilation may be useful as a temporizing measure (not a definitive airway).

- Can be improvised by inserting a 14-gauge angiocatheter through the cricothyroid membrane.
  - 3-0 endotracheal tube adapter will insert into the hub of the angiocath and will allow bagging or connection to oxygen tubing.
- Medications:
  - Racemic epinephrine:
    - Evidence is lacking regarding outcomes.
  - Dexamethasone:
    - Evidence for use is limited in children.
    - Reduces length of stay in adults, but adults are also less likely to need intubation in general [2].
  - If IV access is obtained, antibiotics to cover *H. influenzae, Streptococcus pneumoniae*, and *Staphylococcus aureus* (with or without methicillin-resistant *S. aureus* coverage based on illness severity and risk factors).

Debriefing Plan

Plan for approximately 20 minutes for discussion.

Potential Questions for Discussion

- What is the differential diagnosis for a child with stridor?
- What differences exist between the adult and pediatric airway?
- What options for airway management are relatively or absolutely contraindicated in children?
- What resources does your hospital have for a difficult pediatric airway?

REFERENCES FOR EPIGLOTTITIS

1. Black, A.E., Flynn, P.E., Smith, H.L. et al. (2015). Development of a guideline for the management of the unanticipated difficult airway in pediatric practice. *Paediatr. Anaesth.* 25 (4): 346–362.
2. Lichtor, J.L., Roche Rodriguez, M., Aaronson, N.L. et al. (2016). Epiglottitis: it hasn't gone away. *Anesthesiology* 124 (6): 1404–1407.

SELECTED READING FOR EPIGLOTTITIS

Abdallah, C. (2012). Acute epiglottitis: trends, diagnosis and management. *Saudi J. Anaesth.* 6 (3): 279–281.

Video 13.1 Cardiac ultrasound obtained with phased array. No other abnormal findings present in other views.
Video 13.2 Lung ultrasound obtained with curvilinear probe. Similar findings present in all visualized lung fields.

APPENDIX

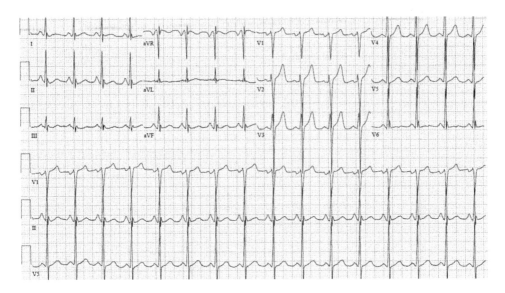

FIGURE 13.1   Electrocardiogram showing sinus tachycardia.

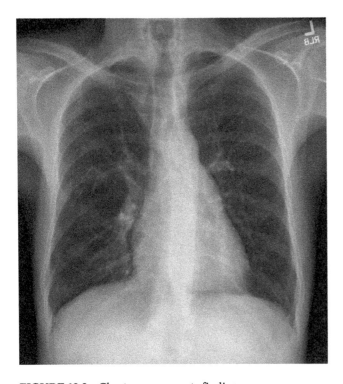

FIGURE 13.2   Chest x-ray, no acute findings.

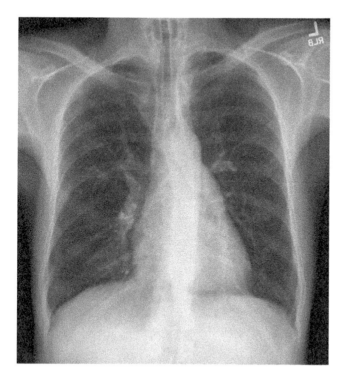

FIGURE 13.3   Post-intubation chest x-ray showing appropriate endotracheal tube placement.

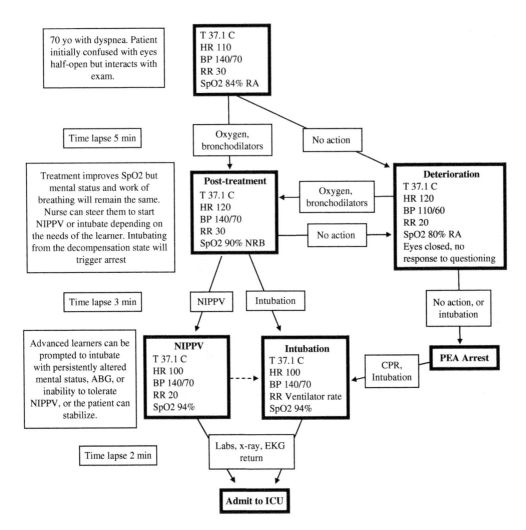

FIGURE 13.4   Flow diagram for chronic obstructive pulmonary disease.

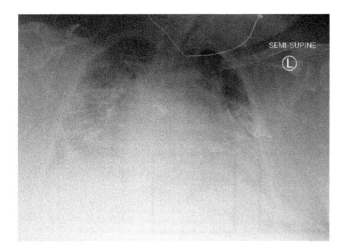

FIGURE 13.5 Chest x-ray, diffuse pulmonary edema.

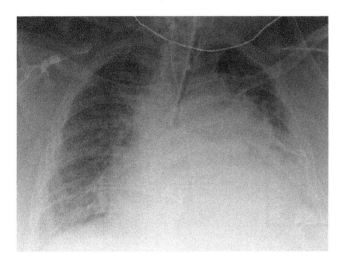

FIGURE 13.6 Post-intubation chest x-ray showing appropriate endotracheal tube placement and improved pulmonary edema.

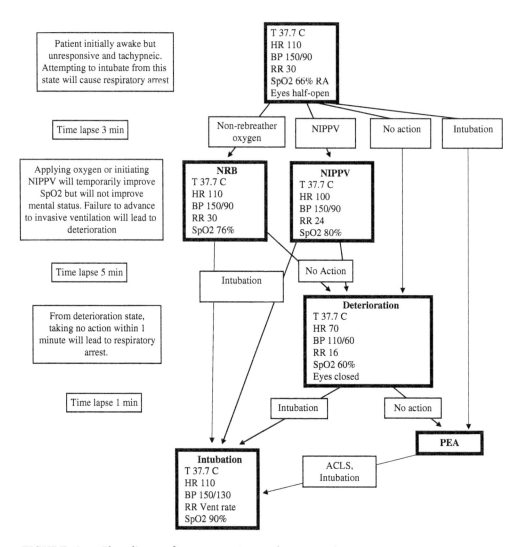

FIGURE 13.7   Flow diagram for acute respiratory distress syndrome.

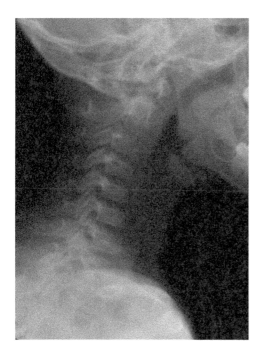

FIGURE 13.8   Lateral neck x-ray showing enlarged epiglottis (thumbprint sign).

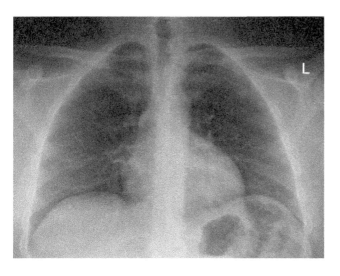

FIGURE 13.9   Chest x-ray, no acute findings.

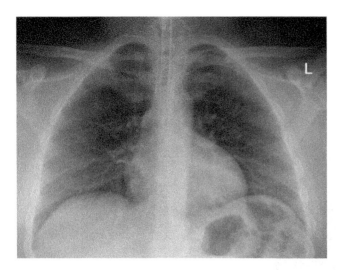

FIGURE 13.10   Post-intubation chest x-ray showing appropriate endotracheal tube placement.

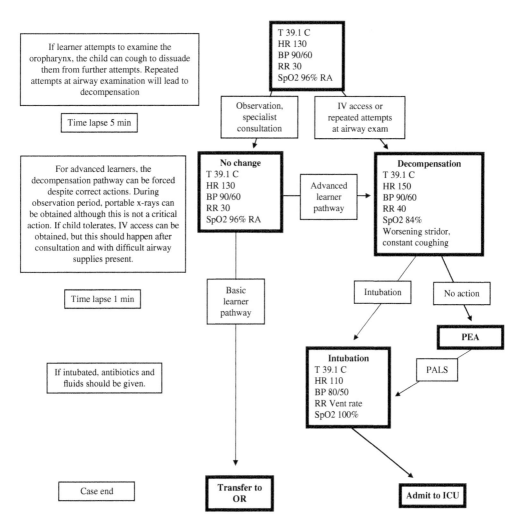

FIGURE 13.11   Flow diagram for epiglottitis.

TABLE 13.1 Complete blood count.

Test	Value	Reference range
White blood cells (k/μl)	5.1	3.5–10.5
Hemoglobin (g/dl)	17.1	12.5–15.5
Hematocrit (%)	51.0	34.9–44.5
Platelets (k/μl)	311	130–400

TABLE 13.2 Basic metabolic panel.

Test	Value	Reference range
Sodium (mmol/l)	140	136–144
Potassium (mmol/l)	4.3	3.7–5.2
Chloride (mmol/l)	106	96–106
CO_2 (mmol/l)	46 (!)	23–29
Blood urea nitrogen (mg/dl)	35	6–20
Creatinine (mg/dl)	1.2	0.8–1.2
Glucose (mg/dl)	151	64–100

TABLE 13.3 Arterial blood gas.

Test	Value	Reference range
pH	7.25 (!)	7.35–7.45
PCO_2 (mmHg)	80 (!)	35–45
Bicarbonate (mmol/l)	44 (!)	22–26
PO_2 (mmHg)	55 (!)	80–100
SpO_2 (%) (calculated)	81 (!)	95–100

TABLE 13.4 Troponin.

Test	Value	Reference range
Troponin (ng/ml)	0.08	< 0.04

TABLE 13.5 B-type natriuretic peptides.

Test	Value	Reference range
B-type natriuretic peptides (pg/ml)	150	< 200

TABLE 13.6   Complete blood count.

Test	Value	Reference range
White blood cells (k/µl)	6.6	3.5–10.5
Hemoglobin (g/dl)	14.2	12.5–15.5
Hematocrit (%)	41.5	34.9–44.5
Platelets (k/µl)	299	130–400

TABLE 13.7   Basic metabolic panel.

Test	Value	Reference range
Sodium (mmol/l)	140	136–144
Potassium (mmol/l)	4.3	3.7–5.2
Chloride (mmol/l)	106	96–106
CO_2 (mmol/l)	31	23–29
Blood urea nitrogen (mg/dl)	51	6–20
Creatinine (mg/dl)	1.4	0.8–1.2
Glucose (mg/dl)	168	64–100

TABLE 13.8   Troponin.

Test	Value	Reference range
Troponin (ng/ml)	0.04	< 0.04

TABLE 13.9   B-type natriuretic peptides.

Test	Value	Reference range
BNP B-type natriuretic peptides (pg/ml)	159	< 200

TABLE 13.10   Arterial blood gas analysis.

Test	Value	Reference range
pH	7.40	7.35–7.45
PCO_2 (mmHg)	35	35–45
Bicarbonate (mmol/l)	28	22–26
PO_2 (mmHg)	**58** (!)	80–100
SpO_2 (%) (calculated)	**64%** (!)	95–100

Bold text = significant result.

CHAPTER 14

Toxicologic Emergencies

Charles Lei, Jeffrey N. Heimiller, and Joseph R. Sikon

Department of Emergency Medicine, Vanderbilt University Medical Center, Nashville, TN, USA

ASPIRIN OVERDOSE

Educational Goals

Learning Objectives

1. Recognize clinical features of aspirin overdose (MK).
2. Demonstrate appropriate treatment of aspirin overdose (MK, PC).
3. Describe indications for hemodialysis in patient with aspirin overdose (MK).
4. Demonstrate proper airway management in patient with aspirin overdose (MK, PC).
5. Demonstrate effective communication skills and professionalism during interactions with Emergency Department (ED) staff and consultants (ICS, P).
6. Direct appropriate disposition of patient (SBP).

Critical Actions Checklist

- ☐ Assess airway, breathing, and circulation (ABC) (PC).
- ☐ Obtain appropriate vascular access (MK, PC).
- ☐ Measure fingerstick glucose and administer dextrose (MK).
- ☐ Perform appropriate fluid resuscitation with crystalloids (MK, PC).
- ☐ Treat hypokalemia (MK, PC).

Emergency Medicine Simulation Workbook: A Tool for Bringing the Curriculum to Life, Second Edition. Edited by Traci L. Thoureen and Sara B. Scott.
© 2022 John Wiley & Sons Ltd. Published 2022 by John Wiley & Sons Ltd.
Companion website: www.wiley.com/go/thoureen/simulation/workbook2e

☐ Initiate urine alkalinization with sodium bicarbonate infusion (MK, PC).
☐ Consult with nephrologist for hemodialysis (MK, ICS, P, SBP).
☐ Communicate with intensive care unit (ICU) for disposition (ICS, P, SBP).

Critical actions can be changed to address learners' educational needs. For example, emergency medical services (*EMS*) learners may be expected to identify evidence of intentional overdose (e.g., empty pill bottles, suicide note).

Simulation Set-Up

Environment: ED treatment area. For EMS learners, the scenario may start on scene and transition to a hospital setting.

Mannequin: Male simulator mannequin on stretcher or hospital bed. Mannequin should be moulaged to show diaphoresis and vomitus on clothing.

Props: To be displayed on screen or distributed on handouts:

- Images (see online component for aspirin overdose, Scenario 14.1 https://www.wiley.com/go/thoureen/simulation/workbook2e):
  - Electrocardiogram showing sinus tachycardia (Figure 14.1).
  - Chest x-ray (normal) (Figure 14.2).
  - Head computed tomography (CT, normal) (Figure 14.3).
- Laboratory tests (see online component as above):
  - Fingerstick glucose (Table 14.1).
  - Complete blood count (Table 14.2).
  - Basic metabolic panel (Table 14.3).
  - Liver function tests (Table 14.4).
  - Lactate (Table 14.5).
  - Arterial blood gases (Table 14.6).
  - Urinalysis (Table 14.7).
  - Urine toxicology screen (Table 14.8).
  - Salicylate level (Table 14.9).
  - Acetaminophen level (Table 14.10).
  - Ethanol level (Table 14.11).

Available supplies:

- Adult airway and code cart.
- Medications:

- Intravenous (IV) fluids in labeled 1l bags: 0.9%, lactated Ringer's solution (LR), 5% dextrose in water (D5W) plus 40 mEq potassium chloride (KCl).
- Pre-labeled syringes:
  - 8.4% sodium bicarbonate.
  - 50% dextrose.
  - Rapid sequence intubation (RSI) medications. Specific induction and paralytic medications typical of your institution.
- Intraosseous (IO) device with insertion trainer.
- Empty aspirin bottle (optional for junior learners).
- Suicide note (optional for junior learners).

Distractor: None.

Actors

- EMS can provide information about the scene. Actor optional if no EMS learner is present.
- Patient is somnolent, confused, not following commands or answering questions, intermittently vomiting.
- Patient's son is available in person or via telephone to provide additional information.
- ED nurse can administer medications, and may cue learners if needed.
- Nephrologist and ICU physician are available via telephone consultation.

Case Narrative

Scenario Background

A 60-year-old man is brought in by EMS from home. Patient's son found him in bed, confused, breathing rapidly, and covered in vomit. According to the son, the patient had been in his usual state of health until today.

Patient's medical history: Hypertension, hyperlipidemia.
Medications: Metoprolol, atorvastatin.
Allergies: None.
Family history: Non-contributory.
Social history: No tobacco, alcohol, or drug use.

Initial Scenario Conditions

Middle-aged man, somnolent, confused, intermittently vomiting.

> Case may start with EMS (learner) receiving this case on scene as presented and performing their objectives to initiate treatment and transport. Alternatively, scenario background may be presented by EMS (actor) on ED arrival.

Vital signs: Temp 102 °F (38.9 °C), HR 115, RR 34, BP 85/50, SpO$_2$ 94% on room air.
Head: Atraumatic.
Eyes: Pupils 2 mm, reactive to light.
Mouth: Airway patent, dry mucous membranes.
Heart: Tachycardic, regular, no murmur, diminished peripheral pulses.
Lungs: Tachypneic, clear breath sounds.
Abdomen: Soft, non-tender, non-distended, normal bowel sounds.
Extremities: No deformities.
Skin: Diaphoretic, delayed capillary refill.
Neurologic: Eyes closed, moaning, arouses to painful stimuli, moving all extremities, confused, not following commands or answering questions.

See flow diagram (Figure 14.4) for further scenario changes described.

Case Narrative, Continued

Learners of all levels should assess ABC. Learners should recognize patient's confusion and vital sign abnormalities. They should measure fingerstick glucose, obtain appropriate vascular access, administer 50% dextrose, and initiate fluid resuscitation. Failure to identify and treat hypoglycemia will lead to the patient having a seizure. Failure to initiate appropriate fluid resuscitation after five minutes will lead to decompensation.

For EMS and postgraduate learners, attempts at IV access will be unsuccessful. Learners should obtain IO access, demonstrating procedure on IO insertion trainer.

> If performance of actual procedure is not a learning objective, then learners can simply verbalize where they would establish IO access.

Following appropriate treatment, the patient will stabilize temporarily. Imaging and laboratory results (except for serum drug levels) can return at this time. Learners should recognize aspirin overdose and initiate bicarbonate infusion. They should correct hypokalemia.

At 10 minutes, if learners have not identified aspirin overdose, the patient's son will inform learners that the patient has been severely depressed due to his wife's recent death. For junior learners, he will provide them with an empty aspirin bottle and patient's suicide note. Serum and urine drug levels will also be available at this time.

For advanced learners, the patient can become more somnolent, tachypneic, and hypoxic. Learners should consider endotracheal intubation in the setting of severe tachypnea and metabolic acidosis. If they attempt intubation before initiating appropriate therapy for aspirin overdose, the patient will develop pulseless electrical activity arrest and case will end.

Case will end after learners have initiated appropriate therapy for aspirin overdose and arranged for hemodialysis and disposition to ICU.

Instructor Notes

Pathophysiology

- Salicylates:
  - Stimulate medullary respiratory center and chemoreceptor trigger zone.
  - Interfere with oxidative phosphorylation.
  - Decrease central nervous system (CNS) glucose concentrations.
  - Cause cerebral edema.
  - Cause hypokalemia.
  - Metabolized by liver, excreted by kidneys.
  - In overdose, metabolic pathways are saturated → elimination depends on pH-sensitive urinary excretion.

Clinical Features

- Initial presentation:
  - Hyperpnea, tachypnea.
  - Tachycardia.
  - Diaphoresis.
  - Nausea, vomiting.
  - Tinnitus.
- As toxicity worsens:
  - Hyperthermia.
  - Confusion, seizures, coma.
  - Pulmonary edema.
  - Cardiovascular collapse.

Diagnosis

- Serum salicylate concentration:
  - May not correlate with symptom severity or degree of toxicity.
  - Nomogram should not be used to predict toxicity or guide therapy.

- Blood gas: primary respiratory alkalosis.
- Metabolic panel:
  - Anion gap metabolic acidosis.
  - Hypokalemia.
  - Hypoglycemia.

Management

- Fluid resuscitation:
  - Initiate aggressive volume repletion with crystalloids unless patient has pulmonary or cerebral edema.
  - Free water deficit may be as high as 4–6 l.
  - Treat fluid-refractory hypotension with vasopressors.
- Hypokalemia:
  - Goal serum potassium level 4.5 mEq/l.
  - Must be corrected before urine alkalinization is possible.
- Urine alkalinization
  - Increases renal elimination of salicylates.
  - Administer 1–2 mEq/kg sodium bicarbonate as IV bolus.
  - Infuse 150 mEq (three 50 ml ampules) sodium bicarbonate in 1 l D5W + 40 mEq KCl at 2–3 ml/kg/hour.
  - Titrate to urine pH of 7.5 to 8.
- Hypoglycemia:
  - In setting of altered mental status, administer dextrose regardless of serum glucose concentration.
- Hemodialysis:
  - Consult with nephrologist early.
  - Indications:
    - Confusion, seizures, coma, cerebral edema.
    - Renal or hepatic failure.
    - Pulmonary edema, respiratory failure.
    - Volume overload preventing adequate bicarbonate administration.
    - Clinical deterioration despite appropriate care.
    - Severe acidosis (e.g., pH < 7.1).
    - Rapidly rising salicylate level.
    - Serum salicylate concentration > 100 mg/dl after acute overdose.
- Airway management:
- Avoid mechanical ventilation unless patient is decompensating:

- Acidemia can acutely worsen during apneic period of intubation (increases CNS toxicity of salicylates).
- Patient's high minute ventilation is difficult to achieve with ventilator.
- If intubation is necessary, maintain high respiratory rate and tidal volume.
- Gastrointestinal decontamination:
  - Consider activated charcoal in alert, cooperative patients or intubated patients.

Debriefing Plan

Plan for around 30 minutes for discussion.

Potential Questions for Discussion

- What is the general approach to a patient with altered mental status?
- What are the clinical features of aspirin overdose?
- What laboratory abnormalities are expected in aspirin overdose?
- Why is urine alkalinization important and how is it accomplished?
- What are the indications for hemodialysis in a patient with aspirin overdose?
- What special considerations should be given to patients who may require intubation?

SELECTED READINGS FOR ASPIRIN OVERDOSE

American College of Medical Toxicology (2015). Guidance document: management priorities in salicylate toxicity. *J. Med. Toxicol.* 11 (1): 149–152.

Hatten, B.W. (2018). Aspirin and nonsteroidal agents. In: *Rosen's Emergency Medicine*, 9e (eds. R.M. Walls, R.S. Hockberger and M. Gausche-Hill), 1858–1862. Philadelphia: Elsevier.

Juurlink, D.N., Gosselin, S., Kielstein, G.M. et al. (2015). Extracorporeal treatment for salicylate poisoning: systematic review and recommendations from the EXTRIP workgroup. *Ann. Emerg. Med.* 66 (2): 165–181.

LITHIUM TOXICITY

Educational Goals

Learning Objectives

1. Demonstrate proper assessment of patient with altered mental status (MK, PC, ICS).
2. Demonstrate appropriate airway management (MK, PC).
3. Demonstrate appropriate resuscitation of patient with undifferentiated shock (MK, PC).
4. Recognize and properly manage lithium toxicity (MK, PC).
5. Describe indications for hemodialysis in patient with lithium toxicity (MK).
6. Demonstrate effective communication skills and professionalism during inter-actions with Emergency Department (ED) staff and consultants (ICS, P).
7. Direct appropriate disposition of the patient (SBP).

Critical Actions Checklist

☐ Obtain appropriate vascular access (MK, PC).
☐ Measure fingerstick glucose or administer empiric dextrose (MK, PC).
☐ Administer intravenous (IV) fluids prior to vasopressors for hypovolemic shock (MK, PC).
☐ Perform endotracheal intubation (MK, PC).
☐ Obtain lithium level and electrocardiogram (ECG) (MK).
☐ Consult with nephrologist for hemodialysis (MK, ICS, P, SBP).
☐ Communicate with intensive care unit (ICU) for disposition (ICS, P, SBP).

Simulation Set-Up

Environment: ED treatment area. For EMS learners, scenario may start on scene and transition to a hospital setting.

Mannequin: Male simulator mannequin, on a stretcher or hospital bed, with emesis on shirt.

Props: To be displayed on screen or distributed on handouts:

- Images (see online component for lithium overdose, Scenario 14.2 https://www.wiley.com/go/thoureen/simulation/workbook2e):
  - ECG showing first degree atrioventricular block and flattened T waves (Figure 14.5).
  - Chest x-ray (normal) (Figure 14.6).

- Post-intubation chest X-ray showing appropriate endotracheal tube position (Figure 14.7).
- Head CT (normal) (Figure 14.8).
- Laboratory tests (see online component as above):
  - Fingerstick glucose (Table 14.12).
  - Complete blood count (Table 14.13).
  - Basic metabolic panel (Table 14.14).
  - Liver function tests (Table 14.15).
  - Lactate (Table 14.16).
  - Lithium level (Table 14.17).
  - Thyroid function tests (Table 14.18).
  - Urinalysis (Table 14.19).
  - Urine toxicology screen (Table 14.20).
  - Salicylate level (Table 14.21).
  - Acetaminophen level (Table 14.22).
  - Ethanol level (Table 14.23).

Available supplies:

- Adult airway and code cart.
- Medications
  - IV fluids in labeled 1 l bags: 0.9% saline, LR.
  - Pre-labeled syringes:
    - 8.4% sodium bicarbonate.
    - RSI medications. Specific induction and paralytic medications typical of your institution.

Distractor: None.

Actors

- EMS can provide information about the scene. Actor optional if no EMS learner is present.
- Patient moans to painful stimuli. Not following commands or answering questions.
- ED nurse can administer medications and may cue learners if needed.
- Nephrologist and ICU physician available via telephone consultation.

Case Narrative

Scenario Background

A 67-year-old man was found semi-conscious by his family. According to family, he has had a "stomach bug" for several days. When he did not answer his phone today, they went to his home and found him confused and covered in vomit.

Patient's medical history: Hypertension, hyperlipidemia, bipolar I disorder, type II diabetes mellitus.

Medications:	Hydrochlorothiazide, metoprolol, amlodipine, metformin, lithium, simvastatin, aspirin.
Allergies:	Penicillin.
Family history:	Non-contributory.
Social historyx:	Occasional ethanol use.

Initial Scenario Conditions

Elderly, disheveled man, moaning to painful stimuli.

> Case may start with EMS (learner) receiving this case on scene as presented and performing their objectives to initiate treatment and transport, including obtaining relevant history from family, assessing medications on scene, and measuring fingerstick glucose. Alternatively, scenario background may be presented by EMS (actor) on ED arrival.

Vital signs:	Temp 96.6 °F (35.6 °C), HR 90, RR 12, BP 70/40, SpO$_2$ 86% on room air.
Head:	Atraumatic.
Eyes:	Pupils 4 mm, reactive to light.
Mouth:	Airway patent, dry mucous membranes
Neck:	Supple, no meningismus.
Heart:	Regular, distal pulses diminished
Lungs:	Clear breath sounds.
Abdomen:	Soft, non-tender, non-distended.
Extremities:	No deformities.
Skin:	Cool, dry, delayed capillary refill, decreased skin turgor.
Neurologic:	Eyes closed, moaning to noxious stimuli, localizing to pain, hyperreflexic in all extremities.

> Physical exam findings not available on your mannequin (e.g., reflexes) can be verbally reported by your nurse, if asked by the leaner.

See flow diagram (Figure 14.9) for further scenario changes described.

Case Narrative, Continued

Learners of all levels should assess ABC, obtain appropriate vascular access, provide supplemental oxygen, and administer IV fluids. They should measure fingerstick glucose and consider empiric dextrose, thiamine, and naloxone administration. If these are administered, there will be no change in patient condition. Learners should recognize the patient's need for intubation and assess for intoxicants with laboratory studies and ECG. They should obtain a head CT and assess for infectious etiologies. Antibiotics may be administered.

For junior learners, EMS may provide the patient's medical history and medication list. For advanced learners, this information may be withheld. If lithium toxicity is not considered by eight minutes, this history may be provided by a family member via telephone. Laboratory results and imaging will be provided at 10 minutes.

Learners should consult with a nephrologist to prepare for hemodialysis. Case will end after learners have arranged for disposition to ICU.

Instructor Notes

Pathophysiology

- Lithium:
  - Narrow therapeutic window.
  - Enters CNS slowly due to blood–brain barrier.
  - Delayed CNS symptoms.
  - Discrepancy between serum levels and CNS symptoms.
  - Excreted by kidneys.
  - Toxicity can be precipitated by dehydration, infection, medication effects.
  - Lithium can directly cause renal injury, worsening toxicity.

Clinical Features

- Gastrointestinal: nausea, vomiting, diarrhea.
  - Dehydration, worsens lithium toxicity.
- Cardiovascular:
  - Hypotension.
  - ECG changes: QTc prolongation, T wave inversion/flattening, first-degree atrioventricular block.
- Neurologic: primary toxicity of concern, develops late:
  - Mild: tremors, hyperreflexia, agitation, ataxia, weakness.
  - Moderate: confusion, hypertonia, dysarthria.
  - Severe: seizures, coma.
- Renal: chronic toxicity: dehydration, hyponatremia.
- Endocrine: hyperthyroidism, hypothyroidism.

Diagnosis

- Primarily clinical:
  - Gastrointestinal distress precedes neurologic signs in acute toxicity.
  - Neurologic abnormalities may be first signs of chronic toxicity.
- Serum lithium concentration:

- Helps guide management, including hemodialysis.
- Not clearly correlated to toxicity.

Management

- Support ABC.
- Fluid resuscitation:
  - Initiate volume repletion with IV crystalloids.
  - Monitor serum sodium, urine output, urine concentration.
- Consider gastrointestinal decontamination.
- Indications for hemodialysis:
  - Serum concentration > 4 mg/dl in acute toxicity.
  - Significant CNS toxicity.
  - Inability to tolerate IV fluid resuscitation.
  - Renal impairment.

Debriefing Plan

Plan for around 30 minutes for discussion.

Potential Questions for Discussion

- What is the general approach to a patient with altered mental status?
- What symptoms and clinical findings in this case suggest lithium toxicity as the cause of this patient's condition?
- What other etiologies should be considered?
- How is the severity of lithium toxicity determined?
- List the indications for hemodialysis in a patient with lithium toxicity.
- What prehospital interventions could have been performed on this patient?

SELECTED READINGS FOR LITHIUM TOXICITY

Baird-Gunning, J., Lea-Henry, T., Hoegberg, L. et al. (2016). Lithium poisoning. *J. Intensive Care Med.* 32 (4): 249–263.

Decker, B.S., Goldfarb, D.S., Dargan, P.I. et al. (2015). Extracorporeal treatment for lithium poisoning: systematic review and recommendations from the EXTRIP workgroup. *Clin. J. Am. Soc. Nephrol.* 10 (5): 875–887.

Han, J.H. and Wilber, S.T. (2013). Altered mental status in older patients in the emergency department. *Clin. Geriatr. Med.* 29 (1): 101–136.

Oruch, R., Elderbi, M.A., Khattab, H.A. et al. (2014). Lithium: a review of pharmacology, clinical uses, and toxicity. *Eur. J. Pharmacol.* 740: 464–473.

ETHYLENE GLYCOL TOXICITY

Educational Goals

Learning Objectives

1. Demonstrate proper assessment of pediatric patient with altered mental status (MK, PC).
2. Recognize and appropriately manage ethylene glycol toxicity (MK, PC).
3. Demonstrate appropriate pediatric airway management (MK, PC).
4. Describe indications for hemodialysis in patient with ethylene glycol toxicity (MK).
5. Demonstrate effective communication skills and professionalism during interactions with patient's parent, ED staff, and consultants (ICS, P).
6. Direct appropriate disposition of pediatric patient with ethylene glycol toxicity (SBP).

Critical Actions Checklist

☐ Obtain appropriate vascular access (MK, PC).
☐ Measure fingerstick glucose or administer empiric dextrose (MK, PC).
☐ Perform endotracheal intubation (MK, PC).
☐ Obtain appropriate toxicology testing (MK).
☐ Administer fomepizole (MK, PC).
☐ Administer sodium bicarbonate for acidosis (MK, PC).
☐ Consult with nephrologist for hemodialysis (MK, ICS, P, SBP).
☐ Communicate with pediatric intensive care unit (PICU) for disposition (ICS, P, SBP).

Simulation Set-Up

Environment: ED treatment area. For EMS learners, the scenario may start on scene and transition to a hospital setting.

Mannequin: Pediatric male simulator mannequin (should be approximately seven years of age) on a stretcher or hospital bed. The mannequin should be moulaged with vomitus on clothing.

Props: To be displayed on screen or distributed on handouts:

- Images (see online component for ethylene glycol overdose, Scenario 14.3 https://www.wiley.com/go/thoureen/simulation/workbook2e):

- ECG showing sinus tachycardia (Figure 14.10).
- Chest X-ray which is normal (Figure 14.11)
- Post-intubation chest X-ray showing appropriate endotracheal tube position (Figure 14.12)
- Head CT interpretation (normal) (Figure 14.13)
- Laboratory tests (see online component as above):
  - Fingerstick glucose (Table 14.24).
  - Complete blood count (Table 14.25).
  - Basic metabolic panel (Table 14.26).
  - Liver function tests (Table 14.27).
  - Lactate (Table 14.28).
  - Arterial blood gases (Table 14.29).
  - Serum osmolality (Table 14.30).
  - Urinalysis (Table 14.31).
  - Urine toxicology screen (Table 14.32).
  - Salicylate level (Table 14.33).
  - Acetaminophen level (Table 14.34).
  - Ethanol level (Table 14.35).
  - Methanol level (Table 14.36).
  - Ethylene glycol level (Table 14.37).
  - Isopropanol level (Table 14.38).

Available supplies:

- Pediatric airway and code cart.
- Medications:
  - Intravenous (IV) fluids in labeled 1 L bags: 0.9% saline, LR.
  - Medications:
    - Liter bags of 0.9% saline, LR, D5W.
    - Pre-labeled syringes:
  - RSI medications, specific induction and paralytic medications typical of your institution.
  - Naloxone.
  - 50% dextrose.
  - 8.4% sodium bicarbonate.
    - Pre-labeled IV bags:
  - Fomepizole.

Distractor: None.

Actors

- EMS can provide information about the scene. Actor optional if no EMS learner is present.
- Patient is somnolent, confused, not following commands or answering questions.
- Patient's parent can provide learners with the patient's medical history.
- ED nurse can administer medications and may cue learners if needed.
- Nephrologist, toxicologist and PICU physician available via telephone consultation.

Case Narrative

Scenario Background

A 7-year-old boy is brought in by EMS from home. He was found obtunded on the couch. He has been unable to answer questions. Patient had been in his usual state of health until today. Parent is en route to hospital.

Patient's medical history: None.
Medications: None.
Allergies: None.
Family history: Non-contributory.
Social history: No tobacco, alcohol, or drug use.

Initial Scenario Conditions

Young boy, somnolent, confused, intermittently moaning.

> Case may start with EMS (learner) receiving this case on scene as presented and performing their objectives to initiate treatment and transport, including questioning family members and looking for bottles of potentially toxic substances that could have been ingested. Alternatively, scenario background may be presented by EMS (actor) on ED arrival.

Vital signs: Temp 98.6 °F (37.0 °C), HR 130, RR 26, BP 90/55, SpO$_2$ 98% on 100% non-rebreather mask.
Head: Atraumatic.
Eyes: Pupils 4 mm, reactive to light.
Heart: Tachycardic, regular.
Lungs: Clear breath sounds.
Abdomen: Soft, non-tender, non-distended, normal bowel sounds.

Extremities: No deformities.
Skin: Warm, dry.
Neurologic: Eyes closed, withdraws and moans to painful stimuli.

See flow diagram (Figure 14.14) for further scenario changes described.

Case Narrative, Continued

Learners of all levels should assess ABC. They should measure fingerstick glucose, obtain appropriate vascular access, and consider empiric naloxone administration. They should order laboratory studies, including drug screens.

Learners should recognize the patient's depressed mental status and need for intubation. Airway equipment should be sized appropriately for a seven-year-old patient. Failure to perform intubation after five minutes will lead to further respiratory deterioration.

Following appropriate airway management, the patient will stabilize temporarily. Imaging and laboratory results can return at this time. Learners should recognize a toxic alcohol ingestion. For junior learners, EMS may report that they found an opened bottle of antifreeze next to the patient. For advanced learners, this information may be withheld. If ethylene glycol toxicity is not considered by 10 minutes, this history may be provided by a family member.

Learners should initiate treatment with IV sodium bicarbonate and fomepizole. They should consult with a nephrologist to prepare for hemodialysis. They should communicate with the patient's parent to keep her/him informed. Case will end after learners have arranged for disposition to PICU.

Instructor Notes

Pathophysiology

- Ethylene glycol:
  - Toxicity caused primarily by metabolites (glycolate, glyoxylate, oxalate).
  - Anion gap metabolic acidosis.
  - CNS depression.
  - Renal failure, slows elimination of ethylene glycol, worsening toxicity.

Clinical Features

- Signs of intoxication.
- Confusion, seizures, coma.
- Hypotension.
- Hematuria, oliguria

Diagnosis

- Metabolic panel:
  - Anion gap metabolic acidosis.
  - Acute kidney injury.
- Serum ethylene glycol concentration:
  - Usually not readily available to guide management.
  - May not reflect level of toxicity or risk of mortality.
- Osmolar gap:
  - Elevated early after ingestion before anion gap develops.
  - Not specific for ethylene glycol.
- Serum ethanol concentration:
  - Ethanol inhibits ethylene glycol metabolism.

Management

- Support ABC.
- Correct acidosis:
  - Degree of acidosis correlates with illness severity and outcome.
  - Administer bicarbonate to patients with pH < 7.3.
  - Initial dose: 1–2 mEq/kg sodium bicarbonate as IV bolus.
  - Infusion: 150 mEq (three 50 ml ampules) sodium bicarbonate in 1 l D5W at 2–3 ml/kg/hour.
  - Titrate to serum pH of 7.35–7.45.
- Fomepizole:
  - Binds alcohol dehydrogenase, inhibits toxic metabolite production.
  - Initiate prior to lab results if there is strong clinical suspicion for ethylene glycol ingestion.
  - Loading dose 15 mg/kg IV.
  - Maintenance dose 10 mg/kg IV every 12 hours for up to 48 hours.
  - Ethanol is an alternative therapy.
  - Difficult to dose appropriately.
  - May worsen CNS and respiratory compromise.
- Hemodialysis:
  - Consult with nephrologist early.
  - Indications:
    - Acidosis (pH < 7.3) regardless of ethylene glycol level.
    - End-organ dysfunction (e.g., vision disturbance, renal failure).
    - Hemodynamic instability.

Debriefing Plan

Plan for around 30 minutes for discussion.

Potential Questions for Discussion

- Describe the general approach to a pediatric patient with altered mental status.
- Describe the clinical features of ethylene glycol toxicity.
- What laboratory abnormalities are expected?
- What is the appropriate therapy for ethylene glycol ingestion?
- List the indications for hemodialysis in a patient with ethylene glycol toxicity.

SELECTED READINGS ETHYLENE GLYCOL TOXICITY

Mcmartin, K., Jacobsen, D., and Hovda, K.E. (2016). Antidotes for poisoning by alcohols that form toxic metabolites. *Br. J. Clin. Pharmacol.* 81 (3): 505–515.

Wu, P.E. and Sivilotti, M.L. (2016). Toxic alcohol calculations and misinterpretation of laboratory results. *JAMA Intern. Med.* 176 (8): 1227–1228.

APPENDIX

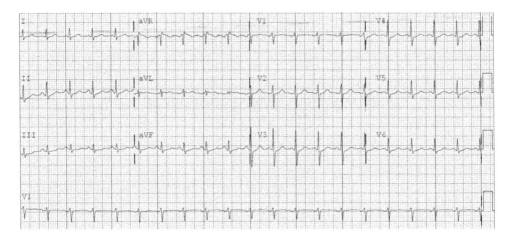

FIGURE 14.1   Electrocardiogram showing sinus tachycardia.

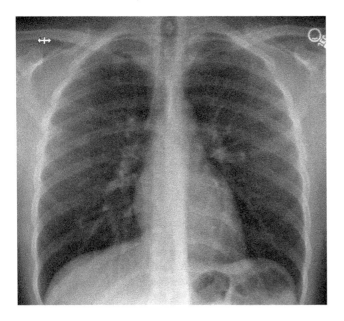

FIGURE 14.2   Chest x-ray showing no acute abnormality.

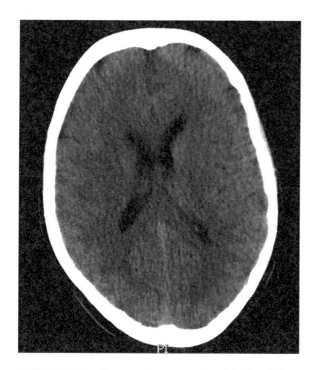

FIGURE 14.3   Computed tomography of the head showing no acute intracranial abnormality.

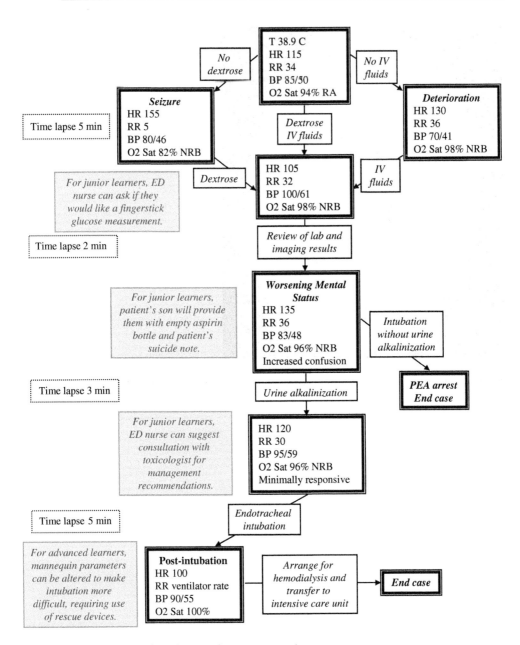

FIGURE 14.4   Scenario flow diagram for aspirin overdose.

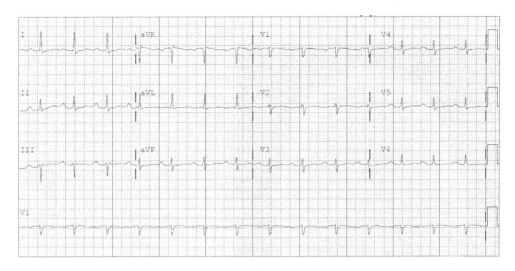

FIGURE 14.5   Electrocardiogram showing first-degree atrioventricular block and flattened T waves.

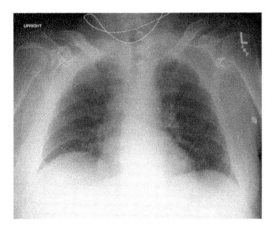

FIGURE 14.6   Chest x-ray showing no acute abnormality.

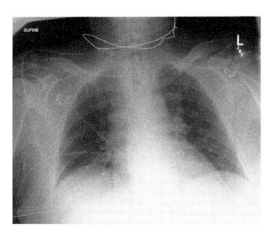

FIGURE 14.7   Post-intubation chest x-ray showing appropriate endotracheal tube position.

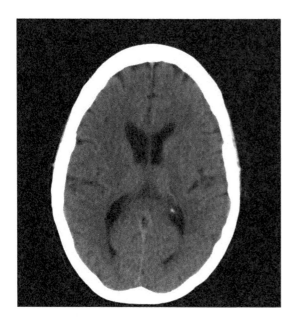

FIGURE 14.8   Computed tomography of the head showing no acute intracranial abnormality.

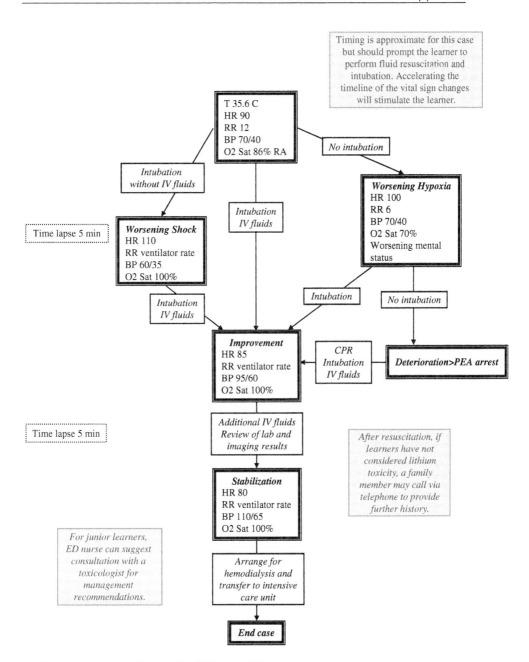

FIGURE 14.9 Flow diagram for lithium toxicity.

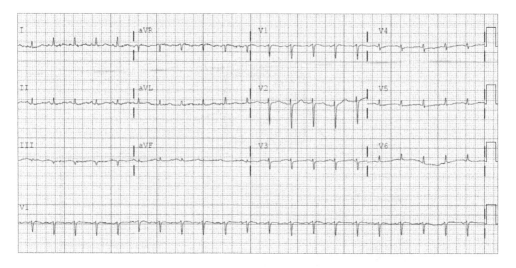

FIGURE 14.10   Ethylene glycol toxicity case: electrocardiogram showing sinus tachycardia.

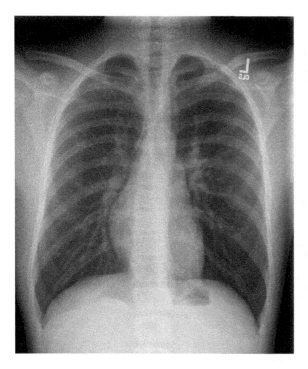

FIGURE 14.11   Chest x-ray showing no acute abnormality.

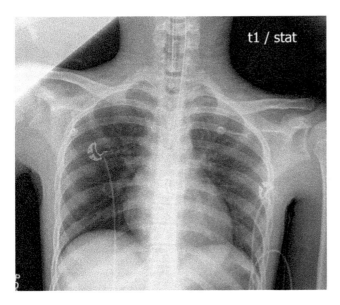

FIGURE 14.12   Post-intubation chest x-ray showing appropriate endotracheal tube position.

CT Head Without Contrast

Impression: No acute intracranial abnormality

FIGURE 14.13   Computed tomography of the head interpretation showing no acute intracranial abnormality.

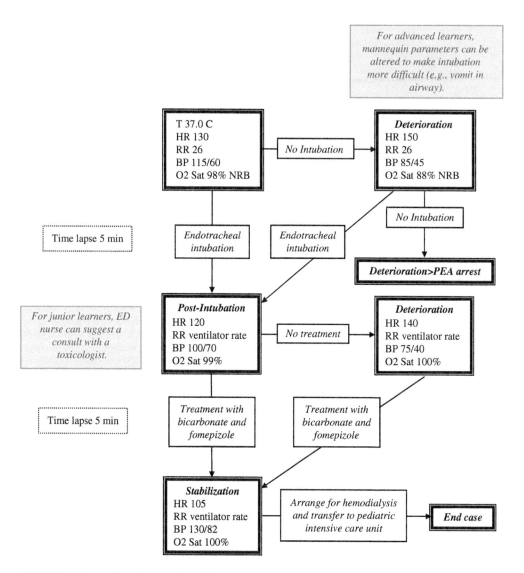

FIGURE 14.14   Flow diagram for ethylene glycol toxicity.

TABLE 14.1 Fingerstick glucose.

Test	Value	Reference range
Fingerstick glucose (mg/dl)	58	70–109

TABLE 14.2 Complete blood count.

Test	Value	Reference range
White blood cells (k/μl)	17.8	3.5–11.0
Hemoglobin (g/dl)	15.1	10.5–15.0
Hematocrit (%)	44	32–45
Platelets (k/μl)	264	150–400

TABLE 14.3 Basic metabolic panel.

Test	Value	Reference range
Sodium (mmol/l)	137	135–145
Potassium (mmol/l)	2.3	3.6–5.1
Chloride (mmol/l)	99	98–110
Bicarbonate (mmol/l)	12	20–30
Blood urea nitrogen	42	6–24
Blood urea nitrogen (mg/dl)	1.6	0.4–1.3
Creatinine (mg/dl)	62	67–109
Glucose (mg/dl)	9.6	8.6–10.3

TABLE 14.4 Liver function tests.

Test	Value	Reference range
Albumin (g/dl)	3.7	3.7–4.8
Total protein(g/dl)	7.6	6.3–8.3
Total bilirubin(mg/dl)	0.5	0.3–0.5
Alkaline phosphatase (iu/l)	56	38–120
Alanine aminotransferase (iu/l)	26	7–52
Aspartate aminotransferase (iu/l)	28	13–39

TABLE 14.5   Lactate.

Test	Value	Reference range
Lactate (mmol/l)	9.4	0.5–2.0

TABLE 14.6   Arterial blood gases.

Test	Value	Reference range
pH	7.32	7.35–7.45
pCO_2 (mmHg)	28	35–45
pO_2 (mmHg)	114	80–100
HCO_3 (mEq/l)	11	22–26
Base excess	−2.7	−4 to +2
SaO_2 (%)	> 95	95–100

TABLE 14.7   Urinalysis.

Test	Value	Reference range
Color	Yellow	Colorless–dark yellow
Appearance	Clear	Clear
Specific gravity	1.021	1.005–1.030
pH	7.0	5.0–8.0
Protein	24	20–30 mmol/l
Glucose	Negative	Negative
Ketones	Negative	Negative
Hemoglobin	Negative	Negative
Urobilinogen (mg/dl)	< 0.2	< 0.2
Red blood cells (/hpf)	0	0–3
White blood cells (/hpf)	0	0–5
Bacteria	None	None
Nitrites	Negative	Negative
Leukocyte esterase	Negative	Negative

TABLE 14.8 Urine toxicology screen.

Test	Value	Reference range
Amphetamines	Negative	Negative
Barbiturates	Negative	Negative
Benzodiazepines	Negative	Negative
Cannabinoids	Negative	Negative
Cocaine	Negative	Negative
Opiates	Negative	Negative
Tricyclics	Negative	Negative
Ethanol	Negative	Negative
Acetaminophen	Negative	Negative
Salicylates	Positive	Negative

TABLE 14.9 Salicylate level.

Test	Value	Reference range
Salicylates (mg/ml)	82	15–30

TABLE 14.10 Acetaminophen level.

Test	Value	Reference range
Acetaminophen (mg/dl)	0	10–30

TABLE 14.11 Ethanol level.

Test	Value	Reference range
Ethanol (mg/dl)	0	–

TABLE 14.12 Fingerstick glucose.

Test	Value	Reference range
Fingerstick glucose (mg/dl)	237	70–109

TABLE 14.13　Complete blood count.

Test	Value	Reference range
White blood cells (k/μl)	15.4	3.5–11.0
Hemoglobin (g/dl)	13.5	10.5–15.0
Hematocrit (%)	40.9	32–45
Platelets (k/μl)	213	150–400

TABLE 14.14　Basic metabolic panel.

Test	Value	Reference range
Sodium (mmol/l)	144	135–145
Potassium (mmol/l)	3.6	3.6–5.1
Chloride (mmol/l)	107	98–110
Bicarbonate (mmol/l)	22	20–30
Blood urea nitrogen	37	6–24
Blood urea nitrogen (mg/dl)	1.7	0.4–1.3
Creatinine (mg/dl)	235	67–109
Glucose (mg/dl)	9.1	8.6–10.3

TABLE 14.15　Liver function tests.

Test	Value	Reference range
Albumin (g/dl)	3.8	3.7–4.8
Total protein (g/dl)	6.8	6.3–8.3
Total bilirubin (mg/dl)	1.2	0.3–0.5
Alkaline phosphatase (iu/l)	71	38–120
Alanine aminotransferase (iu/l)	69	7–52
Aspartate aminotransferase (iu/l)	87	13–39

TABLE 14.16　Lactate.

Test	Value	Reference range
Lactate (mmol/l)	3.2	0.5–2.0

TABLE 14.17 Lithium level.

Test	Value	Reference range
Lithium (mEq/l)	4.7	0.8–1.2

TABLE 14.18 Thyroid function tests.

Test	Value	Reference range
Thyroid stimulating hormone (iu/ml)	2.1	0.530–6.340
Free T4 (iu/ml)	1.5	0.6–1.60

TABLE 14.19 Urinalysis.

Test	Value	Reference range
Color	Yellow	Colorless–dark yellow
Appearance	Clear	Clear
Specific gravity	1.024	1.005–1.030
pH	6.8	5.0–8.0
Protein	25	20–30 mmol/l
Glucose	Negative	Negative
Ketones	Negative	Negative
Hemoglobin	Negative	Negative
Urobilinogen (mg/dl)	< 0.2	< 0.2
Red blood cells (/hpf)	0	0–3
White blood cells (/hpf)	0	0–5
Bacteria	None	None
Nitrites	Negative	Negative
Leukocyte esterase	Negative	Negative

TABLE 14.20 Urine toxicology screen.

Test	Value	Reference range
Amphetamines	Negative	Negative
Barbiturates	Negative	Negative
Benzodiazepines	Negative	Negative
Cannabinoids	Negative	Negative

TABLE 14.20   (Continued)

Test	Value	Reference range
Cocaine	Negative	Negative
Opiates	Negative	Negative
Tricyclics	Negative	Negative
Ethanol	Negative	Negative
Acetaminophen	Negative	Negative
Salicylates	Negative	Negative

TABLE 14.21   Salicylate level.

Test	Value	Reference range
Salicylate (mg/ml)	0	15–30

TABLE 14.22   Acetaminophen level.

Test	Value	Reference range
Acetaminophen (mg/ml)	0	10–30

TABLE 14.23   Ethanol level.

Test	Value	Reference range
Ethanol (mg/ml)	0	–

TABLE 14.24   Fingerstick glucose.

Test	Value	Reference range
Fingerstick glucose (mg/ml)	105	70–109

TABLE 14.25   Complete blood count.

Test	Value	Reference range
White blood cells (k/µl)	15.2	3.5–11.0
Hemoglobin (g/dl)	12	10.5–15.0
Hematocrit (%)	38	32–45
Platelets (k/µl)	420	150–400

TABLE 14.26 Basic metabolic panel.

Test	Value	Reference range
Sodium (mmol/l)	135	135–145
Potassium (mmol/l)	4.2	3.6–5.1
Chloride (mmol/l)	97	98–110
Bicarbonate (mmol/l)	5	20–30
Blood urea nitrogen	18	6–24
Blood urea nitrogen (mg/dl)	0.75	0.4–1.3
Creatinine (mg/dl)	105	67–109
Calcium (mg/dl)	9.6	8.6–10.3

TABLE 14.27 Liver function tests.

Test	Value	Reference range
Albumin (g/dl)	4.0	3.7–4.8
Total protein(g/dl)	7.3	6.3–8.3
Total bilirubin(mg/dl)	0.7	0.3–0.5
Alkaline phosphatase (iu/l)	64	38–120
Alanine aminotransferase (iu/l)	18	7–52
Aspartate aminotransferase (iu/l)	22	13–39

TABLE 14.28 Lactate.

Test	Value	Reference range
Lactate (mmol/l)	5.2	0.5–2.0

TABLE 14.29 Arterial blood gases.

Test	Value	Reference range
pH	7.12	7.35–7.45
pCO_2 (mmHg)	28	35–45
pO_2 (mmHg)	112	80–100
HCO_3 (mEq/l)	5	22–26
Base excess	−1.8	−4 to +2
SaO_2 (%)	>95%	95–100

TABLE 14.30 Serum osmolality.

Test	Value	Reference range
Serum osmolality (mOsm/kg)	345	285–295

TABLE 14.31 Urinalysis.

Test	Value	Reference range
Color	Yellow	Colorless–dark yellow
Appearance	Clear	Clear
Specific gravity	1.016	1.005–1.030
pH	6.7	5.0–8.0
Protein (mmol/l)	24	20–30
Glucose	Negative	Negative
Ketones	Negative	Negative
Hemoglobin	Negative	Negative
Urobilinogen (mg/dl)	< 0.2	< 0.2
Red blood cells (/hpf)	0	0–3
White blood cells(/hpf)	0	0–5
Bacteria	None	None
Nitrites	Negative	Negative
Leukocyte esterase	Negative	Negative

TABLE 14.32 Urine toxicology screen.

Test	Value	Reference range
Amphetamines	Negative	Negative
Barbiturates	Negative	Negative
Benzodiazepines	Negative	Negative
Cannabinoids	Negative	Negative
Cocaine	Negative	Negative
Opiates	Negative	Negative
Tricyclics	Negative	Negative
Ethanol	Negative	Negative
Acetaminophen	Negative	Negative
Salicylates	Negative	Negative

TABLE 14.33   Salicylate level.

Test	Value	Reference range
Salicylate (mg/ml)	0	15–30

TABLE 14.34   Acetaminophen level.

Test	Value	Reference range
Acetaminophen (mg/dl)	0	10–30

TABLE 14.35   Ethanol level.

Test	Value	Reference range
Ethanol (mg/dl)	0	–

TABLE 14.36   Methanol level.

Test	Value	Reference range
Methanol (mg/dl)	0	–

TABLE 14.37   Ethylene glycol level.

Test	Value	Reference range
Ethylene glycol level (mg/dl)	300	–

TABLE 14.38   Isopropanol level.

Test	Value	Reference range
Isopropanol (mg/dl)	0	–

CHAPTER 15

Traumatic Emergencies

Charles Lei, Jeffrey N. Heimiller, and Joseph R. Sikon

Department of Emergency Medicine, Vanderbilt University Medical Center, Nashville, TN, USA

HEMORRHAGIC SHOCK

Educational Goals

Learning Objectives

1. Demonstrate appropriate assessment of trauma patient (MK, PC).
2. Recognize and appropriately manage hemorrhagic shock in setting of trauma (MK, PC).
3. Demonstrate proper use of Focused Assessment with Sonography in Trauma (FAST) examination (MK, PC).
4. Demonstrate appropriate management of open femur fracture (MK, PC).
5. Demonstrate proper airway management in patient with hemorrhagic shock (MK, PC).
6. Demonstrate effective communication skills and professionalism during interactions with Emergency Department (ED) staff and consultants (ICS, P).
7. Direct appropriate disposition of trauma patient with hemorrhagic shock (SBP).

Emergency Medicine Simulation Workbook: A Tool for Bringing the Curriculum to Life,
Second Edition. Edited by Traci L. Thoureen and Sara B. Scott.
© 2022 John Wiley & Sons Ltd. Published 2022 by John Wiley & Sons Ltd.
Companion website: www.wiley.com/go/thoureen/simulation/workbook2e

Critical Actions Checklist

☐ Perform primary and secondary trauma surveys (MK, PC).
☐ Obtain appropriate vascular access (MK, PC).
☐ Perform appropriate fluid resuscitation with crystalloids, blood products (MK, PC).
☐ Perform and interpret FAST examination (MK, PC).
☐ Immobilize femur fracture with splint (MK, PC).
☐ Apply tourniquet proximal to femur fracture (MK, PC).
☐ Initiate massive transfusion protocol (MTP) with balanced blood product administration (MK, PC).
☐ Insert endotracheal tube (MK, PC).
☐ Communicate with trauma service for disposition (ICS, P, SBP).

Critical actions can be changed to address learners' educational needs. For example, emergency medical services (EMS) learners may be expected to fully immobilize patient with cervical collar and backboard.

Simulation Set-up

Environment: ED treatment area. For EMS learners, the scenario may start on scene and transition to a hospital setting.

Mannequin: Male simulator mannequin, with cervical collar, on backboard. Mannequin should be moulaged with bruising across abdomen; a large, bloody, open wound on left mid-thigh; and large amount of blood on sheet under wound.

Props: To be displayed on screen or distributed on handouts:

- Images (see online component for hemorrhagic shock, Scenario 15.1 at https://www.wiley.com/go/thoureen/simulation/workbook2e):
  - FAST images showing intraperitoneal free fluid (Figures 15.1–15.4).
  - Chest x-ray (normal) (Figure 15.5).
  - Post-intubation chest x-ray showing appropriate endotracheal tube position (Figure 15.6).
  - X-ray of the pelvis (normal) (Figure 15.7).
  - X-ray of left femur showing fracture (Figure 15.8).
  - Computed tomography of the head (normal) (Figure 15.9).
  - Computed tomography of the abdomen showing splenic laceration with active extravasation and hemoperitoneum (Figure 15.10).

- Laboratory tests (see online component as above):
  - Complete blood count (Table 15.1).
  - Basic metabolic panel (Table 15.2).
  - Liver function tests (Table 15.3).
  - Lactate (Table 15.4).
  - Coagulation panel (Table 15.5).
  - Type and screen (Table 15.6).

Available supplies:

- Adult airway and code cart.
- Medications:
  - Intravenous (IV) fluids in labeled 1l bags: 0.9% saline, lactated Ringer's solution (LR).
  - Blood products: red blood cells, platelets, fresh frozen plasma.
  - Pre-labeled syringes:
    - Analgesic medications.
    - Rapid sequence intubation medications, typically used at your institution.
    - Tetanus vaccine.
  - Pre-labeled IV bags:
    - Cefazolin
- Intraosseous (IO) device with insertion trainer.
- Cervical collar.
- Backboard.
- Splint or traction device for femur fracture.
- Tourniquet.
- Hemostatic gauze.
- "Blood-soaked" dressings.

Distractor: None.

Actors

- EMS can provide information about the scene. Actor optional if no EMS learner is present.
- Patient in severe pain, confused, agitated, and not following commands or answering questions.
- ED nurse can administer medications. Depending on moulage complexity, may need to cue learners regarding physical exam findings (e.g., abdominal bruising, bony deformity in left thigh, large open thigh wound with brisk bleeding).
- Trauma surgeon and orthopedic surgeon available via telephone consultation.

Case Narrative

Scenario Background

A 30-year-old man was a restrained driver in a motor vehicle collision. He did not lose consciousness but required extrication from the vehicle. EMS immobilized the patient. They were unable to establish IV access.

> Case may start with EMS (learner) receiving this case on scene as presented and performing their objectives to initiate treatment and transport, including patient immobilization. Alternatively, scenario background may be presented by EMS (actor) on ED arrival.

Patient's medical history: None.
Medications: None.
Allergies: None.
Family history: Non-contributory.
Social history: No tobacco, alcohol, or drug use.

Initial Scenario Conditions

Young man moaning in pain.

Vital signs: Temp 97.8 °F (36.6 °C), HR 115, RR 22, BP 80/50, SpO$_2$ 96% on room air.
Head: Atraumatic.
Eyes: Pupils 4 mm, reactive to light.
Mouth: Airway patent.
Heart: Tachycardic, regular rhythm, distal pulses diminished.
Lungs: clear breath sounds.
Chest: Non-tender.
Abdomen: Distended, firm, diffusely tender.
Back: No midline tenderness.
Extremities: Pelvis stable, bony deformity in left mid-thigh with large open wound that is bleeding briskly.
Skin: Bruising across abdomen.
Neurologic: Eyes open, confused, agitated, moaning in pain, does not follow commands or answering questions.

See flow diagram (Figure 15.11) for further scenario changes described.

Case Narrative, Continued

Learners of all levels should perform a primary trauma survey and obtain appropriate IV access. Learners should recognize hypotension and circulatory compromise and perform appropriate fluid resuscitation with crystalloids and blood products. Learners should perform FAST exam and identify intraperitoneal free fluid. Failure to initiate appropriate fluid resuscitation after five minutes will lead to further circulatory decompensation.

For advanced learners, the ED nurse will be unable to establish IV access. Learners should obtain IO access in the right lower extremity or an upper extremity, demonstrating procedure on IO insertion trainer.

> If performance of actual procedure is not a learning objective, then learners can simply verbalize where they would establish IO access.

Following appropriate fluid administration, the patient will stabilize temporarily. Learners should perform a secondary trauma survey and obtain point-of-care imaging studies. Nurse should cue learners that the left thigh wound is continuing to bleed briskly. Learners should immobilize the fracture and perform local hemorrhage control (e.g., direct pressure, hemostatic gauze).

For advanced learners, the leg wound will continue to bleed. This may be cued by the nurse displaying large amounts of "blood-soaked" gauze. Advanced learners should place a tourniquet proximal to the injury site.

The patient will continue to become more hypotensive and tachycardic. Learners should initiate MTP with balanced administration of red blood cells (RBCs), platelets, and fresh frozen plasma (FFP). Laboratory results can return at this time.

For advanced learners, the patient can become increasingly agitated and obtunded. Learners should identify airway compromise and perform intubation in the setting of hemorrhagic shock.

Case will end after learners have arranged appropriate disposition to trauma service.

Instructor Notes

Pathophysiology

- Sites of significant hemorrhage in trauma:
  - Chest.
  - Abdomen.
  - Retroperitoneum.
  - Pelvis.
  - Thigh.
  - External (e.g., scalp).
- Initial physiologic response to hemorrhage:
  - Tachycardia.
  - Increased cardiac contractility.
  - Peripheral vasoconstriction.

- Varies depending on age, cardiovascular function.
- Continuing hemorrhage → hypovolemic shock (cellular hypoxia → multiorgan dysfunction → death).

Clinical Features

- Signs of organ dysfunction:
  - Hypotension.
  - Dyspnea.
  - Tachypnea.
  - Oliguria.
  - Diaphoresis.
  - Cool, clammy skin.
  - Restlessness.
  - Altered mental status.
- Hypotension in setting of trauma should be presumed to be secondary to hemorrhage until proven otherwise.

Diagnosis

- Primarily clinical.
- FAST exam:
- Detects free intraperitoneal and pericardial fluid.
- In supine patients, intraperitoneal fluid first collects in right upper quadrant (Morrison's pouch, paracolic gutter).
- Can detect as little as 200 ml of free fluid in Morrison's pouch.
- Can be performed at bedside.
- CT:
  - Sensitive for intraperitoneal hemorrhage.
  - Identifies other sources of bleeding.
  - Cannot be performed at bedside.
  - More time-consuming than FAST.
- Laboratory studies:
  - Hemoglobin/hematocrit may not reflect degree of acute hemorrhage.

Management of Hemorrhagic Shock

- Primary survey:
  - Diagnose critical, life-threatening injuries requiring immediate intervention.

- Standardized approach:
  - Airway: patency, ability to protect.
  - Breathing: respiratory effort, oxygenation, ventilation.
  - Circulation: heart rate, blood pressure, distal pulses.
- Vascular access:
  - Multiple large-bore IV cannulas.
  - If unable to obtain IV access, promptly establish IO access.
  - Avoid IO placement in or distal to fractured bone.
  - In patients with intra-abdominal injuries, consider humeral IO placement.
  - Consider inserting a large-bore central venous catheter.
- Fluid resuscitation:
  - Goal systolic blood pressure 90 mmHg.
  - Avoid large-volume crystalloid resuscitation (>1l):
    - Can cause hypothermia, acidosis, coagulopathy.
  - Initiate early transfusion of uncrossmatched RBCs:
    - O-negative for pre-menopausal women.
    - O-positive for all other patients.
  - If requiring >2 units of RBCs, initiate MTP:
    - Balanced administration of RBCs, platelets, FFP.
    - Optimal ratio still undetermined.
  - Consider tranexamic acid.
- Secondary survey:
  - Identify and manage any additional significant injuries.
  - Fully expose patient, perform complete exam.
  - Deterioration at any point requires reevaluation of primary survey.

Management of Open Femur Fracture with Active Hemorrhage

- Analgesic medications may worsen hypotension.
- Attempt to reduce displacement by pulling to length.
- Immobilize leg in splint or traction device.
- Apply direct pressure, pressure dressing, and/or hemostatic gauze to bleeding site.
- Apply tourniquet to exposed skin 5 cm proximal to injury site.

Airway Management in Setting of Hemorrhagic Shock

- Positive pressure ventilation may decrease venous return, and worsen shock state.
- Initiate early volume resuscitation.
- Consider push-dose pressors during peri-intubation period.

Debriefing Plan

Plan for around 30 minutes for discussion.

SELECTED READING FOR HEMORRHAGIC SHOCK

Galvagno, S.M., Nahmias, J.T., and Young, D.A. (2019). Advanced trauma life support update 2019: management and applications for adult and special populations. *Anesthesiol. Clin.* 37 (1): 13–32.

Puskarich, M.A. and Jones, A.E. (2018). Shock. In: *Rosen's Emergency Medicine*, 9e (eds. R.M. Walls, R.S. Hockberger and M. Gausche-Hill), 68–76. Philadelphia, PA: Elsevier.

Stephens, C.T., Gumbert, S., and Holcomb, J.B. (2016). Trauma-associated bleeding: management of massive transfusion. *Curr. Opin. Anaesthesiol.* 29 (2): 250–255.

Potential Questions for Discussion

- What are the components of the trauma survey?
- What are the clinical features of hemorrhagic shock?
- What is the appropriate management of hemorrhagic shock in the setting of trauma?
- What is the appropriate treatment for an open femur fracture with continuing external bleeding?
- What special considerations should be given to patients with hemorrhagic shock who require intubation?

NON-ACCIDENTAL TRAUMA

Educational Goals

Learning Objectives

1. Demonstrate ability to obtain history of present illness for an infant (MK, PC, ICS).
2. Demonstrate correct physical exam skills for infant (MK, PC, ICS).
3. Demonstrate appropriate management of pediatric seizure (MK, PC).
4. Demonstrate correct pediatric airway management (MK, PC).
5. Demonstrate appropriate management of infant with intracerebral hemorrhage (ICH) (MK, PC).
6. Recognize clinical features of non-accidental trauma (MK).
7. Demonstrate effective communication skills and professionalism during interactions with patient's parent, ED staff, and consultants (ICS, P).
8. Direct appropriate disposition of pediatric patient with ICH (SBP).

Critical Actions Checklist

☐ Obtain history from patient's parent (MK, PC, ICS).
☐ Perform thorough physical exam (MK, PC, ICS).
☐ Obtain appropriate vascular access (MK, PC).
☐ Measure fingerstick glucose (MK).
☐ Treat seizure with benzodiazepines (MK, PC).
☐ Perform endotracheal intubation (MK, PC).
☐ Obtain and interpret head CT (MK).
☐ Consult with neurosurgery for further management of ICH (ICS, P, SBP).
☐ Communicate with patient's parent regarding concern for non-accidental trauma (ICS, P).
☐ Communicate with designated child abuse specialist to discuss concern for non-accidental trauma (ICS, P).
☐ Communicate with pediatric intensive care unit (PICU) for disposition (ICS, P, SBP).

Simulation Set-up

Environment: ED treatment area. For EMS learners, the scenario may start on scene and transition to a hospital setting.

Mannequin: Infant simulator mannequin. Mannequin should be moulaged with bruising on left chest and left mid-back, seen only if undressed. Bruises should be in different stages of healing.

Props: To be displayed on screen or distributed on handouts:

- Images (see online component for non-accidental trauma, Scenario 15.2 at https://www.wiley.com/go/thoureen/simulation/workbook2e):
  - Post-intubation chest x-ray showing appropriate endotracheal tube position (Figure 15.12).
  - CT of the infant's head showing subdural hematoma (Figure 15.13)
- Laboratory tests (see online component as above):
  - Fingerstick glucose (Table 15.7).
  - Complete blood count (Table 15.8).
  - Basic metabolic panel (Table 15.9).
  - Liver function tests (Table 15.10)
  - Lactate (Table 15.11).
  - Coagulation panel (Table 15.12)
  - Type and screen (Table 15.13).

Available supplies:

- Pediatric airway and code cart.
- Medications:
  - IV fluids in labeled 1 l bags: 0.9% saline, LR.
  - Pre-labeled syringes:
    - Rapid sequence intubation medications typical of your institution.
    - Benzodiazepines (e.g., lorazepam, midazolam).
  - Pre-labeled bags:
    - Antiepileptic medications (e.g., levetiracetam, fosphenytoin).
    - Mannitol.
    - Hypertonic saline.
- Length-based pediatric emergency resuscitation tape.

Distractor: Patient's parent becomes anxious and obstructive if the team does not keep them informed.

Actors

- EMS can provide information about the scene. Actor optional if no EMS learner is present.
- Patient's parent is anxious, but able to provide learners with the patient's medical history. They become aggressive with learners if not kept informed.
- ED nurse can administer medications and may cue learners if needed.
- Neurosurgeon, PICU physician, and social worker available via telephone consultation.

Case Narrative

Scenario Background

A 10-month-old boy brought in by parent for lethargy. Parent had left the patient with a neighbor who watches the child intermittently. When the parent picked the baby up from the neighbors' house, he was less responsive and vomited several times, prompting the ED presentation. Patient had been in a normal state of health until today.

Patient's medical history:	None.
Meds:	None.
Allergies:	None.
Family history:	None.
Social history:	Usually attends daycare.

Initial Scenario Conditions

Infant male child, lethargic, with intermittent crying.

> Case may start with EMS (learner) receiving this case on scene as presented and performing their objectives to initiate treatment and transport, including seizure management. Alternatively, scenario background may be presented by EMS (actor) on ED arrival.

Vital signs:	Temp 98.6 °F (37.0 °C), HR 165, RR 32, BP 85/52, SpO_2 99% on room air.
Head:	Atraumatic.
Eyes:	Open to noxious stimuli, pupils 4 mm, reactive to light.
Neck:	Atraumatic, anterior fontanelle is closed.
Heart:	Regular, tachycardic.
Lungs:	Clear breath sounds.
Chest:	No deformities.
Abdomen:	Soft, non-distended.
Extremities:	No deformities.
Skin:	Bruising on left chest and left mid-back.
Neurologic:	Withdraws and cries in response to noxious stimuli.

See flow diagram (Figure 15.14) for further scenario changes described.

Case Narrative, Continued

Learners of all levels should expose the patient, perform a thorough physical exam, and recognize bruising on the patient's torso. They should consider all causes of the patient's depressed level of consciousness, including the possibility of non-accidental trauma. Learners should obtain additional history from the patient's parent. They should obtain age-appropriate IV access and a fingerstick glucose.

After four minutes, the patient will have generalized tonic–clonic seizure. Learners should treat the patient with benzodiazepines. Learners should identify respiratory compromise and perform intubation.

Following appropriate airway management, the patient will stabilize temporarily. Laboratory results can return at this time. Learners should obtain head CT. Novice learners may be provided with radiology interpretation of head CT. Advanced learners should interpret head CT.

Learners should consult with neurosurgery. They should elevate head of the bed, support patient's oxygenation, ventilation, and blood pressure with appropriate ventilator settings and IV fluid administration, and should consider administering mannitol or hypertonic saline.

Throughout the case, learners should communicate with the patient's parent to express their concerns and keep them informed. Parent may become agitated and aggressive if they are not routinely updated. Learners should discuss their concern for non-accidental trauma with the social worker or other designated child abuse specialist. Case will end after learners have arranged for disposition to PICU.

Instructor Notes

Pathophysiology

- Non-accidental trauma:
  - Child abuse resulting in physical injury.
  - Most common intracranial finding is subdural hematoma.
  - Typically caused by shaking mechanism leading to tearing of bridging veins and bleeding into the subdural space.
  - Can lead to mass effect, increased intracranial pressure, seizures, obtundation.

Clinical Features

- Suspect non-accidental trauma when history is vague, implausible, or inconsistent with child's developmental stage.
- Injuries suspicious for non-accidental trauma:
  - Bruises
    - In a pattern that replicates an object.
    - On ear, neck, or torso.
    - In children who are not mobile.
    - In various stages of healing.
  - Burns:
    - In a pattern that replicates an object.
    - Encircling buttock or extremities.
  - Long-bone fractures in children who cannot walk.
  - Rib fractures, hollow viscus injuries, or subdural hematoma in infants.

Diagnosis

- Head CT.
- Skeletal survey:
  - Fractures in multiple stages of healing.
  - Bucket handle fractures in lower extremities.
- Fundoscopic exam:
  - Retinal hemorrhages.

Management

- ICH:
  - Intubate patients who are hypoxic, obtunded, or otherwise unable to protect airway.
  - In infants, administer atropine pre-intubation to prevent vagal response.
  - Administer IV fluids or vasopressors to support blood pressure.
  - Treat seizures:
  - First line: benzodiazepines.
  - Additional antiepileptics (e.g., levetiracetam, fosphenytoin) may be necessary.
  - Increased intracranial pressure:
  - Elevate head of bed to 15–30 degrees.
  - Maintain head in midline position.
  - Support oxygenation, ventilation, and blood pressure.
  - Consider mannitol or hypertonic saline.
- Non-accidental trauma:
  - Use objective, non-judgmental language when communicating with parent.
  - Educate parent about need for testing.
  - Consult with multidisciplinary child abuse team (if available at your facility).
  - Reporting of suspected child abuse is mandatory for medical providers.

Debriefing Plan

Plan for around 30 minutes for discussion.

Potential Questions for Discussion

- What is the approach to evaluating an infant with altered mental status?
- What is the appropriate management of seizure in a pediatric patient?
- What special considerations should be given when intubating an infant?

- What are the steps to appropriately manage ICH in an infant?
- What clinical features raise your concern for non-accidental trauma?

SELECTED READING FOR NON-ACCIDENTAL TRAUMA

Christian, C.W. (2015). The evaluation of suspected child physical abuse. *Pediatrics* 135 (5): 1337–1354.

Puls, H.T., Anderst, J.D., Bettenhausen, J.L. et al. (2019). Newborn risk factors for subsequent physical abuse hospitalizations. *Pediatrics* 143 (2): e20182108.

Van Horne, B.S., Caughy, M.O., Canfield, M. et al. (2018). First-time maltreatment in children ages 2–10 with and without specific birth defects: a population–based study. *Child Abuse Negl.* 84: 53–63.

PENETRATING CHEST TRAUMA

Educational Goals

Learning Objectives

1. Demonstrate appropriate assessment of trauma patient (MK, PC).
2. Demonstrate appropriate management of hypotension in trauma patient (MK, PC).
3. Recognize and properly manage pneumothorax (MK, PC).
4. Demonstrate proper trauma airway management (MK, PC).
5. Recognize intra-abdominal injury in patient with penetrating thoracic wounds (MK, PC).
6. Demonstrate proper use of extended FAST (eFAST) examination (MK, PC).
7. Demonstrate effective communication skills and professionalism during inter-actions with ED staff and consultants (ICS, P).
8. Direct appropriate disposition of patient penetrating chest trauma (SBP).

Critical Actions Checklist

☐ Perform primary and secondary trauma surveys (MK, PC).
☐ Obtain appropriate vascular access (PC).
☐ Initiate appropriate volume resuscitation prior to endotracheal intubation (MK, PC).
☐ Insrt endotracheal tube (MK, PC).
☐ Perform thoracostomy before or immediately following endotracheal intubation (MK, PC).
☐ Carry out and interpret eFAST examination (MK, PC).
☐ Communicate with trauma service for disposition (ICS, P, SBP).

Simulation Set-up

Environment: ED treatment room in a hospital that is not a trauma center. For EMS learners, scenario may start on scene and transition to a hospital setting.

Mannequin: Male simulator mannequin. Mannequin should be moulaged with two ballistic wounds: (i) in right chest slightly inferior to nipple; and (ii) in right back slightly inferior to scapula. Non-rebreather (NRB) mask is in place. No IV catheters are in place.

Props: To be displayed on screen or distributed on handouts:

- Images (see online component for penetrating chest trauma, Scenario 15.3 at https://www.wiley.com/go/thoureen/simulation/workbook2e):

- chest x-ray showing right pneumothorax (Figure 15.15)
- CXR showing right pneumothorax with thoracostomy tube in place (Figure 15.16)
- CXR showing right pneumothorax with thoracostomy tube in place and appropriate endotracheal tube position (Figure 15.17)
- CXR showing right pneumothorax with appropriate endotracheal tube position (Figure 15.18)
- eFAST videos showing right hemopneumothorax and free fluid in Morrison's pouch (Figures 15.19–15.24 and Videos 15.1–15.5).
- Laboratory tests (see online component as above):
  - Complete blood count (Table 15.14).
  - Basic metabolic panel (Table 15.15).
  - Liver function tests (Table 15.16).
  - Lactate level (Table 15.17).
  - Coagulation panel (Table 15.18).
  - Type and screen (Table 15.19).

Available supplies:

- Adult airway and code cart.
- Medications:
  - IV fluids in labeled 1 l bags: 0.9% saline, LR.
  - Pre-labeled syringes:
    - Analgesic medications.
    - Rapid sequence intubation medications.
- Blood products: RBCs, platelets, FFP.
- Procedure tray with supplies for needle thoracostomy and tube thoracostomy.
- Trauma torso task trainer (optional).
- Ultrasound machine (optional).

Distractor: None.

Actors

- EMS can provide information about the scene. Actor optional if no EMS learner is present.
- Patient moans incoherently to painful stimuli. Not following commands or answering questions.
- ED nurse can administer medications and may cue learners if needed.
- Trauma surgeon is available via telephone consultation.

Case Narrative

Scenario Background

A 19-year-old man has been found semi-conscious following a reported gunshot wound. Patient has a ballistic injury to the right chest wall (wound on back not found by EMS and not disclosed to participants). They were unable to establish IV access.

Patient's medical history:	Unknown.
Medications:	Unknown.
Allergies:	Unknown.
Family history:	Unknown.
Social history:	Unknown.

Initial Scenario Conditions

Young man moaning to painful stimuli.

> Case may start with EMS (learner) receiving this case on scene as presented and performing their objectives to initiate treatment and transport. EMS interventions might include patient immobilization, needle thoracostomy, or treatment of "sucking" chest wound. Alternatively, scenario background may be presented by EMS (actor) on ED arrival.

Vital signs:	Temp 97.3 °F (36.3 °C), BP 70/40, HR 130, RR 26, SpO$_2$ 90% on 100% NRB mask.
Head:	Atraumatic.
Eyes:	Pupils 4 mm, reactive to light.
Mouth:	Airway patent.
Neck:	Atraumatic.
Heart:	Regular, distal pulses diminished.
Lungs:	Shallow, diminished on right.
Chest:	Ballistic injury to right chest inferior to nipple.
Abdomen:	Atraumatic.
Extremities:	Atraumatic.
Back:	Ballistic injury to right back inferior to scapula.
Neurologic:	Eyes closed, moaning incoherently to noxious stimuli, withdraws from pain all extremities; Glasgow Coma Scale (GCS) score: E1, V2, M4.

See flow diagram (Figure 15.25) for further scenario changes described.

Case Narrative, Continued

Learners of all levels should perform a primary trauma survey, obtain appropriate IV access, and administer IV fluids or RBCs. Learners should identify a patient's depressed mental status and need for intubation. They should recognize the patient's right pneumothorax and perform needle decompression or tube thoracostomy in the peri-intubation period. Failure to intubate the patient after five minutes will lead to worsening hypoxia. Failure to perform thoracostomy will lead to worsening tachycardia and hypotension.

Students and postgraduate learners should order appropriate labs and imaging studies. Novice learners should perform needle decompression. Advanced learners may be asked to perform tube thoracostomy on the mannequin or task trainer.

> If performance of actual procedure is not a learning objective, then learners can simply verbalize that tube thoracostomy has been performed.

Following appropriate airway management and tube thoracostomy, the patient will temporarily stabilize. Learners should perform secondary trauma survey, perform point of care imaging such as chest x-ray and eFAST, and identify intraperitoneal free fluid.

> If learners ask for imaging other than point of care studies, they will be told that it will be 20 minutes before that modality is available, and the ED nurse will express concern for the patient's stability.

After five minutes, lab results will be available. For novice learners, the case may end here after consultation with trauma service.

For advanced learners, the patient begins to deteriorate again and requires further volume resuscitation. Learners should assess the volume of blood evacuated via the chest tube (the nurse indicates it is 50 ml) and determine that continuing blood loss is likely arising from a subdiaphragmatic injury. They should continue administration of RBCs and initiate transfusion of platelets and FFP. Case will end after learners have arranged appropriate disposition to trauma service.

Instructor Notes

Pathophysiology

- Penetrating chest trauma may extend below diaphragm or into neck.
- Pneumothorax:
  - Positive pressure ventilation → rapid expansion.
  - Tension pneumothorax:
    - High intrathoracic pressure → cardiopulmonary compromise.
    - Lung collapse → respiratory compromise.
    - Reduced venous return, deviation of vascular structures → decreased blood flow.
- Open pneumothorax:
  - Pleural space open to outside world.
  - Inhalation → air movement through defect.

- Hemothorax:
  - Usually associated with pneumothorax.
  - Each hemithorax can hold 1.51 of blood → hemorrhagic shock, respiratory failure.
- Esophageal and tracheobronchial injuries:
  - Rare in isolation.
  - May cause pneumothorax, pneumomediastinum, mediastinitis, hematemesis, hemoptysis.
- Great vessel injuries:
  - High mortality, most commonly subclavian vessels.
- Cardiac injuries:
  - Rapidly fatal due to hemorrhage, tamponade.
  - Right heart more commonly injured than left heart.
  - Hemopericardium → tamponade → obstructive shock.
- Diaphragmatic injuries:
  - Herniation of abdominal contents may occur acutely or years later.

Clinical Features

- Pneumothorax
  - Common symptoms: pleuritic chest pain, dyspnea.
  - Exam findings:
    - Unilateral decreased breath sounds.
    - Open pneumothorax: "sucking" wound.
    - Tension pneumothorax: tracheal deviation, jugular venous distension.
- Hemothorax:
  - Unilateral decreased breath sounds, dullness to percussion.
- Great vessel injuries:
  - May cause pulse deficit in ipsilateral upper extremity.
- Cardiac injuries:
  - Beck's triad from tamponade: hypotension with narrow pulse pressure, distended neck veins, muffled heart sounds.

Diagnosis

- Depends highly on physical exam and point of care studies.
  - Perform thorough secondary trauma survey:
  - Injuries near infra-mammary crease or inferior scapulae may violate diaphragm.
- Chest x-ray:
  - Tension pneumothorax is a clinical diagnosis and does not require imaging prior to treatment.

- Smaller hemothoraces and pneumothoraces are often missed.
  - eFAST higher sensitivity for pneumothorax than chest x-ray.
  - Assess for pleural, pericardial, or peritoneal free fluid.
- CT:
  - Highly sensitive for hemothorax and pneumothorax.
  - May identify cardiac or vascular injury.
  - CT angiography improves assessment for great vessel injury.

Management
- Primary survey:
  - Diagnose and immediately address life-threatening injuries.
  - Airway: patency, ability to protect.
  - Breathing: pulmonary function, respiratory drive, oxygenation, ventilation.
  - Circulation: heart rate, blood pressure, distal pulses.
  - Disability: calculate GCS.
- Hemorrhagic shock:
  - Hypotension in setting of trauma should be presumed to be secondary to hemorrhage until proven otherwise.
  - Goal systolic blood pressure 90 mmHg.
    - Balances perfusion with risk of exacerbating hemorrhage.
  - Avoid large-volume crystalloid resuscitation (> 1 l).
    - Can cause hypothermia, acidosis, coagulopathy.
  - Initiate early transfusion of uncrossmatched RBCs
    - O-negative for premenopausal females.
    - O-positive for all other patients.
  - Consider tranexamic acid.
  - If requiring > 2 units of RBCs, initiate MTP.
    - Balanced administration of RBCs, platelets, FFP.
- Pneumothorax and hemothorax:
  - Needle thoracostomy for pneumothorax: quick but frequently unsuccessful.
  - Tube thoracostomy: more reliable and lasting.
    - Consider large-diameter tube for hemothorax.
- Esophageal and tracheobronchial injuries:
  - Early antibiotics, likely operative repair.
- ED thoracotomy:
  - Indications vary between groups and institutions.
  - Most successful in penetrating cardiac injury.
  - Allows for pericardiotomy to relieve tamponade, identification of cardiac injury, and tamponade or repair of cardiac injuries.
  - May also clamp great vessel injuries or cross-clamp aorta to slow distal hemorrhage.

Debriefing Plan

Plan for around 30 minutes for discussion.

Potential Questions for Discussion
- What are the components of a trauma survey?
- What are the clinical features of a pneumothorax?
- What is the appropriate management of a pneumothorax?
- How does the presence of a pneumothorax complicate airway management?
- When should you suspect a penetrating chest injury causing extra-thoracic injury?
- What prehospital interventions could have been performed on this patient?

SELECTED READING FOR PENETRATING CHEST TRAUMA

Feinman, M., Cotton, B.A., and Haut, E.R. (2014). Optimal fluid resuscitation in trauma. *Curr. Opin. Crit. Care* 20 (4): 366–372.

Mayglothling, J., Duane, T.M., Gibbs, M. et al. (2012). Emergency tracheal intubation immediately following traumatic injury. *J. Trauma Acute Care Surg.* 73 (5 Suppl 4): S333–S340.

Platz, J.J., Fabricant, L., and Norotsky, M. (2017). Thoracic trauma: injuries, evaluation, and treatment. *Surg. Clin. North Am.* 97 (4): 783–799.

APPENDIX

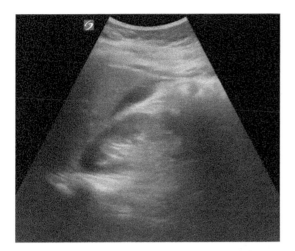

FIGURE 15.1   Right upper quadrant ultrasound showing intraperitoneal free fluid.

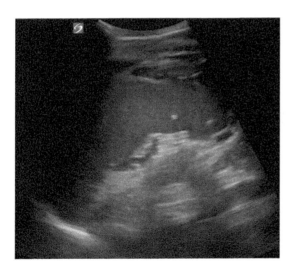

FIGURE 15.2   Left upper quadrant ultrasound showing intraperitoneal free fluid.

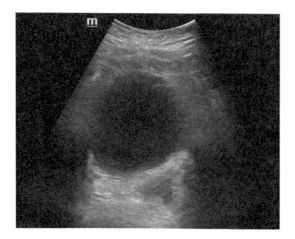

FIGURE 15.3   Suprapubic ultrasound showing intraperitoneal free fluid.

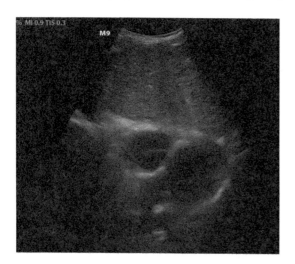

FIGURE 15.4   Subcostal ultrasound still image showing no pericardial free fluid.

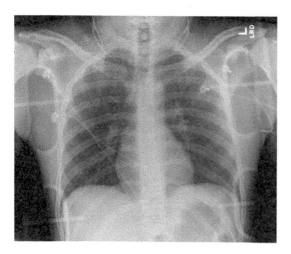

FIGURE 15.5   Chest x-ray showing no acute abnormality.

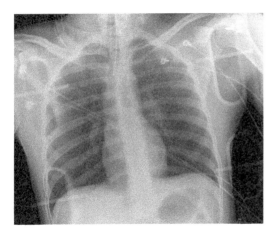

FIGURE 15.6   Post-intubation chest x-ray showing appropriate endotracheal tube position.

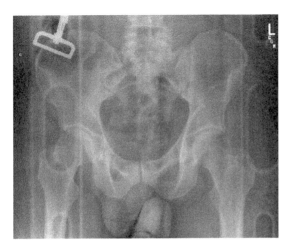

FIGURE 15.7   X-ray of the pelvis showing no acute abnormality.

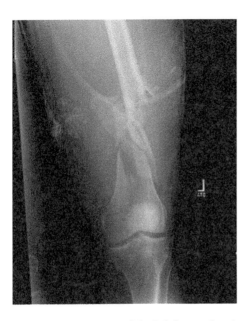

FIGURE 15.8   X-ray of the left femur showing a comminuted mid-shaft femur fracture.

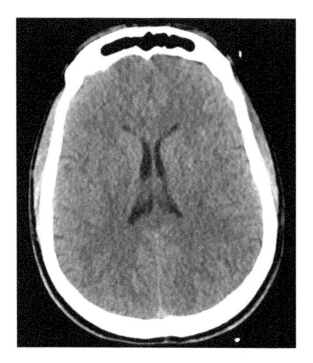

FIGURE 15.9   Head computed tomography showing no acute intracranial abnormality.

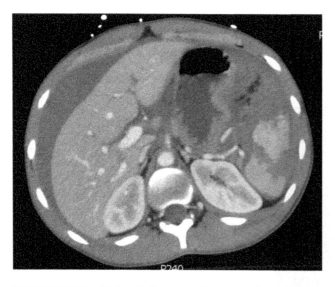

FIGURE 15.10   Abdominal computed tomography showing a grade-4 splenic laceration with active extravasation and hemoperitoneum.

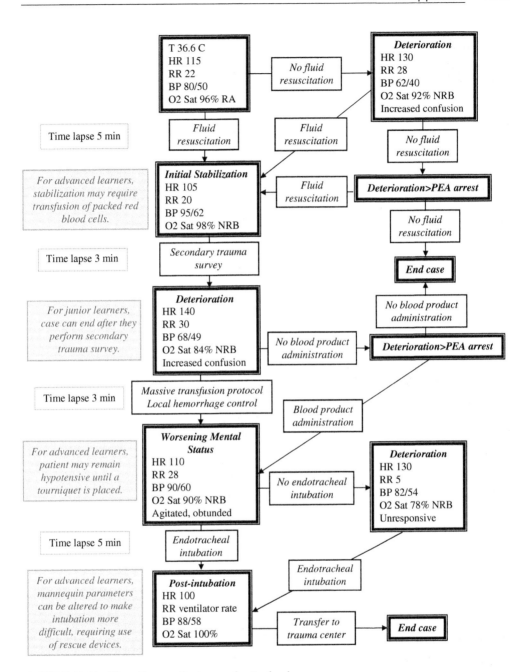

FIGURE 15.11 Flow diagram for hemorrhagic shock.

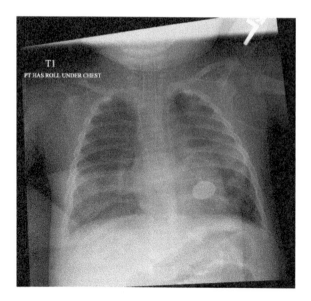

FIGURE 15.12   Post-intubation chest x-ray showing appropriate endotracheal tube position.

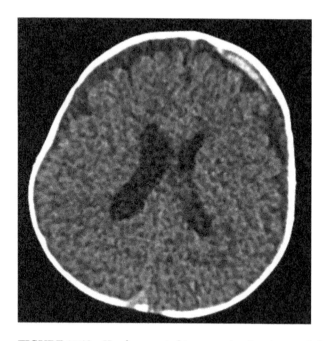

FIGURE 15.13   Head computed tomography showing a subdural hematoma.

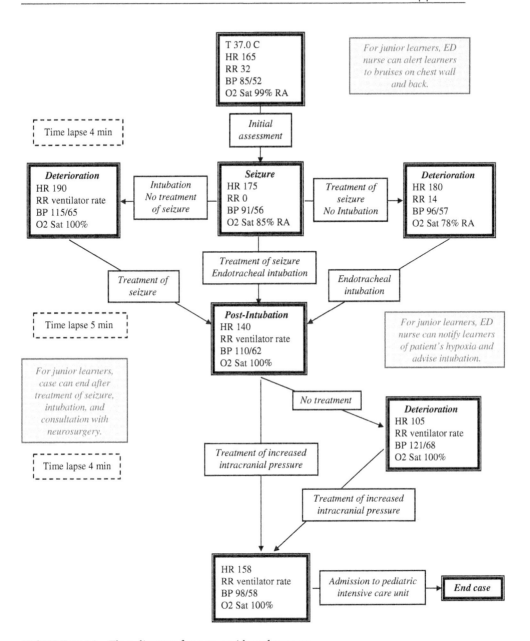

FIGURE 15.14 Flow diagram for non-accidental trauma.

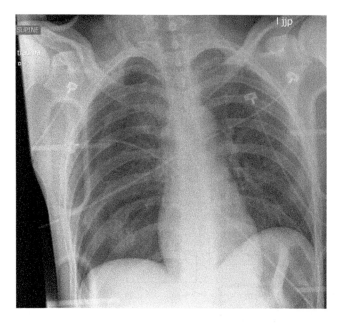

FIGURE 15.15   Chest x-ray showing right pneumothorax.

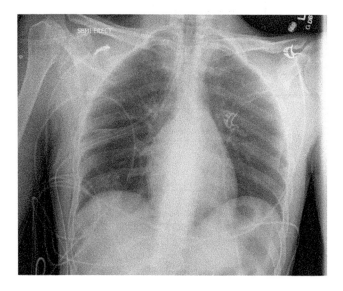

FIGURE 15.16   Chest x-ray showing right pneumothorax with thoracostomy tube in place.

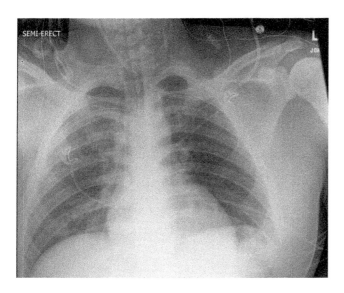

FIGURE 15.17   Chest x-ray showing right pneumothorax with thoracostomy tube in place and appropriate endotracheal tube position.

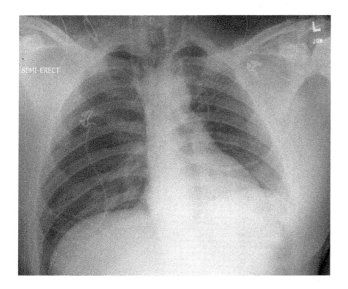

FIGURE 15.18   Chest x-ray showing right pneumothorax with appropriate endotracheal tube position.

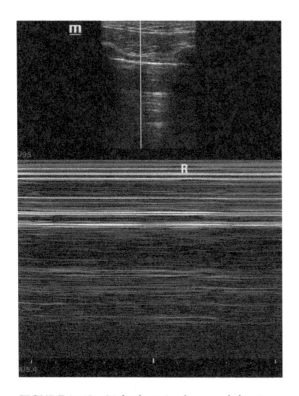

FIGURE 15.19   Right thoracic ultrasound showing normal lung sliding.

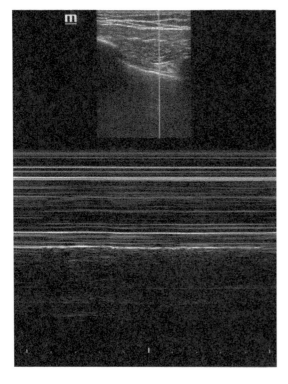

FIGURE 15.20   Left thoracic ultrasound showing normal lung sliding.

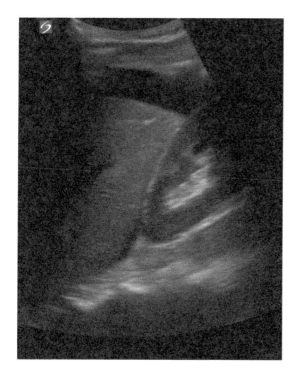

FIGURE 15.21   Right upper quadrant ultrasound showing intraperitoneal free fluid.

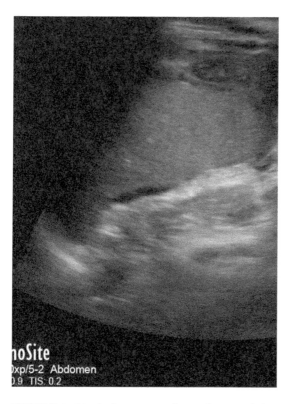

FIGURE 15.22   Left upper quadrant ultrasound showing intraperitoneal free fluid.

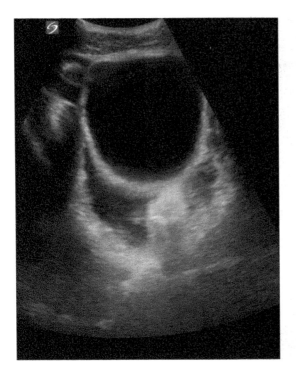

FIGURE 15.23 Suprapubic ultrasound showing intraperitoneal free fluid.

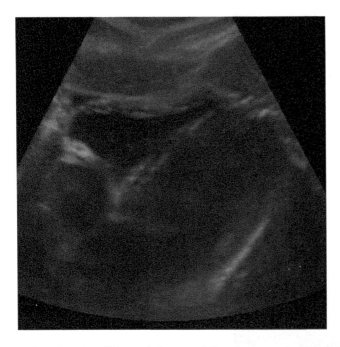

FIGURE 15.24 Subcostal ultrasound showing no pericardial free fluid.

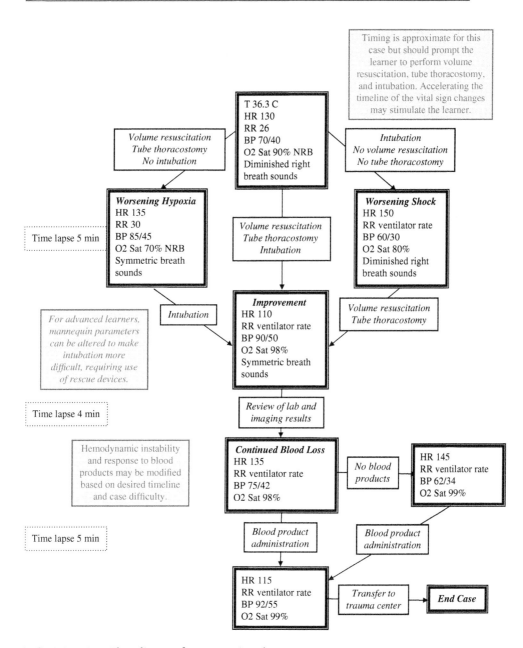

FIGURE 15.25 Flow diagram for penetrating chest trauma.

TABLE 15.1 Complete blood count.

Test	Value	Reference range
White blood cells (k/µl)	17.9	3.5–11.0
Hemoglobin (g/dl)	13.5	10.5–15.0
Hematocrit (%)	42	32–45
Platelets (k/µl)	274	150–400

TABLE 15.2 Basic metabolic panel.

Test	Value	Reference range
Sodium (mmol/l)	139	135–145
Potassium (mmol/l)	3.8	3.6–5.1
Chloride (mmol/l)	106	98–110
Bicarbonate (mmol/l)	22	20–30
Blood urea nitrogen (mg/dl)	17	6–24
Creatinine (mg/dl)	1.43	0.4–1.3
Glucose (mg/dl)	161	67–109
Calcium (mg/dl)	9.1	8.6–10.3

TABLE 15.3 Liver function tests.

Test	Value	Reference range
Albumin (g/dl)	4.1	3.7–4.8
Total protein (g/dl)	7.1	6.3–8.3
Total bilirubin (g/dl)	0.4	0.3–0.5
Alkaline phosphatase (iu/l)	50	38–120
Alanine aminotransferase (iu/l)	62	7–52
Aspartate aminotransferase (iu/l)	88	13–39

TABLE 15.4 Lactate.

Test	Value	Reference range
Lactate (mmol/l)	4.1	0.5–2.0

TABLE 15.5   Coagulation panel.

Test	Value	Reference range
Prothrombin time (seconds)	15.0	9.4–11.5
International normalized ratio	1.2	0.9–1.2
Partial thromboplastin time (seconds)	28.4	24.2–32.0

TABLE 15.6   Type and screen.

Test	Value
ABO type	A
Rh type	Positive

TABLE 15.7   Fingerstick glucose.

Test	Value	Reference range
Fingerstick glucose (mg/dl)	107	70–109

TABLE 15.8   Complete blood count.

Test	Value	Reference range
White blood cells (k/µl)	17.8	3.5–11.0
Hemoglobin (g/dl)	12	10.5–15.0
Hematocrit (%)	38	32–45
Platelets (k/µl)	415	150–400

TABLE 15.9   Basic metabolic panel.

Test	Value	Reference range
Sodium (mmol/l)	135	135–145
Potassium (mmol/l)	3.0	3.6–5.1
Chloride (mmol/l)	94	98–110
Bicarbonate (mmol/l)	24	20–30
Blood urea nitrogen (mg/dl)	18	6–24
Creatinine (mg/dl)	0.53	0.4–1.3
Glucose (mg/dl)	107	67–109
Calcium (mg/dl)	8.9	8.6–10.3

TABLE 15.10 Liver function tests.

Test	Value	Reference range
Albumin (g/dl)	4.3	3.7–4.8
Total protein (g/dl)	6.8	6.3–8.3
Total bilirubin (g/dl)	0.4	0.3–0.5
Alkaline phosphatase (iu/l)	64	38–120
Alanine aminotransferase (iu/l)	17	7–52
Aspartate aminotransferase (iu/l)	18	13–39

TABLE 15.11 Lactate.

Test	Value	Reference range
Lactate (mmol/l)	0.9	0.5–2.0

TABLE 15.12 Coagulation panel.

Test	Value	Reference range
Prothrombin time (seconds)	12.0	9.4–11.5
International normalized ratio	0.9	0.9–1.2
Partial thromboplastin time (seconds)	22.4	24.2–32.0

TABLE 15.13 Type and screen.

Test	Value
ABO type	O
Rh type	Positive

TABLE 15.14 Complete blood count.

Test	Value	Reference range
White blood cells (k/μl)	15.2	3.5–11.0
Hemoglobin (g/dl)	14.7	10.5–15.0
Hematocrit (%)	44	32–45
Platelets (k/μl)	337	150–400

TABLE 15.15 Basic metabolic panel.

Test	Value	Reference Range
Sodium (mmol/l)	142	135–145
Potassium (mmol/l)	4.1	3.6–5.1
Chloride (mmol/l)	105	98–110
Bicarbonate (mmol/l)	21	20–30
Blood urea nitrogen (mg/dl)	18	6–24
Creatinine (mg/dl)	1.2	0.4–1.3
Glucose (mg/dl)	96	67–109
Calcium (mg/dl)	9.3	8.6–10.3

TABLE 15.16 Liver function tests.

Test	Value	Reference range
Albumin (g/dl)	3.9	3.7–4.8
Total protein (g/dl)	7.2	6.3–8.3
Total bilirubin (g/dl)	1.1	0.3–0.5
Alkaline phosphatase (iu/l)	43	38–120
Alanine aminotransferase (iu/l)	136	7–52
Aspartate aminotransferase (iu/l)	127	13–39

TABLE 15.17 Lactate.

Test	Value	Reference range
Lactate (mmol/l)	4.1	0.5–2.0

TABLE 15.18 Coagulation panel.

Test	Value	Reference range
Prothrombin time (seconds)	12.1	9.4–11.5
International normalized ratio	0.9	0.9–1.2
Partial thromboplastin time (seconds)	35	24.2–32.0

TABLE 15.19 Type and screen.

Test	Value
ABO type	AB
Rh type	Positive

Index

Emergency Medicine Simulation Workbook: A Tool for Bringing the Curriculum to Life,
Second Edition. Edited by Traci L. Thoureen and Sara B. Scott.
© 2022 John Wiley & Sons Ltd. Published 2022 by John Wiley & Sons Ltd.
Companion website: www.wiley.com/go/thoureen/simulation/workbook2e